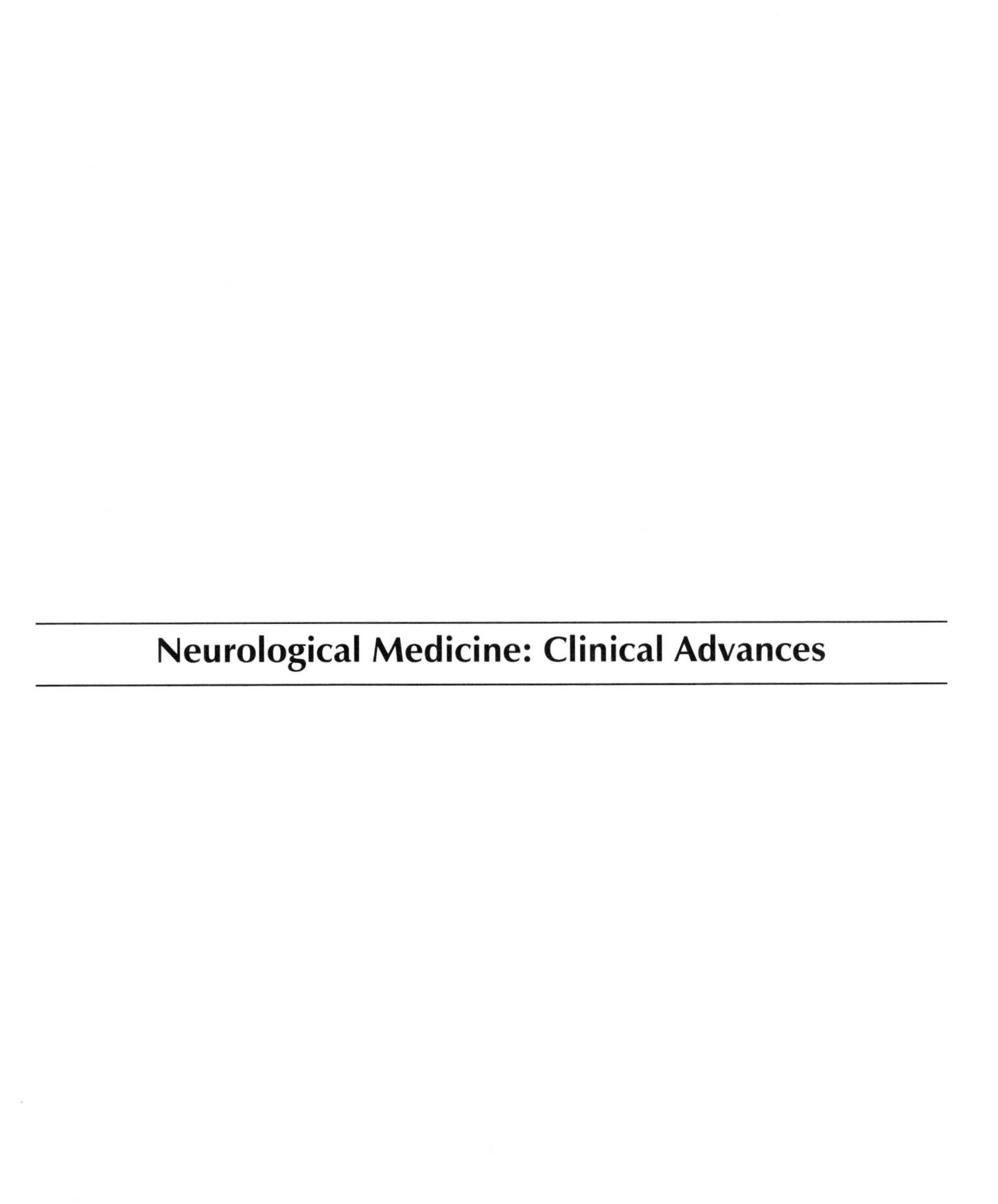

Neurological Medicine: Clinical Advances

Neurological Medicine: Clinical Advances

Editor: Trevor Cornfield

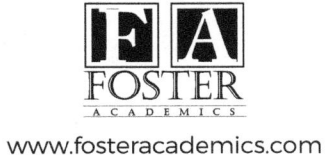

www.fosteracademics.com

www.fosteracademics.com

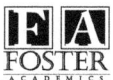

Cataloging-in-Publication Data

Neurological medicine : clinical advances / edited by Trevor Cornfield.
     p. cm.
Includes bibliographical references and index.
ISBN 978-1-63242-721-2
1. Neurology. 2. Nervous system. 3. Nervous system--Diseases. I. Cornfield, Trevor.
RC346 .N48 2019
616.8--dc23

© Foster Academics, 2019

Foster Academics,
118-35 Queens Blvd., Suite 400,
Forest Hills, NY 11375, USA

ISBN 978-1-63242-721-2 (Hardback)

This book contains information obtained from authentic and highly regarded sources. Copyright for all individual chapters remain with the respective authors as indicated. All chapters are published with permission under the Creative Commons Attribution License or equivalent. A wide variety of references are listed. Permission and sources are indicated; for detailed attributions, please refer to the permissions page and list of contributors. Reasonable efforts have been made to publish reliable data and information, but the authors, editors and publisher cannot assume any responsibility for the validity of all materials or the consequences of their use.

Trademark Notice: Registered trademark of products or corporate names are used only for explanation and identification without intent to infringe.

Contents

Preface IX

Chapter 1 **Acute Psychosis as Main Manifestation of Central Pontine Myelinolysis** 1
Mangala Gopal, Melvin Parasram, Harsh Patel, Chike Ilorah and Hrachya Nersesyan

Chapter 2 **Impaired Emotion Recognition after Left Hemispheric Stroke: A Case Report** 8
Hugo P. Aben, Yael D. Reijmer, Johanna M. A. Visser-Meily, Jacoba M. Spikman,
Geert Jan Biessels and Paul L. M. de Kort

Chapter 3 **Bilateral Moyamoya Disease in a 2-Year-Old Pakistani Male Treated with Bilateral Encephaloduroarteriosynangiosis: A Positive Outcome** 14
Shahvaiz Magsi, Adeel Khoja, Mansoor Ali Merchant Rameez,
Ariba Khan and Noman Ishaque

Chapter 4 **Relapsing Polychondritis with Meningoencephalitis Refractory to Immunosuppressant Therapy** 18
Mohammad Mousbah Al-Tabbaa and Hani Habal

Chapter 5 **Central Hyperthermia Treated with Bromocriptine** 22
P. Natteru, P. George, R. Bell, P. Nattanmai and C. R. Newey

Chapter 6 **Could Hallucinogens Induce Permanent Pupillary Changes in (Ab)users?** 27
Ahmed Al-Imam

Chapter 7 **Emotional Lability as a Unique Presenting Sign of Suspected Chronic Traumatic Encephalopathy** 32
Shauna H. Yuan and Sonya G. Wang

Chapter 8 **Comorbid Normal Pressure Hydrocephalus with Parkinsonism: A Clinical Challenge and Call for Awareness** 36
A. Cucca, M. C. Biagioni, K. Sharma, J. Golomb, R. M. Gilbert,
A. Di Rocco and J. E. Fleisher

Chapter 9 **Acute, Nontraumatic Spontaneous Spinal Subdural Hematoma** 44
Leigh A. Rettenmaier, Marshall T. Holland and Taylor J. Abel

Chapter 10 **Familial Hemiplegic Migraine with Severe Attacks: A New Report with *ATP1A2* Mutation** 56
E. Martínez, R. Moreno, L. López-Mesonero, I. Vidriales, M. Ruiz,
A. L. Guerrero and J. J. Tellería

Chapter 11 **Ketamine Infusion used to Successfully Control Refractory Status Epilepticus in a Pregnant Patient** 61
Murad Talahma, Vivek Sabharwal, Yana Bukovskaya and Fawad Khan

Chapter 12 **Bilateral Ganglion Cysts of the Ligamentum Flavum in the Cervical Spine Causing a Progressive Cervical Radiculomyelopathy** 65
Juneki Kim, Jin-gyu Choi and Byung-chul Son

Chapter 13 **Differential Effects of Awake Glioma Surgery in "Critical" Language Areas on Cognition: 4 Case Studies** 70
Djaina Satoer, Elke De Witte, Marion Smits, Roelien Bastiaanse, Arnaud Vincent, Peter Mariën and Evy Visch-Brink

Chapter 14 **Adult Primary Spinal Epidural Extraosseous Ewing's Sarcoma** 80
Mark Bustoros, Cheddhi Thomas, Joshua Frenster, Aram S. Modrek, N. Sumru Bayin, Matija Snuder, Peter B. Schiff and Dimitris G. Placantonakis

Chapter 15 **Retained Glass Fragment in the Cervical Spinal Canal in a Patient with Acute Transverse Myelitis: A Case Report and Literature Review** 88
Simonas Jesmanas, Kristina Norvainytė, Rymantė Gleiznienė and Algirdas Mačionis

Chapter 16 **Simultaneous Combined Myositis, Inflammatory Polyneuropathy and Overlap Myasthenic Syndrome** 94
Stéphane Mathis, LaurentMagy, Philippe Corcia, Karima Ghorab, Laurence Richard, Jonathan Ciron, Mathilde Duchesne and Jean-Michel Vallat

Chapter 17 **CT Perfusion to Guide Placement of Invasive Cerebral Perfusion Monitor in Subarachnoid Hemorrhage Induced Vasospasm** 105
Hosam Al-Jehani, Judith Marcoux, Kawthar Hadhiah, Faisal Alabbas, Mark Angle and Jeanne Teitelbaum

Chapter 18 **Oral High-Dose Thiamine Improves the Symptoms of Chronic Cluster Headache** 108
Costantini Antonio, Tiberi Massimo, Zarletti Gianpaolo, Pala Maria Immacolata and Trevi Erika

Chapter 19 **Uncommon Association of Two Anatomical Variants of Cerebral Circulation: A Fetal-Type Posterior Cerebral Artery and mInferred Artery of Percheron, Complicated with Paramedian Thalamomesencephalic Stroke** 113
Aurelian Anghelescu

Chapter 20 **Primary Sphenoidal Sinus Lymphoma with Initial Presentation as Unilateral Abducens Nerve Palsy Symptom** 122
Xijing Mao, Lifang Jin, Bochi Zhu, Honghua Cui, Min Yao and Gang Yao

Chapter 21 **Acute Ascending Flaccid Paralysis Secondary to Multiple Trigger Factor Induced Hyperkalemia** 127
K. H. D. Thilini Hemachandra, M. B. Kavinda Chandimal Dayasiri and Thamara Kannangara

Chapter 22 **Diagnostic Challenges of *Cryptococcus neoformans* in an Immunocompetent Individual Masquerading as Chronic Hydrocephalus** 131
Kedar R. Mahajan, Amity L. Roberts, Mark T. Curtis, Danielle Fortuna, Robin Dharia and Lori Sheehan

Chapter 23 **Septic Encephalopathy Characterized by Acute Encephalopathy with Biphasic Seizures and Late Reduced Diffusion and Early Nonconvulsive Status Epilepticus** 138
Hiroshi Yamaguchi, Tsukasa Tanaka, Azusa Maruyama and Hiroaki Nagase

Chapter 24 **High-Grade Glioma of the Ventrolateral Medulla in an Adult: Case Presentation and Discussion of Surgical Considerations** 143
Angela Spurgeon, Viet Le, Sanjay Konakondla, Douglas C. Miller, Tamera Hopkins and N. Scott Litofsky

Chapter 25 **Progressive Multifocal Leukoencephalopathy in a Multiple Sclerosis Patient Diagnosed after Switching from Natalizumab to Fingolimod** 152
Tim Sinnecker, Jalal Othman, Marc Kühl, Imke Metz, Thoralf Niendorf, Annett Kunkel, Friedemann Paul, Jens Wuerfel and Juergen Faiss

Chapter 26 **Alzheimer's Dementia due to Suspected CTE from Subconcussive Head Impact** 160
Shauna H. Yuan and Sonya G. Wang

Chapter 27 **Clival Ectopic Pituitary Adenoma Mimicking a Chordoma: Case Report** 164
Constantine L. Karras, Isaac Josh Abecassis, Zachary A. Abecassis, Joseph G. Adel, Esther N. Bit-Ivan, Rakesh K. Chandra and Bernard R. Bendok

Chapter 28 **Friedreich's Ataxia: Clinical Presentation of a Compound Heterozygote Child with a Rare Nonsense Mutation** 172
Vamshi K. Rao, Christine J. DiDonato and Paul D. Larsen

Chapter 29 **Never Too Old? Occurrence of Medulloblastoma in the Elderly beyond the 70th Year of Life** 177
Homajoun Maslehaty, Johannes Van de Nes, Sarah Teuber-Hanselmann, Christoph Moenninghoff, Ulrich Sure and Neriman Oezkan

Chapter 30 **Effect of Spinal Cord Stimulation on Gait in a Patient with Thalamic Pain** 181
Arito Yozu, Masahiko Sumitani, Masahiro Shin, Kazuhiko Ishi, Michihiro Osumi, Junji Katsuhira, Ryosuke Chiba and Nobuhiko Haga

Chapter 31 **Profound Autonomic Instability Complicated by Multiple Episodes of Cardiac Asystole and Refractory Bradycardia in a Patient with Anti-NMDA Encephalitis** 186
Stephanie R. Mehr, Roy C. Neeley, Melissa Wiley and Avinash B. Kumar

Chapter 32 **Acute Stroke due to Electrocution: Uncommon or Unrecognized?** 191
Laxmi Kokatnur and Mohan Rudrappa

Chapter 33 **A Patient with Eight Intracranial Aneurysms: Endovascular Treatment in Two Sessions** 196
Erol Akgul, Hasan Bilen Onan, Huseyin Tugsan Balli and Nuri Eralp Cetinalp

Chapter 34 **Limb Pain as Unusual Presentation of a Parietal Intraparenchymal Bleeding Associated with Crack Cocaine Use: A Case Report** 203
Alan Lucerna, James Espinosa, Taimur Zaman, Risha Hertz and Douglas Stranges

Chapter 35 **Rheumatoid Meningitis Occurring during Etanercept Treatment** 207
Koji Tsuzaki, Takashi Nakamura, Hiroyuki Okumura, Naoko Tachibana and Toshiaki Hamano

Chapter 36 **Advanced Genetic Testing Comes to the Pain Clinic to Make a Diagnosis of
Paroxysmal Extreme Pain Disorder**.. 212
Ashley Cannon, Svetlana Kurklinsky, Kimberly J. Guthrie and
Douglas L. Riegert-Johnson

Permissions

List of Contributors

Index

Preface

The purpose of the book is to provide a glimpse into the dynamics and to present opinions and studies of some of the scientists engaged in the development of new ideas in the field from very different standpoints. This book will prove useful to students and researchers owing to its high content quality.

Neurological medicine is concerned with the diagnosis and treatment of conditions affecting the brain, spinal cord and the peripheral and central nervous system. There are different types of neurological disorders, some of which are common while others are rare. Brain damage and brain dysfunction, spinal cord disorders, neuropsychiatric illnesses, movement disorders, etc. are some examples. They may be assessed through a neurological examination, and treated using techniques developed within the specialties of neurology and clinical neuropsychology. A neurological examination seeks to find any lesions in the central and peripheral nervous systems through an assessment of motor and sensory responses. These findings are then combined to see if they indicate a recognizable medical condition or a neurological disorder. Some of the specializations within neurology are brain injury medicine, hospice and palliative medicine, neuromuscular medicine, sleep medicine, pain medicine, etc. This book is compiled in such a manner, that it will provide in-depth knowledge about the theory and practice of neurological medicine. The ever-growing need of advanced therapeutic strategies is the reason that has fueled the research in the field of neurological medicine in recent times. This book is appropriate for students seeking detailed information in this area as well as for experts.

At the end, I would like to appreciate all the efforts made by the authors in completing their chapters professionally. I express my deepest gratitude to all of them for contributing to this book by sharing their valuable works. A special thanks to my family and friends for their constant support in this journey.

Editor

Acute Psychosis as Main Manifestation of Central Pontine Myelinolysis

Mangala Gopal,[1] Melvin Parasram,[2] Harsh Patel,[3] Chike Ilorah,[4] and Hrachya Nersesyan[4,5]

[1]College of Osteopathic Medicine, Des Moines University, Des Moines, IA, USA
[2]Arizona College of Osteopathic Medicine, Midwestern University, Glendale, AZ, USA
[3]Baroda Medical College, Vadodara, Gujarat, India
[4]Department of Neurology, University of Illinois College of Medicine at Peoria, Peoria, IL, USA
[5]Illinois Neurological Institute, OSF St. Francis Medical Center, Peoria, IL, USA

Correspondence should be addressed to Hrachya Nersesyan; nerses@uic.edu

Academic Editor: Mathias Toft

Central pontine myelinolysis (CPM) is an acute demyelinating neurological disorder affecting primarily the central pons and is frequently associated with rapid correction of hyponatremia. Common clinical manifestations of CPM include spastic quadriparesis, dysarthria, pseudobulbar palsy, and encephalopathy of various degrees; however, coma, "locked-in" syndrome, or death can occur in most severe cases. Rarely, CPM presents with neuropsychiatric manifestations, such as personality changes, acute psychosis, paranoia, hallucinations, or catatonia, typically associated with additional injury to the brain, described as extrapontine myelinolysis (EPM). We present a patient with primarily neuropsychiatric manifestations of CPM, in the absence of focal neurologic deficits or radiographic extrapontine involvement. A 51-year-old female without significant medical history presented with dizziness, frequent falls, diarrhea, generalized weakness, and weight loss. Physical examination showed no focal neurological deficits. Laboratory data showed severe hyponatremia, which was corrected rather rapidly. Subsequently, the patient developed symptoms of an acute psychotic illness. Initial brain magnetic resonance imaging (MRI) was unremarkable, although a repeat MRI two weeks later revealed changes compatible with CPM. This case demonstrates that acute psychosis might represent the main manifestation of CPM, especially in early stages of the disease, which should be taken into consideration when assessing patients with acute abnormalities of sodium metabolism.

1. Introduction

Central pontine myelinolysis (CPM) is a rare neurological syndrome first described in 1959 by Adams et al. [1]. It is an acute demyelinating condition primarily affecting central pons and commonly presenting clinically with spastic quadriparesis, dysarthria, pseudobulbar palsy, and altered mental status. In some patients, parkinsonian features, behavioral manifestations, and neuropsychological symptoms can also be present [2-5]. Pathophysiology of CPM consists of osmotic demyelination in the central pons with relative sparing of axons and neurons and is commonly associated with chronic alcoholism, liver failure, severe burns, malignant neoplasms, hemorrhagic pancreatitis, hemodialysis, and sepsis [6-8]. Rapid correction of hyponatremia has been proven as one of the most common and important etiologic factors [9, 10]. Although central pontine and extrapontine myelinolysis can present with behavioral and neuropsychiatric manifestations, there is limited literature available describing behavioral manifestations (personality changes, labile affect, disinhibition, poor judgment, paranoid delusions, emotional lability, delirium, hallucinations, and catatonia) in patients with CPM without any focal neurological deficits [3-6, 11-13]. Diffusion-weighted MRI (DWI) characteristically shows restricted diffusion in the central pons, and Positron Emission Tomography (PET) scan has been demonstrated to detect central pons hypermetabolism in patients with CPM [14-18].

Here, we describe a case of CPM with delirium and acute psychotic symptoms as the main manifestation of the

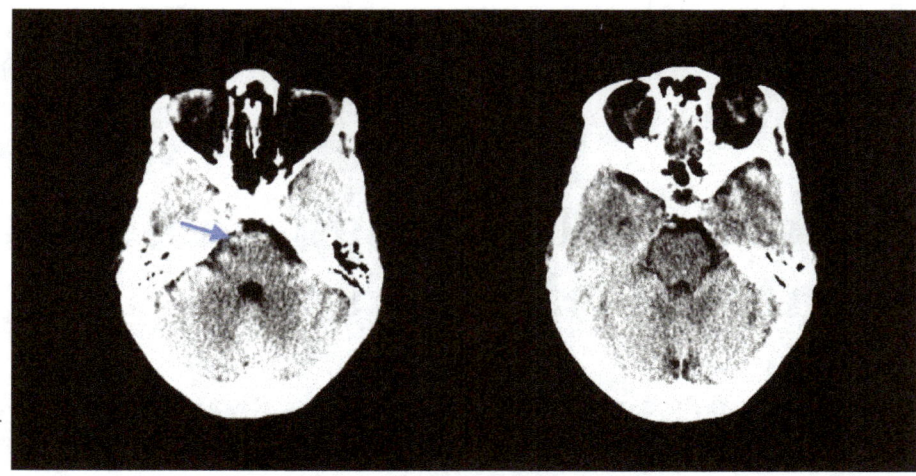

Figure 1: CT scan of the head on admission. Imaging shows no gross acute intracranial abnormality, except for mild bifrontal cerebellar atrophy and a 0.5 × 0.3 cm focal hypodense signal in the right pons (arrow), defined as beam hardening artifact.

syndrome, in the absence of focal neurological deficits, with evident hypermetabolism on PET scan, restricted diffusion on DWI MRI sequence, and minimal signal hyperintensity in the central pons on T2-weighted MRI, which became detectable on neuroimaging only after more than a week from the onset of patient's symptoms.

2. Case Presentation

A 51-year-old female with only medical history of asthma and smoking presented to the emergency department of an outlying hospital for evaluation of dizziness, frequent falls, diarrhea, and generalized weakness, which started about 1 week prior to admission. Review of symptoms was positive for fatigue, three 10-second long syncopal episodes with rapid return to baseline, urinary frequency, weight loss, and recent upper respiratory tract infection treated with azithromycin. Patient also reported to have had associated generalized weakness, lethargy, ataxia, and slurred speech, but no fever, night sweats, chills, and no history of prior neurological or psychiatric disease.

On further investigation into her history, it was found that, six months ago, the patient had a mammogram revealing a breast mass with inconspicuous weight loss. However, she did not follow up with her referral for an ultrasound.

Physical examination in the emergency department showed a somnolent and cachectic appearing female, who was nevertheless alert and oriented to time, place, and person. No focal neurological deficits were detected. Laboratory investigations revealed severe hyponatremia (106 mMol/L), hypokalemia (3 mMol/L), and hypochloremia (54 mMol/L). Treatment was initiated by administration of hypertonic saline, subsequently transitioned to normal saline. Chest X-ray and electrocardiogram were unremarkable. Computed tomography (CT) of the head without contrast showed no acute intracranial abnormality except for a small hypodense area seen at the right portion of the pons, attributed to a beam hardening artifact (Figure 1).

Within 24 hours of admission, the patient's serum sodium was corrected from 106 mMol/L to 121 mMol/L, a 15-point increase (Figure 2). Hypertonic saline was discontinued and replaced with 0.25% normal saline (NS) with 20 mEq KCL to maintain a sodium level in the mid-120s. At 48 hours, patient's sodium level increased to 124 mMol/L. On hospital day 3, she became confused, lethargic, and disorientated to time and place, developed urinary retention, started having intermittent blank stares, and was transferred to our facility for further management. A prompt electroencephalography (EEG) was performed, which showed diffuse background slowing consistent with moderate diffuse cerebral dysfunction, along with infrequent right temporal epileptiform discharges. She was placed on intravenous (IV) fosphenytoin and oral (PO) levetiracetam.

On day 4 of admission, with a sodium level of 120 mMol/L, the patient developed symptoms of acute psychosis: hypervigilance, persistent repetition of words, visual hallucinations, and frenzied speech. Shortly after, she became nonverbal and was unable to follow commands. It was suspected that she could have herpes simplex encephalitis; thus, while screening work-up was initiated, she was started on IV acyclovir.

On day 5, brain MRI was obtained (Figure 3) and lumbar puncture (LP) was performed to evaluate for structural, infectious, inflammatory, demyelinating, vasculitis, and/or autoimmune etiology. Neither neuroimaging nor cerebrospinal fluid (CSF) analysis revealed any significant abnormality. Urine drug screen, thyroid function profile, urinalysis, viral serology, systemic inflammatory and vasculitis markers, and cultures of fluids collected from various sources (blood, urine, and CSF) were all negative. Autoimmune encephalitis panel in blood and CSF also yielded negative results.

On day 7, as sodium level rose to 131 mMol/L, the confusion progressed; the patient was able to state her name but could not follow commands unless repeatedly prompted. She started expressing paranoid delusions, tangential speech, and echolalia. Generalized myoclonic tremor in all

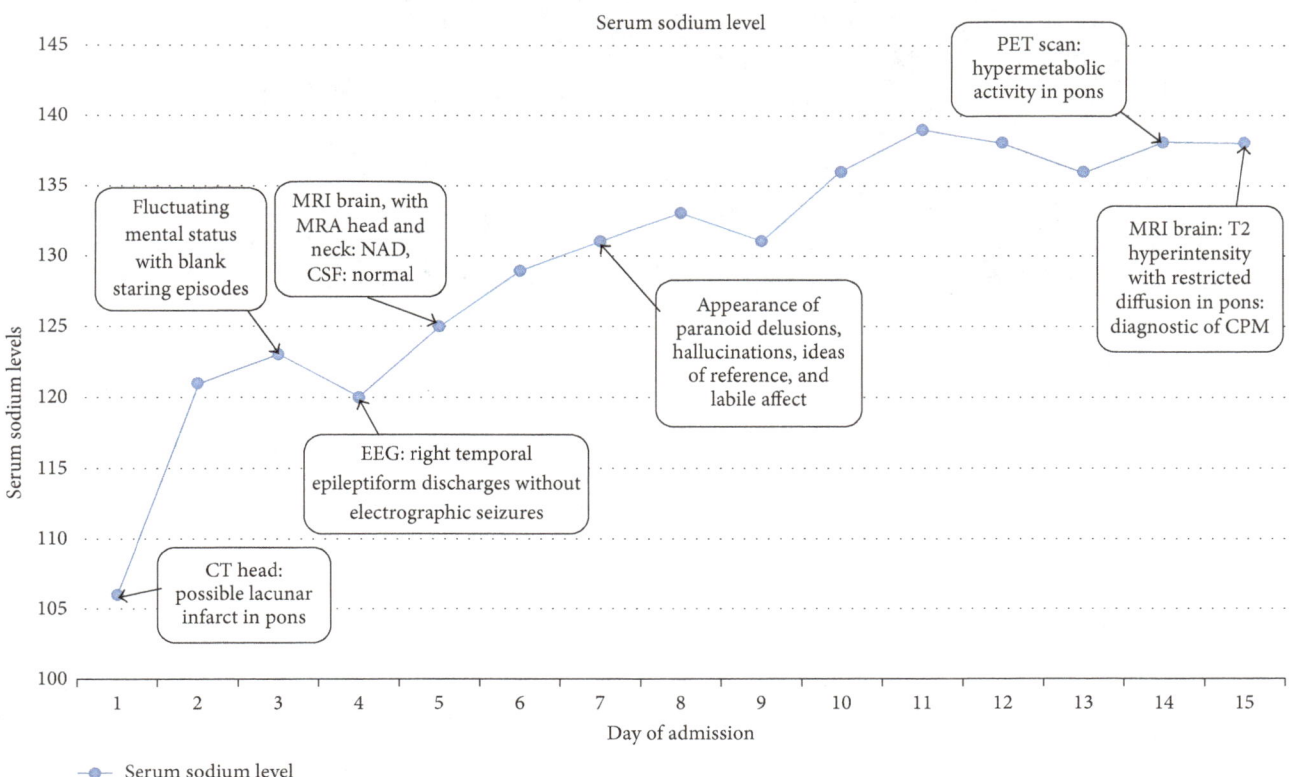

Figure 2: Serum sodium levels (in mMol/L) during hospitalization.

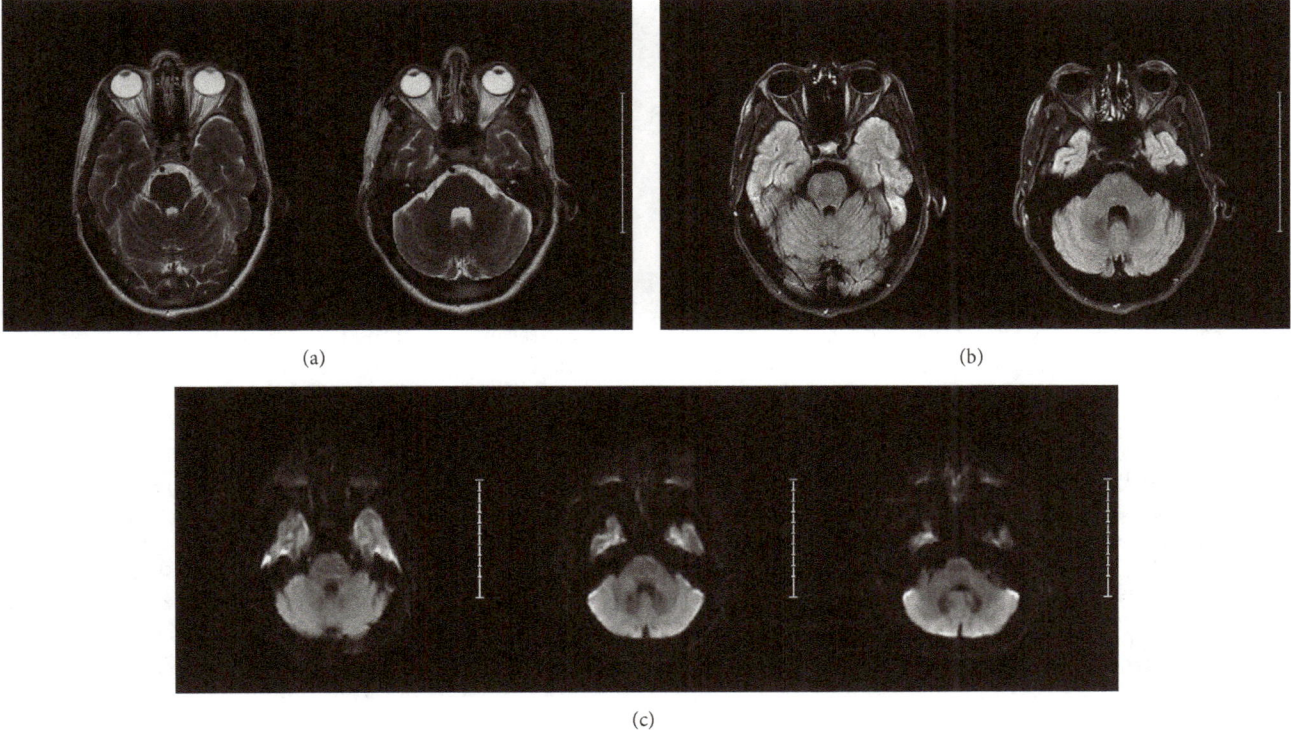

Figure 3: MRI obtained on hospital day 5. T2-weighted images (a), FLAIR (b), and DWI (c) showed no evidence of intracranial pathology.

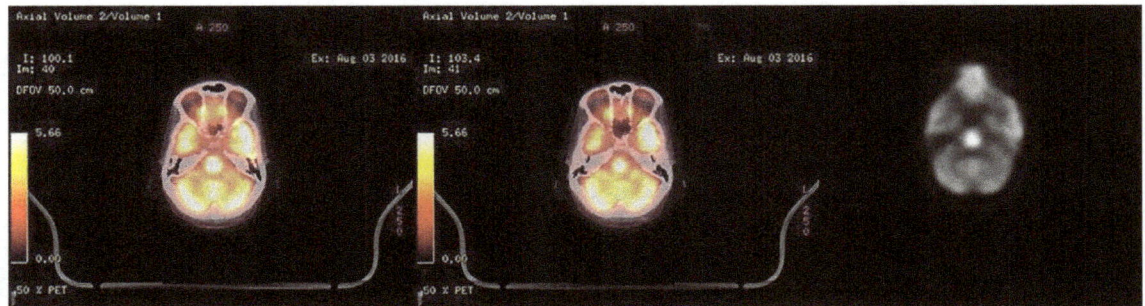

Figure 4: Head PET scan with F-fluorodeoxyglucose tracer on hospital day 14. Scans display focally intense hypermetabolic activity at the pons.

extremities was also noted on examination. A repeat EEG was obtained and showed mild nonspecific encephalopathy with no epileptiform activity. Given progression of patient's acute psychotic illness psychiatry consult was requested, which concluded that her behavioral symptoms were not driven by a primary psychiatric disorder but instead could be secondary to a medical illness.

The patient's sodium level rose to 139 mMol/L on hospital day 11. She continued to have visual hallucinations, paranoia, and persecutory delusions. She spoke to the television, had ideas of reference, and identified hospital staff with members of her family. The nonspecific myoclonic tremor in upper extremities continued with no obvious improvement. No other focal deficits were found on neurologic examination.

On day 14, extending the diagnostic work-up to include paraneoplastic brain syndrome, a full body PET scan was obtained to assess for occult malignancy, especially considering the known breast mass on previous mammogram, a history of smoking, and elevated serum carcinoembryonic antigen (CEA), obtained during this admission. While skeleton, neck, chest, abdomen, and pelvis scans showed no abnormal uptake of the tracer (data not shown), PET scan revealed abnormal hypermetabolic activity in the pons, suggestive of possible central pontine myelinolysis (Figure 4). Follow-up brain MRI with contrast was then obtained on day 15, which showed restricted diffusion in the central pons confirming the diagnosis of CPM (Figure 5).

The patient's clinical status did not change much with neurological treatment, consisting of a combination of antiepileptic medication, benzodiazepine, and atypical antipsychotic; delirium and hallucinations continued; she was still unable to follow complex commands and properly recognize faces and still had mild generalized myoclonic tremor, while all her metabolic and vital parameters were completely normalized. She was eventually discharged to a skilled nursing facility for further symptomatic management and rehabilitation.

3. Discussion

Central pontine myelinolysis (CPM) is a rare neurologic disorder caused by acute demyelination of the central pons. Rapid correction of serum sodium is the most common iatrogenic etiology; others include chronic alcoholism, malnutrition, liver failure, severe burns, and prolonged diuretic use [19]. The most common clinical manifestations of CPM include spastic quadriparesis, dysarthria, pseudobulbar palsy, and altered mental status. These symptoms can be delayed, occurring 2 to 14 days after rapid correction of hyponatremia. In most severe cases, "locked-in syndrome" or even death can occur [20, 21]. Extrapontine myelinolysis (EPM) is a pathophysiologically similar condition affecting 10% of patients with CPM [22]. In EPM, demyelinating lesions occur in brain structures other than the pons, including the basal ganglia (e.g., caudate nucleus), cerebellum, internal capsule, and thalamus. Recent literature has suggested that extrapontine lesions are associated with reversible movement disorders, such as parkinsonism, dystonia, catatonia, mutism, myoclonic jerks, and/or choreoathetosis [2, 9, 11–13]. Both CPM and EPM make up the spectrum of osmotic demyelination syndrome, which affects oligodendrocytes with relative preservation of neuronal axons [9]. The characteristic location of demyelination is thought to occur at the high grey-white matter admixture of the central pons and extrapontine sites in CPM and EPM, respectively.

The work-up of a hyponatremic state initially involves establishing the underlying cause for alteration of sodium metabolism [23]. In our patient, laboratory values for antidiuretic hormone (ADH), urine and serum osmolality, glucose, protein, and lipids were all normal. It is also important to make the distinction between acute and chronic hyponatremia. According to Tzamaloukas et al., while acute hyponatremia (onset less than 48 hours) showed more pronounced brain cell swelling and severity, there is a lower risk of CPM after correction of the sodium level [24]. With chronic hyponatremia, the brain has had the chance to adapt to osmotic fluid shifts; therefore, severe cerebral edema is less likely. However, chronic hyponatremia results in a greater overall loss of brain osmolytes, increasing the risk of CPM after rapid correction of sodium. Unfortunately, it was unknown whether our patient presented to the outlying hospital with acute or chronic hyponatremia.

Our patient's serum sodium level was corrected from 106 mMol/L to 121 mMol/L within the first 24 hours of admission. After 48 hours, the sodium level rose to 124 mMol/L and continued to rise over the following few days to a maximum of 139 mMol/L (Figure 2). According to Martin, a maximum sodium correction of 8 mMol/L within 24 hours,

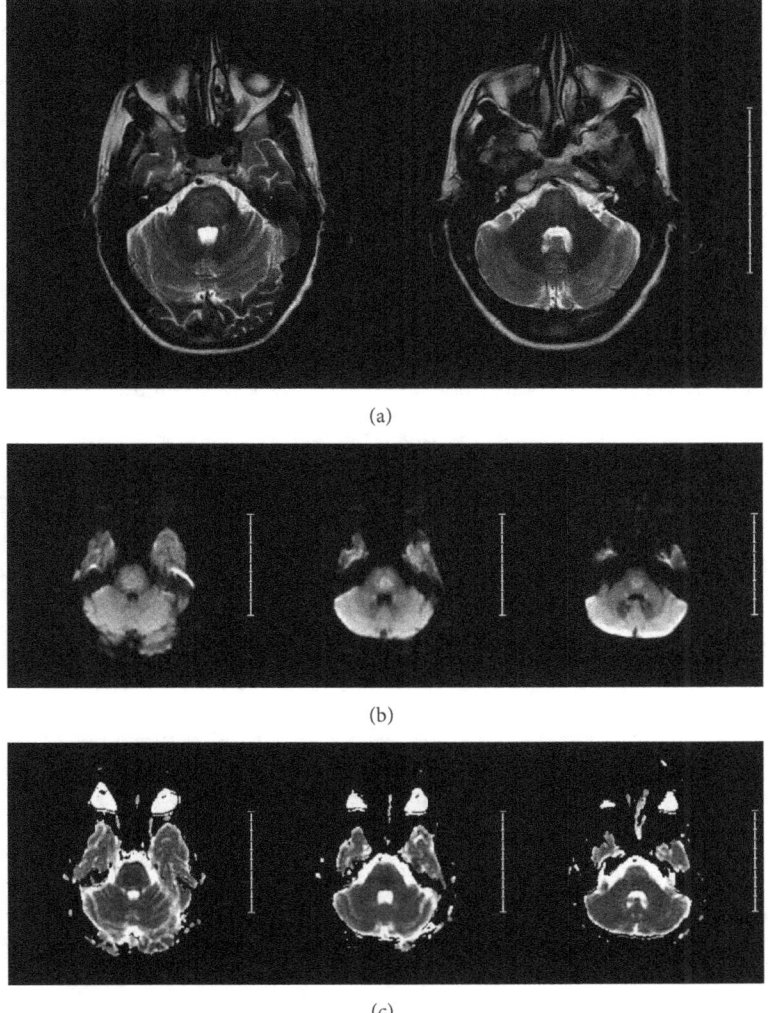

FIGURE 5: MRI with and without contrast on hospital day 15. T2-weighted MRI shows mild diffuse hyperintense signal changes in the pons (a); DWI sequence shows restricted diffusion (b) with corresponding ADC hypointensity (c) in central pons. These findings were not present when compared to MRI on hospital day 5 (Figure 3) and are consistent with central pontine myelinolysis.

not exceeding 1-2 mMol/L/hour, is recommended [9]. It is now apparent that in our patient the serum sodium level was raised too rapidly during the initial 24 hours, causing her to subsequently develop CPM. To date, once CPM has developed, there are no established effective treatments other than supportive therapy. Thus, prevention is the key to avoid iatrogenic CPM via slow correction of hyponatremia.

Psychiatric and behavioral manifestations are rare clinical presentations in patients with CPM and EPM. The psychiatric disturbances reportedly occur with the common motor manifestations of CPM, such as quadriparesis and dysarthria. The timeline for the onset of psychiatric manifestations in CMP/EPM is a conflict between many authors. Some state that psychiatric disturbances occur within two weeks after the onset of motor symptoms, while others report that motor symptoms can present in the two weeks after initial psychiatric disturbance is observed [3, 4, 11, 25]. To date, the exact pathophysiology of the psychiatric and behavioral manifestations in CPM remains to be elucidated. It is hypothesized that demyelination of the ascending fibers of the reticular activating system (RAS) in the pons is the primary etiology [3, 4]. Disruption of the RAS pathway to the thalamic nuclei may affect several neurotransmitter pathways, resulting in an acute change in behavior. Mostly, all case reports of psychiatric symptoms in CPM have demonstrated additional EPM lesions on MRI (basal ganglia, thalamus, etc.), with the exception of two reports by Price and Mesulam and Walterfang et al. [3, 25].

Our patient developed several manifestations of acute psychotic illness, including confusion, personality change, paranoid hallucinations, tangential speech, echolalia, and ideas of reference, within a week of rapid correction of hyponatremia. The most interesting aspect in our case was the lack of any characteristic motor manifestations of CPM, such as spastic quadriparesis, dysarthria, pseudobulbar palsy, or locked-in syndrome. Our patient displayed some motor signs, such as generalized myoclonic tremor and transient slurred speech with ataxia; however, these are not specific for CPM in the absence of the other characteristic motor manifestations. Thus, our case illustrates that acute psychiatric disturbance in the setting of rapid correction of hyponatremia may be the main presenting symptom of CPM.

The initial brain MRI performed two days after the onset of psychiatric symptoms (five days after rapid correction of sodium) was nondiagnostic and showed no changes in T1-weighted, T2-weighted, diffusion-weighted, or FLAIR image sequences (Figure 3). Generally, the appearance of MRI findings lags the clinical picture and could be delayed up to 10–14 days after rapid correction of sodium [9]. Given primarily neuropsychiatric symptoms in our patient and absence of pontine lesions on imaging, we further investigated other potential causes, including paraneoplastic syndrome secondary to an occult malignancy. As a result of such work-up, the full body PET scan showed increased uptake of radioactive glucose tracer in the pontine region (Figure 4), suggestive of possible CPM. Further assessment of the detected hypermetabolic signal in the pons with repeat MRI confirmed the diagnosis of CPM (Figure 5). It should be noted that neither PET scan nor MRI studies showed any extrapontine involvement in our patient, adding this case report to the few cases of primarily psychiatric manifestations of CPM without EPM.

PET scan is not routinely used for the diagnosis of CPM and the lesion was found incidentally while examining our patient for occult malignancy. The hypermetabolic intensity in the setting of CPM represents increased glucose uptake and metabolism of the phagocytic microglial cells and astrocytes following osmotic demyelination of oligodendrocytes in the pons [26]. It has been reported that the hypermetabolic signal is only transient and later scans may show a hypometabolic focus [17, 18]. This is because oligodendrocytes have limited proliferation capacity and the development of residual gliosis after the initial insult will follow.

The hyperintense signals on T2-weighted MRI and hypointense signals on T1-weighted MRI images in areas of pons demyelination are highly sensitive for diagnosis of CPM. While MRI is helpful in diagnosing CPM, the volume of T2-weighted MRI signal abnormality has been demonstrated to have no association with clinical outcomes in retrospective analysis by Graff-Radford et al. [27].

In our case, a repeat brain MRI was performed during the course of diagnostic investigations to confirm suspected CPM based on PET scan results. The repeat MRI revealed an area of diffusion restriction within the pons on DWI sequence and corresponding hyperintensity on T2-weighted imaging sequence confirming the diagnosis, but without evidence of extrapontine lesions (Figure 5). It should be emphasized that the initial MRI was negative on hospital day 5 and these changes were only noted on day 15, delaying the final diagnosis.

Ruzek et al. have reported the ability of DWI to detect changes before conventional MRI in a patient with suspected CPM within 24 hours of the onset of quadriparesis [15]. Since DWI measures the Brownian motion of water, it is hypothesized that the restricted diffusion in CPM is due to osmotic trapping of water in the intravascular space during the state of relative hypernatremia after rapid correction of hyponatremia [15]. The changes observed on DWI in our case, as well as other case reports, support the diagnostic utility of DWI in detecting acute demyelination in CPM, thus, allowing for prompt diagnosis [14], although the radiographic changes may still lag behind clinical manifestation by several days. However, there is no data in the literature on the validity of brain MRI in early diagnosis of CPM with only neuropsychiatric clinical manifestations in the absence of EPM.

The prognosis of recovery from neurological/neuropsychiatric manifestations of CPM is poor and deficit course is commonly thought to be irreversible. However, several case series and reports have demonstrated that some patients can recover with dependency, independency, or completely [6, 20, 27, 28]. Several case reports have shown reversibility of psychiatric symptoms in CPM with atypical antipsychotic medications [6, 11, 29]; hence, it is recommended that psychiatric manifestations in CPM should be treated with atypical antipsychotics and mood stabilizers, once the patient is neurologically stable. Nevertheless, Vermetten et al. have reported that while significant neurologic deficits may be fully reversible, neuropsychological deficits may remain longer after neurological recovery and may even be permanent [4]. Unfortunately, the psychiatric symptoms in our patient persisted despite optimal treatment with atypical antipsychotics and mood stabilizing therapy.

In conclusion, acute psychosis can present as the main manifestation of CPM. When the history of rapid correction of hyponatremia is present in a patient with neuropsychiatric manifestations, without the characteristic neurological abnormalities frequently seen in CPM, a repeat MRI study within 7–10 days after initial negative imaging could be useful in determining timely diagnosis. DWI seems to be the most specific MRI imaging sequence required for establishing the diagnosis. Currently, the only available treatment of neurological and neuropsychiatric manifestations associated with CPM is symptomatic and many patients do not achieve full recovery. Therefore, prevention is the key to proper management, which should consist of careful and gradual correction of serum sodium level in patients presenting with significant hyponatremia.

Disclosure

Mangala Gopal, Melvin Parasram, and Harsh Patel equally share the first authorship.

References

[1] R. D. Adams, M. Victor, and E. L. Mancall, "Central pontine myelinolysis: a hitherto undescribed disease occurring in alcoholic and malnourished patients," *AMA Archives Neuroligal Psychiatry*, vol. 81, no. 2, pp. 154–172, 1959.

[2] A. Seiser, S. Schwarz, M. M. Aichinger-Steiner, G. Funk, P. Schnider, and M. Brainin, "Parkinsonism and dystonia in central pontine and extrapontine myelinolysis," *Journal of Neurology, Neurosurgery, and Psychiatry*, vol. 65, no. 1, pp. 119–121, 1998.

[3] B. H. Price and M. M. Mesulam, "Behavioral manifestations of central pontine myelinolysis," *Archives of Neurology*, vol. 44, no. 6, pp. 671–673, 1987.

[4] E. Vermetten, S. J. E. Rutten, P. J. Boon, P. A. M. Hofman, and A. F. G. Leentjens, "Neuropsychiatric and neuropsychological manifestations of central pontine myelinolysis," *General Hospital Psychiatry*, vol. 21, no. 4, pp. 296–302, 1999.

[5] T. M. C. Lee, C. C. Y. Cheung, E. Y. Y. Lau, A. Mak, and L. S. W. Li, "Cognitive and emotional dysfunction after central pontine myelinolysis," *Behavioural Neurology*, vol. 14, no. 3-4, pp. 103–107, 2003.

[6] R. Gupta, Y. S. Balhara, and R. Sagar, "Acute psychosis with a favorable outcome as a complication of central pontine/extrapontine myelinolysis in a middle aged man," *Journal of Mid-life Health*, vol. 3, no. 2, pp. 103–105, 2012.

[7] J. D. Fleming and S. Babu, "Images in clinical medicine. Central pontine myelinolysis," *The New England Journal of Medicine*, vol. 359, no. 23, p. e29, 2008.

[8] C. Lampl and K. Yazdi, "Central pontine myelinolysis," *European Neurology*, vol. 47, no. 1, pp. 3–10, 2002.

[9] R. J. Martin, "Central pontine and extrapontine myelinolysis: the osmotic demyelination syndromes," *Neurology in Practice*, vol. 75, no. 3, pp. iii22–iii28, 2004.

[10] W.-Y. Huang, W.-C. Weng, T.-I. Peng, L.-S. Ro, C.-W. Yang, and K.-H. Chen, "Central pontine and extrapontine myelinolysis after rapid correction of hyponatremia by hemodialysis in a uremic patient," *Renal Failure*, vol. 29, no. 5, pp. 635–638, 2007.

[11] L. Lim and A. Krystal, "Psychotic disorder in a patient with central and extrapontine myelinolysis," *Psychiatry and Clinical Neurosciences*, vol. 61, no. 3, pp. 320–322, 2007.

[12] J. Chalela and J. Kattah, "Catatonia due to central pontine and extrapontine myelinolysis: case report," *Journal of Neurology, Neurosurgery and Psychiatry*, vol. 67, no. 5, pp. 692–693, 1999.

[13] S. K. Mattoo, P. Biswas, M. Sahoo, and S. Grover, "Catatonic syndrome in central pontine/extrapontine myelinolysis: a case report," *Progress in Neuro-Psychopharmacology and Biological Psychiatry*, vol. 32, no. 5, pp. 1344–1346, 2008.

[14] S. C. Cramer, K. C. Stegbauer, A. Schneider, J. Mukai, and K. R. Maravilla, "Decreased diffusion in central pontine myelinolysis," *American Journal of Neuroradiology*, vol. 22, no. 8, pp. 1476–1479, 2001.

[15] K. A. Ruzek, N. G. Campeau, and G. M. Miller, "Early diagnosis of central pontine myelinolysis with diffusion-weighted imaging," *American Journal of Neuroradiology*, vol. 25, no. 2, pp. 210–213, 2004.

[16] K. Chu, D.-W. Kang, S.-B. Ko, and M. Kim, "Diffusion-weighted MR findings of central pontine and extrapontine myelinolysis," *Acta Neurologica Scandinavica*, vol. 104, no. 6, pp. 385–388, 2001.

[17] J. K. Roh, H. Nam, and M. C. Lee, "A case of central pontine and extrapontine myelinolysis with early hypermetabolism on 18FDG-PET scan," *Journal of Korean Medical Science*, vol. 13, no. 1, pp. 99–102, 1998.

[18] M. Tripathi, A. Jaimini, M. DSouza et al., "Spectrum of brain abnormalities detected on whole body F-18 FDG PET/CT in patients undergoing evaluation for non-CNS malignancies," *Indian Journal of Nuclear Medicine*, vol. 26, no. 2, pp. 123–129, 2011.

[19] R. Abbott, E. Silber, J. Felber, and E. Ekpo, "Lesson of the week: osmotic demyelination syndrome," *British Medical Journal*, vol. 331, no. 7520, pp. 829–830, 2005.

[20] H. Menger and J. Jörg, "Outcome of central pontine and extrapontine myelinolysis ($n = 44$)," *Journal of Neurology*, vol. 246, no. 8, pp. 700–705, 1999.

[21] M. K. Sohn and J. H. Nam, "Locked-in syndrome due to central pontine myelinolysis: case report," *Annals of Rehabilitation Medicine*, vol. 38, no. 5, pp. 702–706, 2014.

[22] D. G. Wright, R. Laureno, and M. Victor, "Pontine and extrapontine myelinolysis," *Brain*, vol. 102, no. 2, pp. 361–385, 1979.

[23] G. Spasovski, R. Vanholder, B. Allolio et al., "Clinical practice guideline on diagnosis and treatment of hyponatraemia," *European Journal of Endocrinology*, vol. 170, no. 3, pp. G1–G47, 2014.

[24] A. H. Tzamaloukas, D. Malhotra, B. H. Rosen, D. S. C. Raj, G. H. Murata, and J. I. Shapiro, "Principles of management of severe hyponatremia," *Journal of the American Heart Association*, vol. 2, no. 1, Article ID e005199, 2013.

[25] M. Walterfang, A. Goh, R. Mocellin, A. Evans, and D. Velakoulis, "Peduncular hallucinosis secondary to central pontine myelinolysis," *Psychiatry and Clinical Neurosciences*, vol. 66, no. 7, pp. 618–621, 2012.

[26] S. Takefuji, T. Murase, Y. Sugimura et al., "Role of microglia in the pathogenesis of osmotic-induced demyelination," *Experimental Neurology*, vol. 204, no. 1, pp. 88–94, 2007.

[27] J. Graff-Radford, J. E. Fugate, T. J. Kaufmann, J. N. Mandrekar, and A. A. Rabinstein, "Clinical and radiologic correlations of central pontine myelinolysis syndrome," *Mayo Clinic Proceedings*, vol. 86, no. 11, pp. 1063–1067, 2011.

[28] R. N. Kallakatta, A. Radhakrishnan, R. K. Fayaz, J. P. Unnikrishnan, C. Kesavadas, and S. P. Sarma, "Clinical and functional outcome and factors predicting prognosis in osmotic demyelination syndrome (central pontine and/or extrapontine myelinolysis) in 25 patients," *Journal of Neurology, Neurosurgery and Psychiatry*, vol. 82, no. 3, pp. 326–331, 2011.

[29] R. Goggin, N. Nguyen, P. Tibrewal, R. Dhillon, B. Finlay, and D. Law, "Central pontine myelinolysis-induced mania: a case study," *Asian Journal of Psychiatry*, vol. 14, pp. 73–74, 2015.

Impaired Emotion Recognition after Left Hemispheric Stroke: A Case Report and Brief Review of the Literature

Hugo P. Aben,[1,2] Yael D. Reijmer,[2] Johanna M. A. Visser-Meily,[3] Jacoba M. Spikman,[4] Geert Jan Biessels,[2] Paul L. M. de Kort,[1] and PROCRAS Study Group[1,2,3,4]

[1]Department of Neurology, Elisabeth Tweesteden Hospital, Tilburg, Netherlands
[2]Department of Neurology, Brain Center Rudolf Magnus, University Medical Center Utrecht, Utrecht, Netherlands
[3]Department of Rehabilitation Medicine, Brain Center Rudolf Magnus, University Medical Center Utrecht, Utrecht, Netherlands
[4]Department of Clinical and Experimental Neuropsychology, University of Groningen, Groningen, Netherlands

Correspondence should be addressed to Hugo P. Aben; h.aben@etz.nl

Academic Editor: Majaz Moonis

Impaired recognition of emotion after stroke can have important implications for social competency, social participation, and consequently quality of life. We describe a case of left hemispheric ischemic stroke with impaired recognition of specifically faces expressing fear. Three months later, the patient's spouse reports that the patient was irritable and slow in communication, which may be caused by the impaired emotion recognition. The case is discussed in relation to the literature concerning emotion recognition and its neural correlates. Our case supports the notion that emotion recognition, including fear recognition, is regulated by a network of interconnected brain regions located in both hemispheres. We conclude that impaired emotion recognition is not uncommon after stroke and can be caused by dysfunction of this emotion-network.

1. Introduction

Social cognition concerns the psychological processes by which we perceive, process, and interpret social information [1]. Nowadays, neurologists are increasingly aware of the importance of screening for deficits in social cognition [2]. For example, screening for impaired social cognition has become more common in patients with traumatic brain injury [2, 3]. After stroke, impaired social cognition is prevalent, with a reported prevalence rate of 49% [4]. Despite the high prevalence, deficits in social cognition after stroke are often overlooked by the neurologist, and it is generally not spontaneously mentioned by the patient or his caregiver.

After stroke, impaired social cognition is partly reflected by worse emotion recognition in studies that compared patients to healthy controls in tasks examining facial, prosodic, and lexical emotional stimuli [5, 6]. These studies show that impaired emotion recognition after stroke is not limited to one modality: a stroke affects general processing of emotion for different modalities.

Impaired emotion recognition after stroke has a negative influence on social participation, and it can have important implications for a patient's quality of life [7]. Moreover, it can affect social competence [8], it predicts social behavior disorders [9], and it is negatively correlated with maintenance of personal and professional relations [10, 11].

We present a case with a profound difficulty in the recognition of faces expressing fear after insular stroke. Furthermore, the case is discussed in relation to the literature concerning emotion recognition and its neural correlates.

2. Case Description

A sixty-five-year-old, right-handed man, who had just retired from his work as a detective, presented with global aphasia, agitation, and a mild paresis of his right arm, which started acutely 5 hours before admission. He had no known vascular risk factors, and he had a degree in higher vocational education. The admission CT scan of his brain revealed no signs of ischemia or hemorrhage. One day after admission, the total

TABLE 1: The patient's results for the "Ekman 60 Faces Test."

Emotion	Nr correct answers	Mean scores reference sample (SD)	Cutoff values
Anger	8/10	7.33 (1.90)	4
Disgust	6/10	9.00 (1.62)	6
Fear	1/10*	6.47 (2.03)	3
Happiness	10/10	9.93 (0.42)	9
Sadness	5/10	8.03 (1.66)	5
Surprise	5/10*	8.66 (1.44)	6
Total	35/60*	49.41 (4.88)	41

The mean scores, standard deviations, and cutoff values for the reference sample (aged 61–70) are derived from the FEEST manual. This sample consisted of 58 healthy participants with an IQ > 90. Cutoff values have been calculated by using the nearest integer value to a z-value of 1.65 below average [12]. *Scores below the cutoff value.

TABLE 2: Neuropsychological assessment of the patient.

Domain	T-score	Tests	T-scores
Attention and processing speed	46.6	Reaction Time Test, Vienna Test System, S1, S2	50.5
		Symbol Digit Modalities Test	44.2
		Trail Making Test A	41.0
(Working) memory and learning	39.2	WAIS Digit Span Forward and Backward	41.7
		The Rey Auditory Verbal Learning Test	38.0
Frontal-Executive functions	39.8	Controlled Oral Word Association Test	30.0*
		Hayling Test	40.0
		Reaction time test, Vienna Test System, S3	47.0
		Trail Making Test B	44.0
Language	31.6*	Boston Naming Test	23.1*
		Semantic fluency	40.0
Visuospatial function	NA	Bells Test, no T-score available, 1 omission	NA

This table shows the T-scores of the patient for each of the tested domains in the neuropsychological assessment. *Scores below 1.5 standard deviations.

score on the Montreal Cognitive Assessment (MoCA) was 20 out of a maximum of 30 points, mainly failing the subdomains language (0/3), delayed recall (2/5), and visuospatial function (2/5). The patient correctly copied the cube and made no mistake in the contour of the clock. However, he did not add numbers to the clock and placed the hands at ten to eleven, instead of ten past eleven. Two days after admission, the patient did not report any complaints. The aphasia, paresis, and agitation had resolved quickly, and the patient was discharged home. As part of an observational study, the PROCRAS study, see Additional Points for more information, the patient underwent a detailed neuropsychological assessment and MRI scan of his brain 4 weeks after the stroke. Apart from complaining of being tired more quickly, he had no other complaints at that point. As part of the neuropsychological assessment, the "Ekman 60 Faces Test," part of the Facial Expressions of Emotion: Stimuli and Tests (FEEST), was performed [12]. Interestingly, out of 10 presented fearful faces, he recognized only 1 facial expression correctly. For his performance on other emotions, see Table 1. His total score on the FEEST was nearly 3 standard deviations below the norm. There were no symptoms of depression or anxiety on the Hospital Anxiety and Depression Scale (HADS). Moreover, there were no signs of prosopagnosia, and the Bells Test revealed no visuospatial dysfunction. Further extensive neuropsychological testing revealed problems with naming objects on the Boston Naming Test but no impaired performance on the verbal fluency test. In Table 2, the T-scores for each domain and the subtests that constitute these domains are presented. The MRI showed a lesion of the posterior part of the left insula but also of a part of the left temporal cortex and the left parietal cortex as can be seen in Figure 1. In order to investigate potential impairments in brain connectivity, the brain network of the patient was reconstructed from the diffusion weighted MR images as described in Reijmer et al. [13]. The mean fractional anisotropy of the white matter tracts connected to each of the 90 cortical and subcortical brain regions was calculated. The brain networks of 25 age-matched healthy control participants served as a reference group. Results showed that the connectivity strength of the patient was markedly reduced (>1.5 SD lower compared to the reference sample) in several parietal, temporal, and subcortical regions, primarily in the left hemisphere (Figure 2), indicating disconnection of a network of brain regions.

Three months after the stroke, the patient felt no restrictions in his ability to perform hobbies such as gardening and reading, and he experienced no difficulties in social

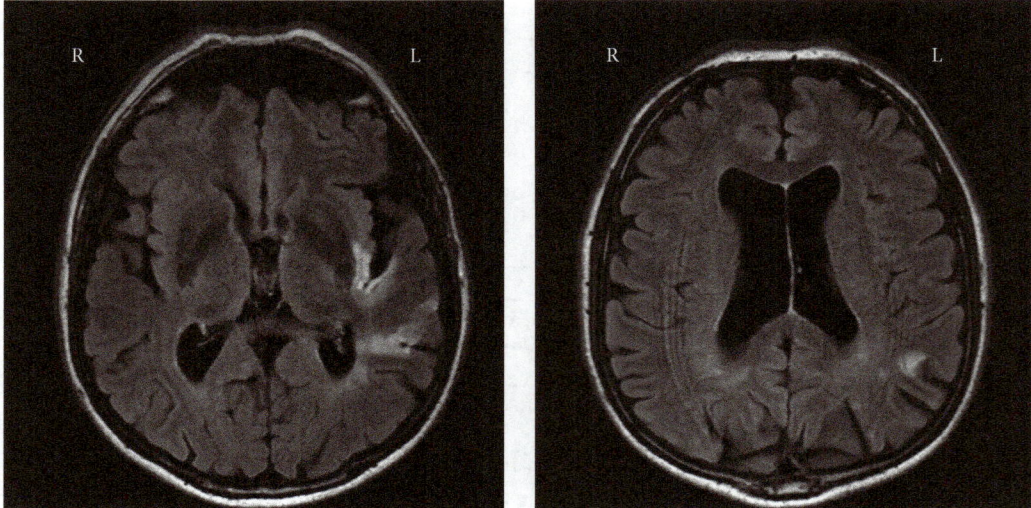

Figure 1: Transversal fluid attenuated inversion recovery (FLAIR) images of the patient, revealing a lesion to the posterior part of the insula and part of the left temporal cortex and left parietal cortex.

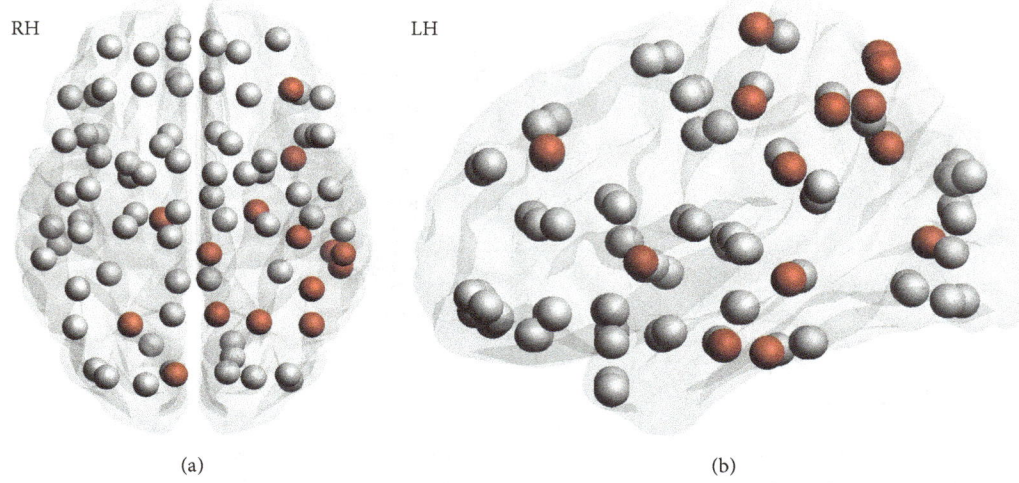

Figure 2: Axial (a) and lateral (b) view of the disconnectivity profile of the patient (obtained from analyzing the DTI-MRI data). Nodes represent 90 cortical and subcortical brain regions [38]. The red nodes indicate regions with more than 1.5 standard deviations of decreased connectivity strength compared to 25 age-matched healthy controls. Note that nodes surrounding the ischemic zone are affected. In addition, however, nodes in the contralesional hemisphere and a frontal node are affected. This suggests that the stroke affected a network of brain regions.

contact. However, his wife reported that he has been slower in communication and manifests slight irritability ever since the stroke.

3. Discussion

In this article, we present a case with a profound deficit in the recognition of facial emotions expressing fear after enduring a stroke of the posterior part of the left insula and parts of the left temporal and parietal cortex. There was no evidence of depressive or anxious symptoms on follow-up, suggesting that the difficulty in recognition of fearful faces was not caused by a depressive or anxiety disorder. It has not been ruled out that visuospatial dysfunction caused the impaired recognition of facial emotions. However, the score of 2/5 for the MoCA's visuospatial subdomain might have been caused by a language disorder rather than a visuospatial disorder. Moreover, the Bells Test revealed no abnormalities at the neuropsychological examination 4 weeks after stroke, making a neglect very unlikely. It was not clear whether our patient had difficulties in emotion recognition before the stroke, for example, due to an autism spectrum disorder or traumatic brain injury in the past. However, we think that his higher education level and his work as a detective require at least adequate social cognitive skills. Therefore, it is plausible to attribute the profound deficit in fear recognition to the stroke. This case stood out because of two reasons. First, the stroke involved the left hemisphere, while emotion recognition is generally attributed to the right hemisphere [5]. Secondly, the deficit in recognition of fearful faces after ischemia of the posterior part of the insula seems to contradict earlier findings in the literature [14–16]. Recognition of fear has been strongly linked to activity in the amygdala [16], whereas the insula is thought to be specifically engaged in the recognition of disgust [14, 15]. We will discuss the literature in relation to the case and these two findings.

3.1. Laterality in Emotion Recognition.

Researchers have still not reached consensus on the specific contribution of the right and left hemisphere to emotion recognition. A recent review of many studies examining emotion recognition after stroke found more support for the hypothesis that emotion recognition seems to be largely lateralized to the right hemisphere, independent of valence [5, 17]. Several studies report that left hemispheric stroke patients perform as good as healthy controls in the recognition of emotions [18–21]. However, other studies do reveal differences in emotion recognition between patients with a left hemispheric stroke and healthy controls [22–24]. The left hemispheric stroke of our patient is in line with these studies and adds to the theory that the left hemisphere also contributes to the process of emotion recognition. According to the motoric direction theory, the left hemisphere is specialized in "approach" emotions (i.e., happiness, anger, and surprise), whereas the right hemisphere is responsible for recognizing "withdrawal" emotions (i.e., sadness, fear, and disgust) [25]. The patient had relative ease in recognizing anger and happiness, although he scored below the cutoff score for surprise. He scored relatively low for the withdrawal emotions: fear, sadness, and disgust. Although the patient does partly fit the pattern of this hypothesis, the location of the stroke would suggest that the specialization of both hemispheres is just the opposite of what the motoric direction theory suggests. Possibly, disconnectivity between both hemispheres (Figure 2) could explain this mismatch.

3.2. Neural Correlates of Emotion Recognition.

Several brain structures have been suggested to be involved in emotion recognition. For example, lesions to left or right temporal cortex lead to impaired emotion recognition [26]. However, lesions to the basal ganglia [27, 28], the cerebellum [29], the thalamus [30], the right inferior parietal cortex, and the anterior infracalcarine cortex [18] can have the same consequence. It is well known that activity in the amygdala has been strongly linked to recognition of fear [16], and a lesion of the amygdala causes an impairment in fear recognition [31–33]. However, this does not imply that lesions of the amygdala are the unique cause of impaired fear recognition. For example, a study reported that a lesion to the right infracalcarine cortex also seems to lead to a specific impairment in the recognition of fear [18]. This suggests that even the recognition of one single emotion, in this case the emotion fear, is a process that involves, like all cognitive functions [34], a network of brain structures.

A meta-analysis of fMRI and PET studies [16] in healthy controls concluded that the neural network involved in recognition of emotion consists of three important structures. The first is the medial prefrontal cortex (MPFC), which has a general role in emotional processing. The other two are the anterior cingulate cortex (ACC) and the insula, which are more specifically involved in emotion recognition, especially in more cognitive demanding tasks [16].

3.3. The Insula and Emotion Recognition.

Because our patient had a stroke involving, among others, the posterior part of the left insula, this specific lesion might have caused the difficulty in recognition of emotion. In behavioral and imaging studies, the insula is found to be engaged in the recognition of disgust [14, 15]. However, less is known about the consequences of a lesion to the insula. Several case studies describe different responses to an acute lesion of the left insula. In one study, a patient had impairments in global cognitive functioning as reflected by cognitive screening with the MoCA [35], comparable with the case we described. In a double case report, one patient with insular stroke had only slightly slower response times but no impaired emotion recognition [36]. The second case that is described had a subcortical stroke, disconnecting the connections from the insula to the frontal cortex. In this case, an impaired recognition of all negative emotions was found. Another study reported on a patient with behavioral changes after an isolated stroke of the anterior part of the right insula [37]. Although emotion perception was not assessed, an additional SPECT scan showed hypoperfusion in several right anterior brain structures, most of which are thought to be involved in an emotion-network.

3.4. A Matter of (Dis)connection?

As stated earlier, the left insula plays a role in a network of structures involved in emotion recognition. This can be supported by a recent study in which direct electrical stimulation was applied to the left insula during awake surgery in thirteen patients causing a decreased recognition of all negative emotions [39]. Another study found that impaired emotion recognition was associated with dysfunction of a bilateral fronto-temporal-limbic network in 180 patients with traumatic brain injury (TBI) [40]. A different study found that damage anywhere to the inferior frontooccipital fasciculus or the inferior longitudinal fasciculus is associated with impaired emotion recognition [41]. The seemingly contradicting evidence of different presentations after insular stroke can be better interpreted as the consequence of disconnection to frontal or a variety of contralateral regions [42]. This implies that the process of emotion recognition is not confined to a specific location, a lesion anywhere in this "emotion-network" may lead to a deficit in emotion recognition [43].

We hypothesize that in our patient the stroke caused damage to the network involved in emotion recognition, which is supported by the analysis of the DTI-MRI data (Figure 2). Although this analysis does not provide direct evidence for emotion recognition being a network-function, it does support this theory by showing disconnection in more brain structures than those directly affected by the stroke. We propose that the profound impairment of recognition of fear can be explained by a disconnection of fibers to this emotion-network.

3.5. Impact of Impaired Emotion Recognition after Stroke. Impaired emotion recognition has been found to negatively impact social participation and quality of life after stroke [44]. For deficits in emotion regulation, the same consequences have been established [45]. The patient's spouse reported that the patient showed slight irritability and slowness in communication after the stroke, although the patient himself stated having no difficulties in social interaction. We hypothesize that the deficit in emotion recognition could partly contribute to these symptoms, and this deficit could consequently lead to restrictions in social participation.

4. Conclusions

Impaired emotion recognition is prevalent after stroke. However, it is not often reported by the patient or the caregiver, it is not easily recognized, and it is not routinely investigated in clinical practice. This is unfortunate, since impaired emotion recognition negatively impacts social participation. Detection of impaired emotion recognition may help in guidance of the patient and his caregiver. In turn, this should help people better reintegrate into daily life and increase quality of life.

Emotion recognition is a complex process involving many neural structures. A lesion anywhere in this emotion-network can lead to dysfunction. Further research on emotion recognition should shift its focus from the specific localization of emotion recognition to identifying the brain regions and the functional and structural connections that form part of this emotion-network.

Additional Points

In the Prediction of Cognitive Recovery After Stroke (PROCRAS) study, we aim to investigate the additional value of measures of structural connectivity derived from diffusion tensor imaging- (DTI-) MRI in the prediction of cognitive recovery after stroke. Patients with the clinical diagnosis of a stroke with a MoCA total score below 26 undergo a neuropsychological assessment and DTI-MRI 3-6 weeks after stroke. One year after stroke the neuropsychological assessment is repeated to assess the primary endpoint.

Acknowledgments

The names of the PROCRAS study group are as follows: H. Aben, M.D. (author); P. de Kort MD, Ph.D. (author); G. J. Biessels, M.D., Ph.D. (author); A. Meily-Visser M.D., Ph.D. (author); J. Spikman, Ph.D. (author); Y. Reijmer, Ph.D. (author); J. Smetsers, M.S.; L. Luijten, M.D.; P. van de Sande; J. de Bresser, M.D., Ph.D.; M. de Groot, Ph.D.; B. Jakobs, Ph.D. The PROCRAS study is funded by ZonMW (Grant no. 842003011); Y. Reijmer receives funding from Alzheimer Nederland and ZonMw/Memorabel (Grant no. 733050503).

References

[1] J. D. Henry, W. von Hippel, P. Molenberghs, T. Lee, and P. S. Sachdev, "Clinical assessment of social cognitive function in neurological disorders," *Nature Reviews Neurology*, vol. 12, no. 1, pp. 28–39, 2016.

[2] M. R. Benedictus, J. M. Spikman, and J. Van Der Naalt, "Cognitive and behavioral impairment in traumatic brain injury related to outcome and return to work," *Archives of Physical Medicine and Rehabilitation*, vol. 91, no. 9, pp. 1436–1441, 2010.

[3] J. M. Spikman, M. E. Timmerman, M. V. Milders, W. S. Veenstra, and J. van der Naalt, "Social cognition impairments in relation to general cognitive deficits, injury severity, and prefrontal lesions in traumatic brain injury patients," *Journal of Neurotrauma*, vol. 29, no. 1, pp. 101–111, 2012.

[4] S. E. Starkstein, R. C. Leiguarda, J. P. Federoff, T. R. Price, and R. G. Robinson, "Neuropsychological and neuroradiologic correlates of emotional prosody comprehension," *Neurology*, vol. 44, no. 3, pp. 515–522, 1994.

[5] R. Yuvaraj, M. Murugappan, M. I. Norlinah, K. Sundaraj, and M. Khairiyah, "Review of emotion recognition in stroke patients," *Dementia and Geriatric Cognitive Disorders*, vol. 36, no. 3-4, pp. 179–196, 2013.

[6] J. C. Borod, L. K. Obler, H. M. Erhan et al., "Right hemisphere emotional perception: evidence across multiple channels," *Neuropsychology*, vol. 12, no. 3, pp. 446–458, 1998.

[7] K. Kim, Y. M. Kim, and E. K. Kim, "Correlation between the activities of daily living of stroke patients in a community setting and their quality of life," *Journal of Physical Therapy Science*, vol. 26, no. 3, pp. 417–419, 2014.

[8] S. L. Langer, L. C. Pettigrew, J. F. Wilson, and L. X. Blonder, "Personality and social competency following unilateral stroke," *Journal of the International Neuropsychological Society*, vol. 4, no. 5, pp. 447–455, 1998.

[9] P. Narme, M. Roussel, H. Mouras, P. Krystkowiak, and O. Godefroy, "Does impaired socioemotional functioning account for behavioral dysexecutive disorders? Evidence from a transnosological study," *Aging, Neuropsychology, and Cognition*, pp. 1–14, 2016.

[10] G. Yeates, M. Rowberry, S. Dunne et al., "Social cognition and executive functioning predictors of supervisors' appraisal of interpersonal behaviour in the workplace following acquired brain injury," *NeuroRehabilitation*, vol. 38, no. 3, pp. 299–310, 2016.

[11] L. X. Blonder, L. C. Pettigrew, and R. J. Kryscio, "Emotion recognition and marital satisfaction in stroke," *Journal of Clinical and Experimental Neuropsychology*, vol. 34, no. 6, pp. 634–642, 2012.

[12] A. Young, D. Perrett, A. Calder, R. Sprengelmeyer, and P. Ekman, *Facial Expressions of Emotion—Stimuli and Tests (FEEST)*, v.1.0, Thames Valley Test Company, v.1.0 edition, 2002.

[13] Y. D. Reijmer, A. Leemans, K. Caeyenberghs, S. M. Heringa, H. L. Koek, and G. J. Biessels, "Disruption of cerebral networks and cognitive impairment in Alzheimer disease," *Neurology*, vol. 80, no. 15, pp. 1370–1377, 2013.

[14] P. Krolak-Salmon, M.-A. Hénaff, J. Isnard et al., "An attention modulated response to disgust in human ventral anterior insula," *Annals of Neurology*, vol. 53, no. 4, pp. 446–453, 2003.

[15] R. Adolphs, D. Tranel, and A. R. Damasio, "Dissociable neural systems for recognizing emotions," *Brain and Cognition*, vol. 52, no. 1, pp. 61–69, 2003.

[16] K. L. Phan, T. Wager, S. F. Taylor, and I. Liberzon, "Functional neuroanatomy of emotion: a meta-analysis of emotion activation studies in PET and fMRI," *NeuroImage*, vol. 16, no. 2, pp. 331–348, 2002.

[17] J. C. Borod, "Interhemispheric and intrahemispheric control of emotion: a focus on unilateral brain damage," *Journal of Consulting and Clinical Psychology*, vol. 60, no. 3, pp. 339–348, 1992.

[18] R. Adolphs, H. Damasio, D. Tranel, and A. R. Damasio, "Cortical systems for the recognition of emotion in facial expressions," *Journal of Neuroscience*, vol. 16, no. 23, pp. 7678–7687, 1996.

[19] D. Bowers, R. M. Bauer, H. B. Coslett, and K. M. Heilman, "Processing of faces by patients with unilateral hemisphere lesions. I. Dissociation between judgments of facial affect and facial identity," *Brain and Cognition*, vol. 4, no. 3, pp. 258–272, 1985.

[20] S. Charbonneau, B. P. Scherzer, D. Aspirot, and H. Cohen, "Perception and production of facial and prosodic emotions by chronic CVA patients," *Neuropsychologia*, vol. 41, no. 5, pp. 605–613, 2003.

[21] J. J. Schmitt, W. Hartje, and K. Willmes, "Hemispheric asymmetry in the recognition of emotional attitude conveyed by facial expression, prosody and propositional speech," *Cortex*, vol. 33, no. 1, pp. 65–81, 1997.

[22] K. Kucharska-Pietura, M. L. Phillips, W. Gernand, and A. S. David, "Perception of emotions from faces and voices following unilateral brain damage," *Neuropsychologia*, vol. 41, no. 8, pp. 1082–1090, 2003.

[23] M. K. Mandal, J. C. Borod, H. S. Asthana, A. Mohanty, S. Mohanty, and E. Koff, "Effects of lesion variables and emotion type on the perception of facial emotion," *Journal of Nervous and Mental Disease*, vol. 187, no. 10, pp. 603–609, 1999.

[24] M. Peper and E. Irle, "The decoding of emotional concepts in patients with focal cerebral lesions," *Brain and Cognition*, vol. 34, no. 3, pp. 360–387, 1997.

[25] R. J. Davidson, P. Ekman, C. D. Saron, J. A. Senulis, and W. V. Friesen, "Approach-withdrawal and cerebral asymmetry: emotional expression and brain physiology I," *Journal of Personality and Social Psychology*, vol. 58, no. 2, pp. 330–341, 1990.

[26] C. Xi, Y. Zhu, C. Zhu, D. Song, Y. Wang, and K. Wang, "Deficit of theory of mind after temporal lobe cerebral infarction," *Behavioral and Brain Functions*, vol. 9, no. 1, article 15, 2013.

[27] J. Kemp, M.-C. Berthel, A. Dufour et al., "Caudate nucleus and social cognition: neuropsychological and SPECT evidence from a patient with focal caudate lesion," *Cortex*, vol. 49, no. 2, pp. 559–571, 2013.

[28] C. C. Y. Cheung, T. M. C. Lee, J. T. H. Yip, K. E. King, and L. S. W. Li, "The differential effects of thalamus and basal ganglia on facial emotion recognition," *Brain and Cognition*, vol. 61, no. 3, pp. 262–268, 2006.

[29] M. Adamaszek, K. C. Kirkby, F. Dagata et al., "Neural correlates of impaired emotional face recognition in cerebellar lesions," *Brain Research*, vol. 1613, pp. 1–12, 2015.

[30] E. Wilkos, T. J. B. Brown, K. Slawinska, and K. Akucharska, "Social cognitive and neurocognitive deficits in inpatients with unilateral thalamic lesions—pilot study," *Neuropsychiatric Disease and Treatment*, vol. 11, pp. 1031–1038, 2015.

[31] R. Adolphs, F. Gosselin, T. W. Buchanan, D. Tranel, P. Schyns, and A. R. Damasio, "A mechanism for impaired fear recognition after amygdala damage," *Nature*, vol. 433, no. 7021, pp. 68–72, 2005.

[32] D. R. Bach, R. Hurlemann, and R. J. Dolan, "Impaired threat prioritisation after selective bilateral amygdala lesions," *Cortex*, vol. 63, pp. 206–213, 2015.

[33] D. Dellacherie, D. Hasboun, M. Baulac, P. Belin, and S. Samson, "Impaired recognition of fear in voices and reduced anxiety after unilateral temporal lobe resection," *Neuropsychologia*, vol. 49, no. 4, pp. 618–629, 2011.

[34] H.-J. Park and K. Friston, "Structural and functional brain networks: from connections to cognition," *Science*, vol. 342, no. 6158, Article ID 1238411, 2013.

[35] P. Julayanont, D. Ruthirago, and J. C. DeToledo, "Isolated left posterior insular infarction and convergent roles in verbal fluency, language, memory, and executive function," *Proceedings (Baylor University Medical Center)*, vol. 29, no. 3, pp. 295–297, 2016.

[36] B. Couto, L. Sedeño, L. A. Sposato et al., "Insular networks for emotional processing and social cognition: comparison of two case reports with either cortical or subcortical involvement," *Cortex*, vol. 49, no. 5, pp. 1420–1434, 2013.

[37] H.-J. Cho, S.-J. Kim, S. J. Hwang et al., "Social-emotional dysfunction after isolated right anterior insular infarction," *Journal of Neurology*, vol. 259, no. 4, pp. 764–767, 2012.

[38] N. Tzourio-Mazoyer, B. Landeau, D. Papathanassiou et al., "Automated anatomical labeling of activations in SPM using a macroscopic anatomical parcellation of the MNI MRI single-subject brain," *NeuroImage*, vol. 15, no. 1, pp. 273–289, 2002.

[39] C. Papagno, A. Pisoni, G. Mattavelli et al., "Specific disgust processing in the left insula: new evidence from direct electrical stimulation," *Neuropsychologia*, vol. 84, pp. 29–35, 2016.

[40] O. Dal Monte, F. Krueger, J. M. Solomon et al., "A voxel-based lesion study on facial emotion recognition after penetrating brain injury," *Social Cognitive and Affective Neuroscience*, vol. 8, no. 6, pp. 632–639, 2013.

[41] C. L. Philippi, S. Mehta, T. Grabowski, R. Adolphs, and D. Rudrauf, "Damage to association fiber tracts impairs recognition of the facial expression of emotion," *Journal of Neuroscience*, vol. 29, no. 48, pp. 15089–15099, 2009.

[42] R. Limongi, A. Tomio, and A. Ibanez, "Dynamical predictions of insular hubs for social cognition and their application to stroke," *Frontiers in Behavioral Neuroscience*, vol. 8, article 380, 2014.

[43] D. P. Kennedy and R. Adolphs, "The social brain in psychiatric and neurological disorders," *Trends in Cognitive Sciences*, vol. 16, no. 11, pp. 559–572, 2012.

[44] C. L. Cooper, L. H. Phillips, M. Johnston, B. Radlak, S. Hamilton, and M. J. McLeod, "Links between emotion perception and social participation restriction following stroke," *Brain Injury*, vol. 28, no. 1, pp. 122–126, 2014.

[45] C. L. Cooper, L. H. Phillips, M. Johnston, M. Whyte, and M. J. Macleod, "The role of emotion regulation on social participation following stroke," *British Journal of Clinical Psychology*, vol. 54, no. 2, pp. 181–199, 2015.

Bilateral Moyamoya Disease in a 2-Year-Old Pakistani Male Treated with Bilateral Encephaloduroarteriosynangiosis: A Positive Outcome

Shahvaiz Magsi,[1] Adeel Khoja,[1] Mansoor Ali Merchant Rameez,[2] Ariba Khan,[2] and Noman Ishaque[1]

[1]*Aga Khan University, Karachi, Pakistan*
[2]*DOW University of Health Sciences, Karachi, Pakistan*

Correspondence should be addressed to Shahvaiz Magsi; magsi.shahvaiz@gmail.com

Academic Editor: Majaz Moonis

Background. We present a rare case of bilateral moyamoya disease presenting as multiple strokes and neurological deficits, treated with the neurosurgical procedure, encephaloduroarteriosynangiosis (EDAS), in a 2-year-old male Pakistani minor. A positive outcome was achieved and the patient recovered fully. *Case Summary*. Our patient presented with a history of seizures and multiple episodes of hemiparesis (on and off weakness) at the age of 2 years. He had a delayed speech development and could not speak more than a few words. He had a slight slurring of speech too. He was diagnosed with bilateral moyamoya disease on Computed Tomography Angiography (CTA). Bilateral EDAS was done in the same year, after which his symptoms improved and patient had moderate functional recovery. *Conclusion*. A rare disease, moyamoya has been left unexplored in Pakistan; physicians and surgeons when dealing with cases in the pediatric population presenting with symptoms of stroke, signs of generalized weakness, and seizures should consider moyamoya disease as a possibility. Furthermore, this case demonstrates the effectiveness of EDAS procedure for the treatment of moyamoya disease.

1. Background

First described in 1957, moyamoya disease, a rare cerebrovascular disorder, is defined as a disease of progressive stenosis involving the terminal portions of internal carotid arteries as well as the anterior and middle cerebral vasculature, associated with formation of collateral vessels at the base of the brain [1]. The diagnosis of moyamoya is mainly based on angiographic findings and a majority of these cases are reported in Asia [2].

There has not been much studied regarding moyamoya in our population as there are only two case series with a total of 17 patients, of which 10 were of less than 12 years of age [3, 4]. Few studies reported higher incidence of stroke in younger age group in our part of the world as compared to western population, which probably indicate underdiagnosis of moyamoya [5].

Surgical treatments such as EDAS involve revascularization of underperfused areas by creating an indirect anastomosis between external and internal carotid circulation by transposition of a segment of scalp artery onto the surface of the brain leading to proliferation of collateral blood vessel development [6]. The ability to develop collateral blood vessels after EDAS procedure has shown a better result in pediatric age group as compared to the adult population [6].

2. Case Report

We report a case of 2-year-old male patient, resident of Punjab, Pakistan, presenting with high grade fever along with seizures and left sided weakness of face, arm, and leg. An MRI was recommended along with a CSF culture; the MRI did not show any signs of stroke; it was deduced to be an episode of a transient ischemic attack (TIA) or an infection.

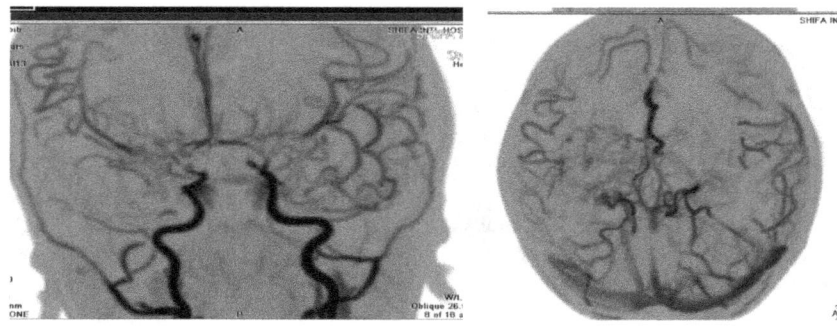

Figure 1: Preoperative CTA head showing stenosis of supraclinoid parts of bilateral ICA.

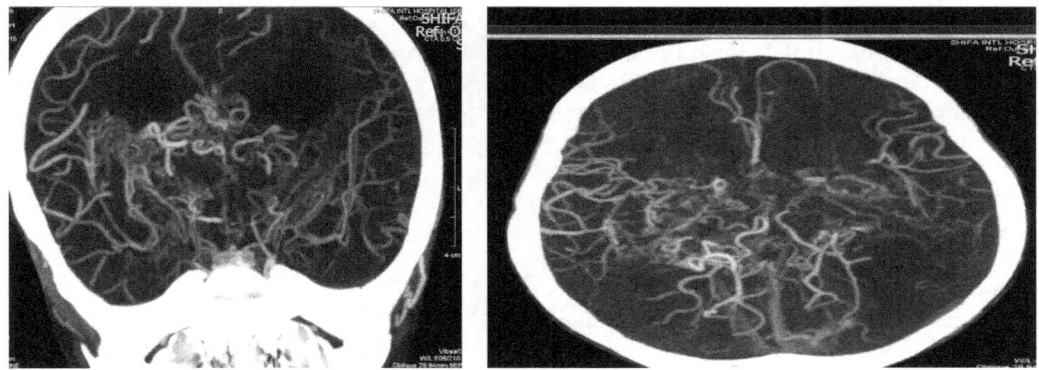

Figure 2: Postoperative CTA head showing good collateral supply to both cerebral hemispheres.

The CSF culture also was negative; the patient was treated for meningoencephalitis and recovered in 10 days. Six months after this initial presentation, he suffered another stroke-like episode, this time affecting the middle cerebral artery/right temporal artery regions with hemiparesis in the right upper and lower extremities.

An MRI was recommended, which was positive for the ischemic changes in the regions supplied by the abovementioned arterial regions. Blood biochemistries for Protein C and S deficiencies were negative.

This continued when he suffered 3 more stroke-like episodes within the following three months, which affected his speech and vision along with right sided facial and limb weakness. He underwent all his lab investigations such as Hepatitis B titers, VZV titers, and poliovirus which were negative for viral illnesses. Lupus anticoagulant was negative, refuting presence of lupus disorders, and Hb electrophoresis was done showing normal electrophoresis negating presence of sickle cell disease. His coagulation profile was with normal PT/APTT and INR values; no abnormality was seen on echocardiogram. It is pertinent to mention that the patients' mother had suffered tuberculosis during her pregnancy with the patient; the TB was negative however in the patient upon testing. He was screened for Protein C and S deficiencies, which were negative. The patient was finally diagnosed as the case of bilateral moyamoya disease based on CT angiogram, which showed severe bilateral stenosis and occlusion of supraclinoid segments of bilateral internal carotid artery (ICA), middle cerebral artery (MCA), and proximal A1 and bilateral Anterior Cerebral Arteries (ACAs), with an extensive collateral formation and enhanced vascularity in both cerebral hemispheres (please refer to Figure 1). Patient was recommended for surgery and was started on Carbamazepine and aspirin.

He was listed for bilateral EDAS, first on the right side of the brain to preserve the better functioning hemisphere and four months later for the left side of the brain. He has shown considerable improvement with no new stroke reported after the EDAS. CT angiography was repeated after 6 months from his second surgery and showed improved patency of collateral vessels and better anastomoses (please refer to Figure 2). He is currently undergoing physiotherapy and has shown continued progress in his functional recovery. With only slight residual weakness in fine motor movements of the right hand and some drooling and slurring of speech, the patient is progressively getting better. He is now able to move his limbs and can speak few words.

Patient has been seizure-free for more than a year and is now being maintained on Carbamazepine.

3. Discussion

Moyamoya is a rare cerebrovascular disease characterized by unilateral or bilateral progressive occlusion of internal carotid and the proximal portion of anterior and middle carotid arteries. The name "moyamoya" refers to "puff of smoke" in Japanese and defines the appearance on cerebral angiogram of the web of collaterals formed to compensate for the blockage [1].

The incidence of moyamoya is relatively higher in Asia compared to Europe and North America; the disease has also been reported from China, India, and other parts of Asia [7]. The disease predominantly affects children and often presents with stroke or recurrent transient ischemic attacks that are commonly accompanied by paralysis affecting one side of the body, muscle weakness, and seizures [8]. Medical management may involve drugs such as antiplatelet agents which are generally given to prevent thrombosis, but the mainstay of treatment remains surgery [9].

Revascularization procedures are preferred currently and are aimed to reestablish blood flow to the hypoxic brain tissue by opening occluded blood vessels [10]. Many surgical procedures have been described to restore blood flow, among them two are mostly discussed in literature; first is known as the indirect procedure, including encephaloduroarteriosynangiosis (EDAS), while the second is the direct method which includes superficial temporal artery and middle cerebral artery (STA-MCA) bypass. Combined approaches including both direct and indirect methods have shown good results and are of prime significance [9].

The accepted first choice of treatment is the direct method which includes superficial temporal artery and middle cerebral artery (STA-MCA) anastomosis combined with indirect revascularization [11]. The treatment of choice among young children suffering from moyamoya disease who presents with reversible ischemic changes, transient ischemic attack, and/or minor stroke is an indirect revascularization surgery, termed as encephaloduroarteriosynangiosis (EDAS) [12]. There are certain limitations related to direct revascularization procedure in the management of pediatric moyamoya disease patients. Major reasons are tiny recipient and donor vessels and requisite for temporary blockage of blood in the cortical artery [12]. The indirect revascularization technique is comparatively easier and results in fewer complications such as postoperative infarctions in pediatric moyamoya disease patients [13]. Having said that, indirect surgeries offer poorer collateral circulation compared to direct procedures [12].

Indirect surgical methods have a higher success rate and are used more often for pediatric moyamoya disease patients that present with ischemic symptoms and perfusion defects in territory of middle cerebral artery [14]. Still under debate is the ideal treatment method for severely ischemic pediatric moyamoya disease patients due to poor circulation in anterior or middle cerebral arteries and those presenting with epilepsy [15]. In a Japanese study, EDAS has proved an efficacious procedure benefitting 75% of patients suffering from transient ischemic attacks within one year [16]. Clinical symptoms have been observed to improve even before angiographic evidence of reperfusion.

Moyamoya being a rare disorder does not get much clinical attention and often remains underdiagnosed as it requires trained neurophysician and sound quality of neuroimaging techniques for its diagnosis. Even if diagnosed, the treatment demands skillful expertise to perform this complex intervention and even the slightest mishandling can worsen the condition.

4. Conclusion

This case highlights the presence of the elusive and rare moyamoya disease in a pediatric subset of Pakistani population. Due to the lack of proper health resources, diagnostic modalities, and trained health care professionals in Pakistan along with a deficiency of dedicated stroke centers and tertiary care centers, it is often misdiagnosed and seldom brought to attention among neurosurgeons and physicians. Moyamoya disease should be on the differential diagnosis for stroke in a minor showing symptoms like focal neurological deficits. A keen eye and timely intervention by the surgeons and physicians may be beneficial for the patient, allowing a proper diagnosis and subsequent management for better outcomes.

Competing Interests

The authors declare that they have no competing interests.

References

[1] M. Fukui, "Current state of study on moyamoya disease in Japan," *Surgical Neurology*, vol. 47, no. 2, pp. 138–143, 1997.

[2] Y. Natori, K. Ikezaki, T. Matsushima, and M. Fukui, "'Angiographic moyamoya' its definition, classification, and therapy," *Clinical Neurology and Neurosurgery*, vol. 99, supplement 2, pp. S168–S172, 1997.

[3] K. B. Asumal, N. Akhtar, N. A. Syed, S. Shafqat, and S. M. Baig, "Moyamoya disease: an elusive diagnosis," *JPMA. The Journal of the Pakistan Medical Association*, vol. 53, no. 4, pp. 160–162, 2003.

[4] S. Shoukat, A. Itrat, A. M. Taqui, M. Zaidi, and A. K. Kamal, "Moyamoya disease: a clinical spectrum, literature review and case series from a tertiary care hospital in Pakistan," *BMC Neurology*, vol. 9, article no. 15, 2009.

[5] M. Wasay, I. A. Khatri, and S. Kaul, "Stroke in South Asian countries," *Nature Reviews Neurology*, vol. 10, no. 3, pp. 135–143, 2014.

[6] T. Matsushima, K. Inoue, M. Kawashima, and T. Inoue, "History of the development of surgical treatments for moyamoya disease," *Neurologia Medico-Chirurgica*, vol. 52, no. 5, pp. 278–286, 2012.

[7] J. C. Takahashi and S. Miyamoto, "Moyamoya disease: recent progress and outlook," *Neurologia Medico-Chirurgica*, vol. 50, no. 9, pp. 824–832, 2010.

[8] R. M. Scott and E. R. Smith, "Moyamoya disease and moyamoya syndrome," *The New England Journal of Medicine*, vol. 360, no. 12, pp. 1226–1237, 2009.

[9] J. Piao, W. Wu, Z. Yang, and J. Yu, "Research progress of moyamoya disease in children," *International Journal of Medical Sciences*, vol. 12, no. 7, pp. 556–575, 2015.

[10] R. Guzman, M. Lee, A. Achrol et al., "Clinical outcome after 450 revascularization procedures for moyamoya disease: clinical article," *Journal of Neurosurgery*, vol. 111, no. 5, pp. 927–935, 2009.

[11] T. Ishikawa, K. Houkin, H. Kamiyama, and H. Abe, "Effects of surgical revascularization on outcome of patients with pediatric moyamoya disease," *Stroke*, vol. 28, no. 6, pp. 1170–1173, 1997.

[12] A. Veeravagu, R. Guzman, C. G. Patil, L. C. Hou, M. Lee, and G. K. Steinberg, "Moyamoya disease in pediatric patients: outcomes of neurosurgical interventions," *Neurosurgical Focus*, vol. 24, no. 2, article E16, 2008.

[13] P. Tripathi, V. Tripathi, R. J. Naik, and J. M. Patel, "Moya Moya cases treated with encephaloduroarteriosynangiosis," *Indian Pediatrics*, vol. 44, no. 2, pp. 123–127, 2007.

[14] A. A. Abla, G. Gandhoke, J. C. Clark et al., "Surgical outcomes for moyamoya angiopathy at barrow neurological institute with comparison of adult indirect encephaloduroarteriosynangiosis bypass, adult direct superficial temporal artery-to-middle cerebral artery bypass, and pediatric bypass: 154 revascularization surgeries in 140 affected hemispheres," *Neurosurgery*, vol. 73, no. 3, pp. 430–439, 2013.

[15] J.-I. Choi, S.-K. Ha, D.-J. Lim, and S.-D. Kim, "Differential clinical outcomes following encephaloduroarteriosynangiosis in pediatric moyamoya disease presenting with epilepsy or ischemia," *Child's Nervous System*, vol. 31, no. 5, pp. 713–720, 2015.

[16] T. Matsushima, M. Fukui, K. Kitamura, K. Hasuo, Y. Kuwabara, and T. Kurokawa, "Encephalo-duro-arterio-synangiosis in children with Moyamoya disease," *Acta Neurochirurgica*, vol. 104, no. 3-4, pp. 96–102, 1990.

Relapsing Polychondritis with Meningoencephalitis Refractory to Immunosuppressant Therapy

Mohammad Mousbah Al-Tabbaa[1] and Hani Habal[2]

[1] Visiting MD, University of Illinois College of Medicine at Peoria, Peoria, IL, USA
[2] Clinical Assistant Professor, University of Illinois College of Medicine at Peoria, Peoria, IL, USA

Correspondence should be addressed to Mohammad Mousbah Al-Tabbaa; mmrt1989@gmail.com

Academic Editor: Peter Berlit

Meningoencephalitis is a rare complication of relapsing polychondritis. We report a case of a 25-year-old male who presented with visual hallucinations and symptoms of depression and anxiety, white matter changes on MRI, and CSF lymphocytosis, along with inflammatory chondritis seen in his auricle cartilage biopsy. Eventually he was given the diagnosis of RP presenting with meningoencephalitis based on CSF analysis, brain MRI findings, negative serologies, and neurologic exam findings. The patient's clinical state did not improve despite being on IV methylprednisolone for a period of 7 days; afterwards he was switched to oral prednisone with no clinical improvement. As a result, he was given cyclophosphamide and rituximab, respectively, without benefit. He also underwent craniectomy with VP shunt due to worsening hydrocephalus and a brain biopsy was done to confirm the diagnosis. He is currently on methotrexate and steroid dependent with a goal to taper down. Even though all 19 reported cases of meningoencephalitis with RP in the literature did respond to immunosuppressive therapy, in our case, however the patient did not respond to immunosuppressive treatment and currently is in mute dementia status after three years of treatment.

1. Introduction

RP is a rare connective tissue disease in which recurrent bouts of inflammation involve the cartilage of the ears, nose, larynx, tracheobronchial tree, and cardiovascular system [1]. Involvement of the peripheral or central nervous system occurs in 3% of patients, sometimes in relation to concomitant vasculitis. Palsies of the cranial nerves (V and VII) are the most common neurological manifestations. Hemiplegia, ataxia, myelitis, and polyneuropathy have been reported. More rarely, aseptic meningitis, meningoencephalitis, stroke, focal or generalized seizures, and cerebral aneurysms may develop [2]. All of the 19 reported cases of meningoencephalitis secondary to RP in the literature did respond to immunosuppressants and most patients age ranges between the 4th and the 5th decade. Here we report a case of a young 25-year-old Caucasian male with a diagnosis of meningoencephalitis secondary to RP that did not respond to different kinds of high potent immunosuppressants. Ultimately, he is being treated palliatively.

2. Case Report

This is a case of a 25-year-old Caucasian male who presented to the ED of St. Francis medical center on 12/2015 with visual hallucinations and symptoms of depression and anxiety, bilateral ear warmth, and swelling and eye redness. His behavioral symptoms have been going for six months prior to presentation. His initial brain MRI showed diffuse, patchy foci of increased FLAIR signal in the periventricular, deep, and subcortical white matter (Figure 1). Right ear lobe biopsy was done and showed a mixed inflammatory infiltrate of the perichondrium composed of plasma cells, lymphocytes, histiocytes and neutrophils, and loss of the cartilage basophilia. GMS and AFB were negative for fungal and mycobacterial organisms. Those findings were consistent with RP.

CSF analysis on admission showed lymphocytosis (21 WBCs, 81% lymphocytes) and admission labs showed lymphocytosis and mildly elevated inflammatory markers (Table 1).

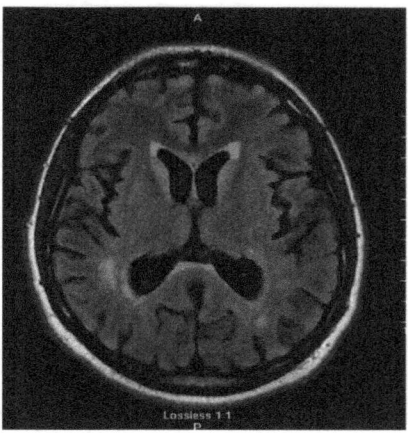 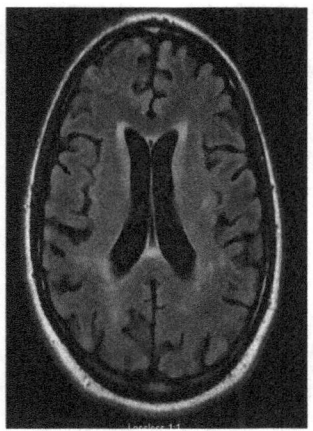

Figure 1: Initial MRI showed diffuse, patchy foci of increased FLAIR signal in the periventricular, deep, and subcortical white matter.

Based on his neurological presentation, his ear lobe biopsy finding, brain MRI findings [3], and negative serologies, he was given a diagnosis of RP with meningoencephalitis.

He was started on IV 1-gram methylprednisolone for 7 days starting in 12/3/15 and then switched to oral prednisone 60 mg/day with a goal to taper off gradually.

The patient's clinical condition did not improve and repeat brain MRI did not show any significant interval change in white matter foci. As a result, the patient was given intravenous cyclophosphamide 1000 mg for total of 5 doses (first 3 doses 3 weeks apart, and another 2 doses 2 weeks apart) between 1/14/2016 and 3/17/2016.

Unfortunately, subsequent MRI after cyclophosphamide on 4/2016 showed progressive periventricular, mid, and also a component of superficial/juxtacortical white matter T2/FLAIR hyperintensity, the latter of which is more apparent within the frontal lobes. There has been further progression of hydrocephalus with diffuse ventricular enlargement (Figure 2).

He was admitted in 5/2016 at SFMC for status epilepticus. Head CT done in the ED showed worsening hydrocephalus. VP shunt was placed and right frontal brain biopsy was done and showed infiltration of the dura and leptomeninges by a mixed chronic inflammatory infiltrate consisting of primarily histiocytes, but also lymphocytes and a few plasma cells. The brain parenchyma shows diffuse gliosis and scant perivascular infiltrates comprised of histiocytes and lymphocytes. No granulomas or vasculitis was identified. Special stains for fungal (GMS and PAS), acid fast (AFB), and bacterial (Gram) organisms are negative. Immunostains for HSV-1/2, CMV, and EBV are also negative. No parasitic organisms are seen on H&E or any of the special stains either. While these morphologic features are nonspecific, they could be consistent with CNS involvement by the patient's known RP. Repeat CSF analysis on the same admission showed 180 RBC, 468 nucleated cells (68% neutrophils, 17% monocytes, and 15% lymphocytes), and normal glucose and protein.

The patient was continued on oral prednisone treatment. A repeat MRI on 12/5/2016 did not show any improvement, so the decision was made to start rituximab and he got 2 doses in January 2017.

Table 1: Labs on admission.

ESR	22 mm/hr (ref. 0-15)
Urine drug screen	negative
CRP	1.76 mg/dl (ref. less than 0.50)
CSF, cell count	RBCs: 7 Nucleated cells: 21
CSF, differential	Neutrophils: 3% Lymphocytes: 81% Monocytes: 16%
CSF, VDRL	Negative
CSF, autoimmune encephalopathy panel	Negative
CSF, Lactic acid	WNL
Paraneoplastic panel	Negative
HIV 1&2 antibody	Negative
ASO	Negative
AFP	Negative
RPR	Non-reactive
ANA	Negative
ENA panel	Negative
VIT b12	WNL
Cryoglobulin	Negative
Hepatitis B and C	Negative
ANCA MPO PR3	Negative
C3&C4	WNL
SPEP (check)	No abnormal protein band detected

WNL: within normal limit, SPEP: serum protein electrophoresis, ref: reference.

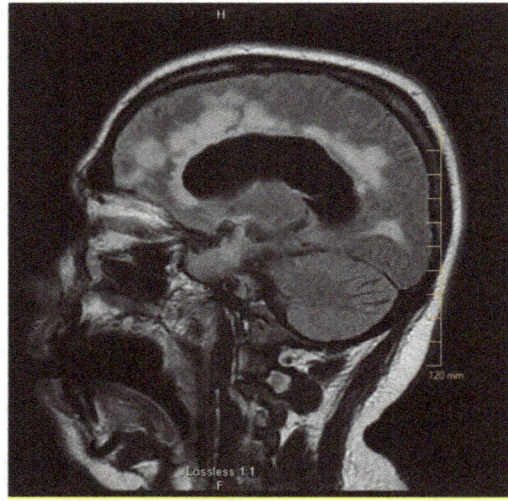

Figure 2: Post-cyclophosphamide MRI showed progressive periventricular, mid, and also a component of superficial/juxtacortical white matter T2/FLAIR hyperintensity, the latter of which is more apparent within the frontal lobes. There has been further progression of hydrocephalus with diffuse ventricular enlargement.

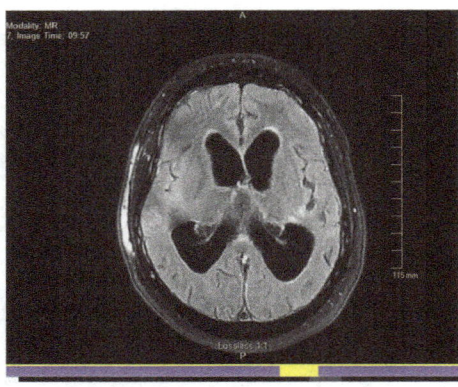

Figure 3: Post-rituximab MRI did not show any significant interval change in findings suggesting leptomeningitis/pachymeningitis, and foci of prolonged T2 values within the white matter.

Subsequent brain MRI on 5/26/17 did not show any significant interval change in findings suggesting leptomeningitis/pachymeningitis, and foci of prolonged T2 values within the white matter (Figure 3).

Currently the patient is in stable mute dementia status. He is alert. Language skills are very limited (up to one or two words mostly). He is relatively distractible. He can follow commands, but this is usually when demonstrated to him. He is currently on prednisone 15 mg/day which is being tapered off, and he is on methotrexate 25 mg/week since 4/2018 which was added as a steroid sparing agent to help taper down the prednisone dose.

3. Discussion

Neurologic complications of RP are rare in general; in the literature limbic encephalitis was reported and the patient presented with cognitive dysfunction [4]. Another case reported rhombencephalitis in which the patient presented with severe occipital headache and this resulted in brain edema and death in two months [5]. Most of the reported cases in the literature reported vasculitic encephalitis, limbic encephalitis, and rarely aseptic meningoencephalitis.

Neurologic presentation of meningoencephalitis with RP varied between cases; reported presentations were hearing loss, unsteadiness, personality changes, generalized tonic-clonic seizure, impaired cognitive function, impaired visual acuity, confusion, memory loss, unstable gait, ataxia, hydrocephalus, delirium, cerebral infarction, coordination problems, distraction, word finding difficulty, emotional lability, abducens nerve palsy, anxiety, insomnia, memory loss, deafness, gait change, urinary incontinence, expressive and receptive aphasia, dullness, acalculia, and papilledema [6].

In the literature all cases of RP-related meningoencephalitis were in the older patient population than our patient and had responded well to immunosuppressive therapy. There are no current guidelines for meningoencephalitis due to RP, because of its rarity. Corticosteroids were the main therapy along with other immunosuppressants. The choice of immunosuppressant varies in the literature, although azathioprine and cyclophosphamide were most commonly used. The choice of immunosuppressant was empirical, with no specific immunosuppressant reported for meningoencephalitis due to RP, due to the lack of clinical trials and cohorts for this specific complication.

Treatment trends differed between cases. 10 of 19 cases improved on glucocorticoids and 5 out of those 10 showed a relapse of disease. Cyclophosphamide was added to glucocorticoids in 3 cases, one case died [7], one improved with no relapse [8, 9], and the most recent case had to add cyclosporin A to relieve symptoms, even though the patient relapsed [6]. Azathioprine was added to glucocorticoids in 4 cases all of which showed improvement, but three of those cases relapsed [6].

Currently, there are no guidelines for treatment of meningoencephalitis in RP; all the reported cases responded to immunosuppressive therapy with glucocorticoids alone or with other high potent immunosuppressants like cyclophosphamide and azathioprine. Our case did not show any improvement to two high potent immunosuppressive therapies (cyclophosphamide and rituximab). Currently he has irreversible dementia and is dependable on steroids with the goal of tapering off his prednisone as a palliative measure.

4. Conclusion

Although meningoencephalitis due to RP usually responds to immunosuppresive therapy, our case is an example of a severe case of RP-related meningoencephalitis that is refractory to any treatment regimen.

Abbreviations

RP: Relapsing polychondritis
MRI: Magnetic resonance imaging
ED: Emergency department
VP: Ventriculoperitoneal.

Authors' Contributions

Both authors contributed equally to this manuscript.

References

[1] L. Longo, G. Antonio, R. Andrea et al., *RP: a clinical update, Autoimmunity Reviews*, Elsevier, Autoimmunity Reviews, 2016.

[2] X. Puéchal, B. Terrier, L. Mouthon, N. Costedoat-Chalumeau, L. Guillevin, and C. Le Jeunne, "Polychondrite chronique atrophiante," *Revue du Rhumatisme*, vol. 81, no. 3, pp. 213–219, 2014.

[3] S. Appenzeller, E. Kobayashi, T. L. L. Costallat, V. DE. A. ZANARDI et al., "Magnetic resonance imaging in the evaluation of patients with aseptic meningoencephalitis and connective tissue disorders," *Arquivos de Neuro-Psiquiatria*, vol. 58, no. 1, pp. 45–51, 2000.

[4] T. Kondo, M. Fukuta, A. Takemoto et al., "limbic encephalitis associated with relapsing polychondritis responded to infliximab and maintained its condition without recurrence after discontinuation: a case report and review of the literature," *Nagoya Journal of Medical Science*, vol. 76(3-4), pp. 361–368, 2014.

[5] C. H. Jeon, "Relapsing Polychondritis with Central Nervous System Involvement: Experience of Three Different Cases in a Single Center," *Journal of Korean Medical Science*, vol. 31, no. 11, pp. 1846–1850, 2016.

[6] K. Shen, G. Yin, C. Yang et al., "Aseptic meningitis in relapsing polychondritis: a case report and literature review," *Clinical Rheumatology*, vol. 37, no. 1, pp. 251–255, 2018.

[7] D. Erten-Lyons, B. Oken, R. L. Woltjer, and J. Quinn, "Relapsing polychondritis: an uncommon cause of dementia," *Journal of Neurology, Neurosurgery & Psychiatry*, vol. 79, no. 5, pp. 609-610, 2008.

[8] J. Kingdon, J. Roscamp, S. Sangle, and D. D'Cruz, "Relapsing polychondritis: a clinical review for rheumatologists," *Rheumatology*, vol. 57, no. 9, pp. 1525–1532, 2018.

[9] K. Hatti and V. Giuliano, "Central nervous system involvement in relapsing polychondritis," *JCR: Journal of Clinical Rheumatology*, vol. 20, pp. 396-397, 2014.

Central Hyperthermia Treated with Bromocriptine

P. Natteru,[1] P. George,[2] R. Bell,[3] P. Nattanmai,[1] and C. R. Newey[1]

[1]*Department of Neurology, University of Missouri, 5 Hospital Drive, CE 540, Columbia, MO 65211, USA*
[2]*Department of Neurology, Cerebrovascular Center, Cleveland Clinic, 9500 Euclid Avenue, Cleveland, OH 44125, USA*
[3]*Department of Surgery, Division of Neurosurgery, University of Missouri, 1 Hospital Drive, Columbia, MO 65211, USA*

Correspondence should be addressed to C. R. Newey; neweyc@health.missouri.edu

Academic Editor: Isabella Laura Simone

Introduction. Central hyperthermia is common in patients with brain injury. It typically has a rapid onset with high temperatures and marked fluctuations and responds poorly to antibiotics and antipyretics. It is also associated with worse outcomes in the brain injured patient. Recognizing this, it is important to aggressively manage it. *Case Report.* We report a 34-year-old male with a right thalamic hemorrhage extending to the midbrain and into the ventricles. During his admission, he developed intractable fevers with core temperatures as high as 39.3°C. Infectious workup was unremarkable. The fever persisted despite empiric antibiotics, antipyretics, and cooling wraps. Bromocriptine was started resulting in control of the central hyperthermia. The fever spikes were reduced to minor fluctuations that significantly worsened with any attempt to wean off the bromocriptine. *Conclusion.* Diagnosing and managing central hyperthermia can be challenging. The use of bromocriptine can be beneficial as we have reported.

1. Introduction

In general, hyperthermia is considered secondary to an infectious etiology [1, 2]. However, in neurologically injured patients, hyperthermia may be related to the underlying brain injury and is associated with worse outcomes [3, 4]. Central hyperthermia has a rapid onset of temperature with marked fluctuations [5]. It may be a result of damage or dysfunction to central fever control centers, such as at the level of the diencephalon [6, 7]. This region regulates core temperatures [6, 7]. Any damage to this area can disrupt the thermoregulatory apparatus of the body, as evidenced in about 42% of autopsies in brain injured patients [6, 7]. Theories have been suggested to explain the role of the hypothalamus in central hyperthermia [6–8]. It may be the selective loss of warm-sensitive neurons, the osmotic changes detected by the organum vasculosum laminae terminalis (OVLT), or the humoral changes (progesterone, prostaglandin) modifying the firing rate of heat sensitive neurons in the medial preoptic nucleus (MPO) [8].

There has been increasing evidence to show that central hyperthermia is a poor responder to antipyretics [9]. Thus, it may require a multimodal approach to management that includes additional medications such as bromocriptine and/or surface or intravascular cooling device [10].

In this paper, we present a 34-year-old male with prolonged central fever after intracerebral hemorrhage of the thalamus and midbrain. The prolonged fever was controlled with the administration of bromocriptine which we graphically represent along with a review of the literature.

2. Case

A 34-year-old Hispanic male was found by his family unresponsive to verbal and noxious stimulation. His arms were asymmetrically extended. Emergency medical service was called. He was intubated in the field for airway protection and transported to the emergency department. His initial Glasgow Coma Scale (GCS) score was 5 (eyes: 1, verbal: 1, motor: 3). His computed tomography (CT) scan of the head showed a right thalamic hemorrhage (10.4 cc) with extension into the upper midbrain along with intraventricular extension resulting in obstructive hydrocephalus (Figure 1(a)).

The initial blood pressure (BP) was 163/115 mmHg. He was started on a nicardipine infusion to achieve systolic BP of <140 mmHg. His right pupil was dilated (4 mm) and

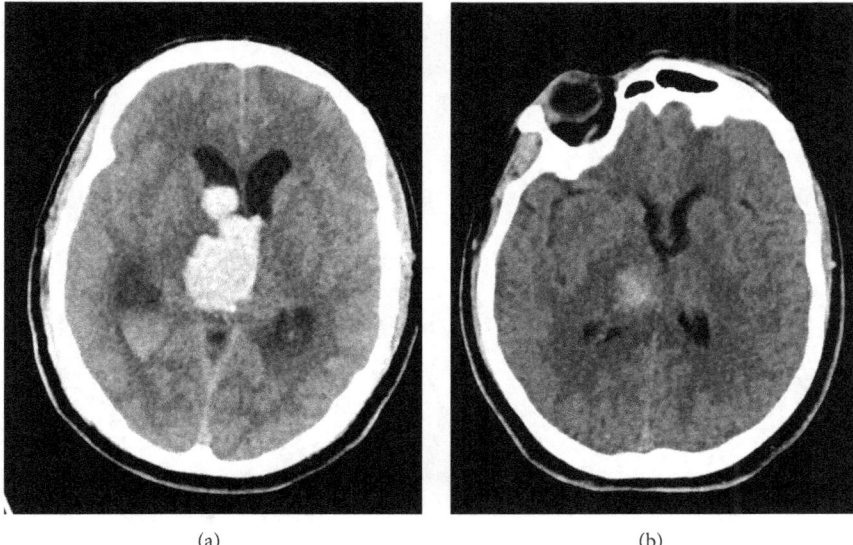

(a) (b)

Figure 1: Computed tomography (CT) of the head. (a) CT head on admission showing a right thalamic hemorrhage with intraventricular extension. Note the obstructive hydrocephalus. (b) CT head on hospital day 9 showing evolution of the right thalamic hemorrhage and resolution of the obstructive hydrocephalus with external ventricular drainage (not shown) and after intraventricular tissue plasminogen activator (tPA).

nonreactive. He had extensor posturing of all extremities. An emergent external ventricular drain (EVD) was placed. Cerebral angiography was performed to evaluate for underlying aneurysm, vertebral dissection, arteriovenous malformation, or dural arteriovenous fistula. The cerebral angiography was negative. Magnetic resonance imaging (MRI) confirmed the hemorrhage without identifying any additional abnormality. Electroencephalogram (EEG) was negative for seizures. He was subsequently treated with intraventricular tissue plasminogen activator (t-PA; 1 mg q8 h) for three days (total 9 doses). The intraventricular hemorrhage improved significantly by day 9 of hospitalization (Figure 1(b)). His neurological examination, however, remained poor. EVD weaning was attempted. After multiple failed attempts, a ventriculoperitoneal shunt was placed.

During his admission, his core temperature rose to 39.3°C (102.7°F). Acetaminophen and cooling wraps (Gaymar Medi-Therm Hyper/Hypothermia System, Stryker, Kalamazoo, MI, USA) were initiated to control the fever. He was also on a fentanyl infusion for light sedation. A complete fever workup only showed leukocytosis. He was treated for presumed aspiration pneumonia. His fevers persisted with marked fluctuations despite antibiotic therapy. Other differential diagnoses such as malignant hyperthermia and neuroleptic malignant syndrome were ruled out due to normal creatinine kinase level (81 units/L; normal 20–200 units/L) and lack of causative medication.

He was started on bromocriptine in addition to the antipyretics and cooling wraps for treatment of his central hyperthermia. The fever spikes reduced to minor fluctuations that worsened with each attempt to wean off the bromocriptine (Figure 2). Cultures remained negative. Figure 2 is a graph of the average core temperature (+/− standard error of the mean) and association of bromocriptine initiation and discontinuation. Note the significant improvement with initiation of bromocriptine and the significant worsening of fever with discontinuation of bromocriptine. There was no correlation with the resolution of the intracerebral and intraventricular hemorrhages and the administration of intraventricular tPA with the fever. Statistical analysis was performed using analysis of variance (ANOVA) on GraphPad Prism 7 (La Jolla, CA, USA). A p value of <0.05 was considered significant.

He required a tracheostomy and percutaneous gastrostomy tube. Neurologically, he remained in a coma with asymmetric posturing of the upper extremities and extension of the lower extremities. He was eventually transferred to a long term acute care facility.

3. Discussion

This case highlights the effectiveness of bromocriptine to treat fever of central origin. Neurogenic fever can occur alone or in conjunction with other autonomic (e.g., tachycardia, tachypnea, diaphoresis, and pupillary changes) and motor findings (e.g., extensor posturing) [11]. These are collectively termed paroxysmal sympathetic hyperactivity (PSH).

Hyperthermia of central origin has a rapid onset, high temperature, marked fluctuation, and poor to no response to antipyretics [9]. Fever is an independent variable in patients with neurologic injury and usually suggests worse outcomes [12]. In a retrospective study of 74 patients in the neurosciences intensive care unit with poststroke central hyperthermia, nearly 70% of the patients with fever expired within a month, especially those with temperatures > 39°C [5].

The features of central hyperthermia are hypothesized to be due to the compression of hypothalamic and brain stem thermoregulatory centers [13]. Several physiological pathways contribute to the central thermoregulation and are

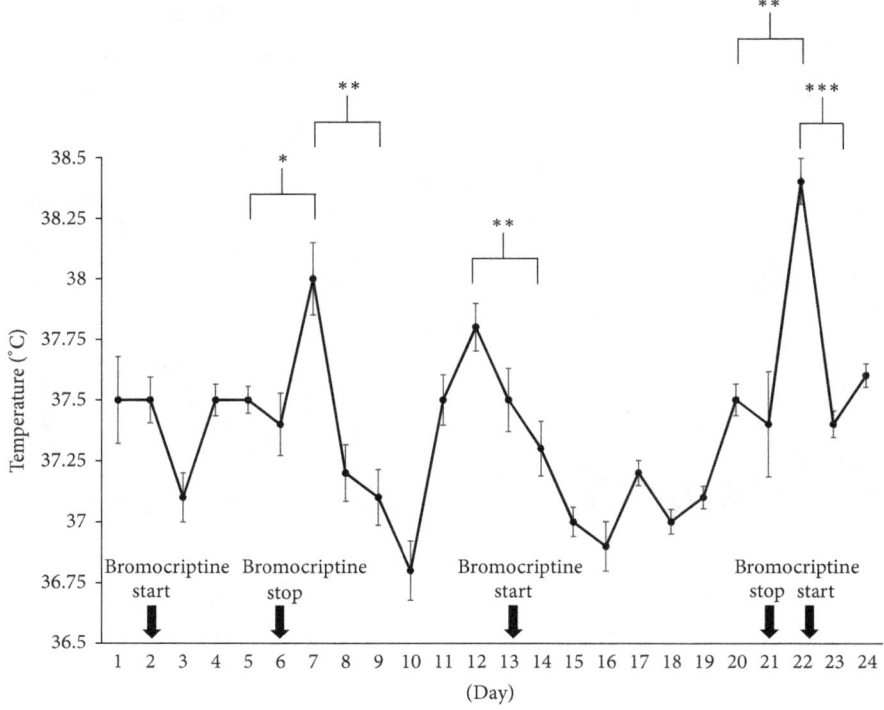

FIGURE 2: Temperature graph. Average core temperature for each day during hospital course is graphically shown. Error bars are standard errors of the mean. Bromocriptine was started on days 2, 13, and 22. It was stopped on days 6 and 21. Immediately after discontinuation of bromocriptine, there was a significant increase in core temperature. After resuming bromocriptine, there was a significant decrease in core temperature. $^*p < 0.05$, $^{**}p < 0.001$, and $^{***}p < 0.0001$.

coordinated by the hypothalamus [14]. These areas include the lateral parabrachial nucleus at the junction of the pons and medulla, inputs from spinothalamocortical relay pathways, and the preoptic area (POA) of the hypothalamus [15]. The median preoptic nucleus within the POA is temperature sensitive, especially to heat [14]. In addition to the hypothalamus, the brainstem also plays a significant role in central thermoregulation through brown adipose thermogenesis (BAT) [10]. The rostral ventromedial medulla augments BAT, whereas the ventrolateral medulla (nucleus of the solitary tract) and the ventromedial midbrain (periaqueductal gray) inhibit BAT [16, 17]. These anatomical considerations are the reason why injury to the brainstem significantly alters the homeostasis and can lead to central hyperthermia, as seen in 64% of patients [5]. We suspect that disruption of the hypothalamus and/or ventromedial midbrain resulted in the central fever in our patient given the location of his hemorrhages.

Criteria for diagnosing central hyperthermia have been suggested: (a) high fever with temperatures > 39°C within 24 hours after onset of stroke, (b) no prior infections or fevers at least 1 week prior to onset of stroke, and (c) negative workup for fever of infectious origin [18]. Our patient met all the criteria for diagnosis of central hyperthermia.

Treatment of central hyperthermia typically requires a multimodal approach. Options include medications like bromocriptine or baclofen with or without surface or intravascular cooling devices [9, 19–22]. In our patient, we added bromocriptine to surface cooling and antipyretic to treat the central fever. In addition to bromocriptine, the patient did receive fentanyl infusion for mild sedation to allow for frequent neurological assessments.

Bromocriptine is a dopamine D2 agonist that acts on the corpus striatum and the hypothalamus [23]. It has been known to help in PSH, because of its action on dopaminergic transmission [24, 25]. Unfortunately, there is no systematic study on the efficacy and safety of dopamine agonists in traumatic brain injury [26]. Much of the current literature are case reports and small studies with inherent bias [26]. It may be best to individualize the therapy for each patient. In clinical practice, the use of bromocriptine has been less robust for the treatment of the constellation of findings associated with PSH except for central hyperthermia [11].

Other treatment options for central hyperthermia include baclofen, a GABA agonist, which acts on the raphe nuclei and inhibits BAT which in turn can suppress the core body temperature [21]. Baclofen use in the neurocritical care unit, however, is limited by side effects such as drowsiness, tiredness, and muscle weakness of the affected or unaffected limbs [27]. Lastly cooling devices are effective in reaching normothermia [28]. However, these devices have risks such as infection and thrombosis with intravascular cooling and skin breakdown with the cooling wraps [29]. Both increase risk of shivering [28, 30].

4. Conclusion

Our case report illustrates that bromocriptine is an effective treatment option for central hyperthermia. Future studies should evaluate improvement in temperature management and outcomes in patients treated with bromocriptine in the setting of neurogenic fever.

Competing Interests

The authors have no conflict of interests to report.

Authors' Contributions

P. Natteru, P. George, R. Bell, P. Nattanmai, and C. R. Newey contributed equally to the writing of the case and formatting the images.

References

[1] K. Georgilis, A. Plomaritoglou, U. Dafni, Y. Bassiakos, and K. Vemmos, "Aetiology of fever in patients with acute stroke," *Journal of Internal Medicine*, vol. 246, no. 2, pp. 203–209, 1999.

[2] E. J. Roth, L. Lovell, R. L. Harvey, A. W. Heinemann, P. Semik, and S. Diaz, "Incidence of and risk factors for medical complications during stroke rehabilitation," *Stroke*, vol. 32, no. 2, pp. 523–529, 2001.

[3] G. Azzimondi, L. Bassein, F. Nonino et al., "Fever in acute stroke worsens prognosis: a prospective study," *Stroke*, vol. 26, no. 11, pp. 2040–2043, 1995.

[4] J. Castillo, A. Dávalos, J. Marrugat, and M. Noya, "Timing for fever-related brain damage in acute ischemic stroke," *Stroke*, vol. 29, no. 12, pp. 2455–2460, 1998.

[5] C.-Y. Sung, T.-H. Lee, and N.-S. Chu, "Central hyperthermia in acute stroke," *European Neurology*, vol. 62, no. 2, pp. 86–92, 2009.

[6] C. B. Saper, J. Lu, T. C. Chou, and J. Gooley, "The hypothalamic integrator for circadian rhythms," *Trends in Neurosciences*, vol. 28, no. 3, pp. 152–157, 2005.

[7] M. R. Crompton, "Hypothalamic lesions following closed head injury," *Brain*, vol. 94, no. 1, pp. 165–172, 1971.

[8] M. Rango, A. Arighi, L. Airaghi, and N. Bresolin, "Central hyperthermia, brain hyperthermia and low hypothalamus temperature," *Clinical Autonomic Research*, vol. 22, no. 6, pp. 299–301, 2012.

[9] K.-W. Yu, Y.-H. Huang, C.-L. Lin, C.-Z. Hong, and L.-W. Chou, "Effectively managing intractable central hyperthermia in a stroke patient by bromocriptine: a case report," *Neuropsychiatric Disease and Treatment*, vol. 9, pp. 605–608, 2013.

[10] N. Samudra and S. Figueroa, "Intractable central hyperthermia in the setting of brainstem hemorrhage," *Therapeutic Hypothermia and Temperature Management*, vol. 6, no. 2, pp. 98–101, 2016.

[11] A. A. Rabinstein, "Paroxysmal sympathetic hyperactivity in the neurological intensive care unit," *Neurological Research*, vol. 29, no. 7, pp. 680–682, 2007.

[12] D. M. Greer, S. E. Funk, N. L. Reaven, M. Ouzounelli, and G. C. Uman, "Impact of fever on outcome in patients with stroke and neurologic injury: a comprehensive meta-analysis," *Stroke*, vol. 39, no. 11, pp. 3029–3035, 2008.

[13] A. Deogaonkar, M. De Georgia, C. Bae, A. Abou-Chebl, and J. Andrefsky, "Fever is associated with third ventricular shift after intracerebral hemorrhage: pathophysiologic implications," *Neurology India*, vol. 53, no. 2, pp. 202–207, 2005.

[14] K. Nakamura, T. Kaneko, Y. Yamashita et al., "Immunocytochemical localization of prostaglandin EP3 receptor in the rat hypothalamus," *Neuroscience Letters*, vol. 260, no. 2, pp. 117–120, 1999.

[15] S. F. Morrison and K. Nakamura, "Central neural pathways for thermoregulation," *Frontiers in Bioscience*, vol. 16, no. 1, pp. 74–104, 2011.

[16] S. F. Morrison, K. Nakamura, and C. J. Madden, "Central control of thermogenesis in mammals," *Experimental Physiology*, vol. 93, no. 7, pp. 773–797, 2008.

[17] J. A. Rathner and S. F. Morrison, "Rostral ventromedial periaqueductal gray: a source of inhibition of the sympathetic outflow to brown adipose tissue," *Brain Research*, vol. 1077, no. 1, pp. 99–107, 2006.

[18] H. C. Lee, J. M. Kim, J. K. Lim, Y. S. Jo, and S. K. Kim, "Central hyperthermia treated with baclofen for patient with pontine hemorrhage," *Annals of Rehabilitation Medicine*, vol. 38, no. 2, pp. 269–272, 2014.

[19] S. A. Mayer, R. G. Kowalski, M. Presciutti et al., "Clinical trial of a novel surface cooling system for fever control in neurocritical care patients," *Critical Care Medicine*, vol. 32, no. 12, pp. 2508–2515, 2004.

[20] G. Broessner, R. Beer, P. Lackner et al., "Prophylactic, endovascularly based, long-term normothermia in icu patients with severe cerebrovascular disease: bicenter prospective, randomized trial," *Stroke*, vol. 40, no. 12, pp. e657–e665, 2009.

[21] Y.-S. Huang, M.-C. Hsiao, M. Lee, Y.-C. Huang, and J.-D. Lee, "Baclofen successfully abolished prolonged central hyperthermia in a patient with basilar artery occlusion," *Acta Neurologica Taiwanica*, vol. 18, no. 2, pp. 118–122, 2009.

[22] S. Muehlschlegel and J. R. Sims, "Dantrolene: mechanisms of neuroprotection and possible clinical applications in the neurointensive care unit," *Neurocritical Care*, vol. 10, no. 1, pp. 103–115, 2009.

[23] S. H. Kang, M. J. Kim, I. Y. Shin, D. W. Park, J. W. Sohn, and Y. K. Yoon, "Bromocriptine for control of hyperthermia in a patient with mixed autonomic hyperactivity after neurosurgery: a case report," *Journal of Korean Medical Science*, vol. 27, no. 8, pp. 965–968, 2012.

[24] R. N. Russo and S. O'Flaherty, "Bromocriptine for the management of autonomic dysfunction after severe traumatic brain injury," *Journal of Paediatrics and Child Health*, vol. 36, no. 3, pp. 283–285, 2000.

[25] D. E. Bullard, "Diencephalic seizures: responsiveness to bromocriptine and morphine," *Annals of Neurology*, vol. 21, no. 6, pp. 609–611, 1987.

[26] A. J. Frenette, S. Kanji, L. Rees et al., "Efficacy and safety of dopamine agonists in traumatic brain injury: a systematic review of randomized controlled trials," *Journal of Neurotrauma*, vol. 29, no. 1, pp. 1–18, 2012.

[27] A. Hulme, W. J. MacLennan, R. T. Ritchie, V. A. John, and P. A. Shotton, "Baclofen in the elderly stroke patient its side-effects and pharmacokinetics," *European Journal of Clinical Pharmacology*, vol. 29, no. 4, pp. 467–469, 1985.

[28] G. S. Aujla, P. Nattanmai, K. Premkumar, and C. R. Newey, "Comparison of two surface cooling devices for temperature management in a neurocritical care unit," *Therapeutic Hypothermia and Temperature Management*, 2016.

[29] N. Badjatia, J. O'Donnell, J. R. Baker et al., "Achieving normothermia in patients with febrile subarachnoid hemorrhage: feasibility and safety of a novel intravascular cooling catheter," *Neurocritical Care*, vol. 1, no. 2, pp. 145–156, 2004.

[30] V. Scaravilli, G. Tinchero, and G. Citerio, "Fever management in SAH," *Neurocritical Care*, vol. 15, no. 2, pp. 287–294, 2011.

Could Hallucinogens Induce Permanent Pupillary Changes in (Ab)users? A Case Report from New Zealand

Ahmed Al-Imam[1,2]

[1] Novel Psychoactive Substances Unit, Doctoral College, Hertfordshire University, Hertfordshire, UK
[2] College of Medicine, University of Baghdad, Baghdad, Iraq

Correspondence should be addressed to Ahmed Al-Imam; tesla1452@gmail.com

Academic Editor: Norman S. Litofsky

An eighteen-year-old female patient of the Caucasian ethnicity from Australasia presented with a persistently dilated pupil causing her discomfort and occasional burning sensation when she is outdoors due to oversensitivity to sunlight. However, her pupillary reaction to light (pupillary light reflex) was intact. The patient is a known user of psychedelic substances (entheogens) including LSD, NBOMe, psilocybin, and DMT. The condition affects both eyes to the same extent. Thorough medical, neurological, and radiological examinations, including an EEG and an MRI of the head and neck region, were completely normal. All these tests failed to detect any pathophysiological or anatomical abnormalities. The patient is a known case of chronic endogenous depression in association with attention deficit hyperactivity disorder, for which she is taking citalopram and Ritalin, respectively. There was neither a family history nor a similar congenital condition in her family.

1. Introduction

Novel psychoactive substances (NPS), also known as research chemicals or designer drugs, are a group of substances, including chemicals that can either stimulate (stimulants) or inhibit (depressants) the nervous system, particularly the central nervous system [1, 2]. According to the classification scheme reported by the *European Monitoring Centre for Drugs and Drug Addiction* (EMCDDA), NPS can be categorised into cannabis and cannabimimetic, phenethylamines, cathinones, tryptamines, piperazine, and pipradrol derivatives and a 7th miscellaneous group which is composed predominantly of CNS stimulants [2, 3]. This taxonomy is based on the structural chemistry of 252 substances that were reported to the EMCDDA in between 1997 and 2012. The exponential rise in of the NPS phenomenon is considered to be correlated with the logarithmic growth of information and communication technology [4, 5].

The majority of these substances possess addictive properties. Hence, substance users and misusers may develop dependence syndrome, withdrawal manifestations, or adverse reactions [6]. These substances act on various neurotransmitters within the nervous system, including the central nervous system (CNS) and the peripheral nervous system (PNS) [2, 7]. The key neurotransmitters are monoamines including dopamine, serotonin, and catecholamine. In fact, NPS exert their effects via their highly selective affinity towards monoamine transporters (MATs); MATs include serotonin transporter (SERT), dopamine transporter (DAT), and norepinephrine (NET) [8, 9].

MATs are located just around the synaptic cleft (perisynaptically); they are responsible for the reuptake of monoamines back from the synaptic cleft into the cytoplasm of the presynaptic neurons [10, 11]. Therefore, the action of NPS on the body systems, both centrally and peripherally, can be attributed to changes achieved via MATs. NPS can induce several physiologic changes including ocular alterations [12], for example, morphometric variations in the dimension (diameter) of the pupillary aperture leading to either pupillary constriction (miosis) or dilation (mydriasis).

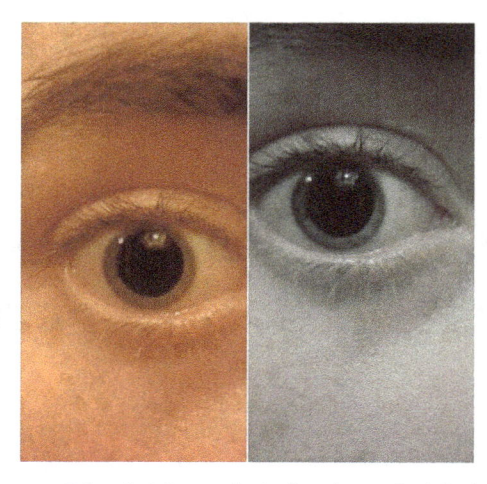

Figure 1: Dilated right pupil of a female psychedelics' user.

2. Case Report

The patient is an 18-year-old female of the Caucasian ethnicity; she is from Australasia, specifically New Zealand; she has light coloured skin of Fitzpatrick type-1 category [13, 14]. She is a right-handed artist and of a potentially left-hemispheric cerebral dominance. She has a past history of substance use and misuse starting at the age of eleven years, smoking cannabis and hashish; at that age she developed an abnormally and continuously dilated pupil (Figure 1) leaving a thin rim of blue iridial tissue; the condition is affecting both eyes (bilaterally) though both pupils still react to light, including sunlight (i.e., pupillary light reflex is intact).

She had no complaints except for intolerance to sunlight, both direct and indirect, which mandates wearing *UV sunglasses* for optimal protection of the retina as advised by a specialist optometrist. Hence, the patient is almost unbothered by her condition; she described it by saying "*my eyes always look like this, I have constantly dilated pupils, haha, not even tripping.*" In fact, she considers her overall eye appearance as *sexier* than the normal eye. However, she was bothered of the potential eye and retinal damage from overexposure to sunlight.

The patient has correlated her eye condition with the use of hallucinogens, primarily with LSD (acid) and psilocybin mushrooms. Furthermore, her condition started at the age of eleven years in association with substance use. Hence, it is not congenital. In 1992, the 1st case of a bilateral congenital mydriasis was reported in the literature [15]. The patient has a past medical history, being treated with citalopram and Ritalin for the management of her chronic endogenous depression and attention deficit hyperactivity disorder (ADHD); she has been on these medications for several years. She also admitted using tramadol, opium, and opioid derivatives; these substances induce a paradoxical effect on her pupil leading to pupillary constriction. The patient had no prior history of head trauma, brain tumors, or any other neurological conditions. Furthermore, a thorough neurological and radiological exam was done; an MRI of the head and neck region was also entirely normal.

3. Discussion

In Renaissance Italy, Italian ladies used to apply a purified extract from the berries of *Atropa belladonna* as eye drops to both eyes; the purpose was to create artificially dilated pupils; it was considered a sign of beauty; *belladonna* is Italian for a *beautiful lady* [16, 17]. The extract contains anticholinergic substances including atropine, scopolamine, and hyoscyamine [16, 17]. In this case presentation, the pupillary changes (mydriasis) were brought by the pathophysiologic effect of possibly more than one substance, primarily hallucinogenic agents that own sympathomimetic or parasympathomimetic-related properties [18]. Though it may still be considered as a sign of beauty, it increases the sensitivity towards sunlight (photosensitivity) particularly in fair skin individuals and Caucasians of *Fitzpatrick skin type*-1 and type-2 [19].

Changes in the pupillary dimensions are brought up by either an increment or a decrement in its diameter via the action of iridial smooth muscles, both longitudinal (dilator pupillae) and circular (sphincter pupillae) [7]. The autonomic nervous system (ANS), an integral component of the PNS, is responsible for the automatic (visceral) control of the pupillary aperture [20]. The sympathetic nervous system (SNS) usually mediates pupillary dilation (mydriasis), while the parasympathetic nervous system, via the oculomotor nerve (cranial nerve III) and its modulatory effect over the ciliary autonomic ganglion, mediates pupillary constriction (miosis) [20, 21]. Changes in the sympathetic or parasympathetic tone (neuronal activity) are brought up by changes via reflex mechanism (as in pupillary light reflex), emotional changes affecting the limbic system and the diencephalon specifically the hypothalamus, and the modulation of the neuronal activity in the midbrain specifically pretectal region and the Edinger–Westphal nucleus (accessory oculomotor nucleus). The last nucleus houses the presynaptic (preganglionic) parasympathetic motor neurons of the oculomotor nerve which innervate the sphincter pupillae iridial muscles [7, 22]. Hence, this pathway, pretectal-accessory oculomotor nucleus, is a critical constituent of the pupillary light reflex; the afferent and efferent nerves of this pathway are the optic nerve and the oculomotor nerve, respectively; the reflex is considered to be a four-neuronal reflex pathway [23]. Accordingly, this reflex neuronal pathway controls the momentary changes *(pupillary unrest under ambient light)* in the pupillary aperture with a high accuracy and an ultimate speed (milliseconds) in response to variations in the illumination level of the surrounding environment [24, 25].

Certain pathophysiological changes can influence the pupillary aperture; these include the pupillary light reflex mechanism, the tone of SNS or PNS including their autonomic ganglion, and pathologies of the midbrain around the regions of the *cerebral aqueduct of Sylvius* including the regions of tectum and tegmentum, hypothalamic region, limbic system, and higher centres. For instance, *Horner's syndrome* is a condition in which damage affects the function of the upper segments (cervicothoracic) of the paravertebral sympathetic chain, leading to dilated pupil on the ipsilateral side in addition to ipsilateral eyelid ptosis and hemifacial anhidrosis [26]. Several conditions may result in Horner's syndrome, including central (CNS) and peripheral (PNS and ANS), including syringomyelia, multiple sclerosis, brain tumors, encephalitis, lateral medullary syndrome, cervical rib, thyroid tumors and thyroidectomy, bronchogenic carcinoma, tube thoracostomy, carotid artery dissection, cavernous sinus thrombosis, middle ear infections, sympathectomy, and nerve block procedures [26, 27]. All these pathological conditions operate either centrally at the level of the hypothalamospinal tract or at the presynaptic sympathetic neurons, or peripherally at the postsynaptic sympathetic neurons. Horner's syndrome can occur either unilaterally or bilaterally; several tests are used to diagnose this syndrome as in the *cocaine drop test* [28].

Several conditions and agents can cause mydriasis; these are injury to the eye and associated neural elements, anticholinergic medications and chemicals such as atropine and scopolamine, the elevated level of oxytocin hormone, and drug use and misuse [15, 29]. Drugs include cocaine (crack), MDMA (ecstasy), hallucinogens, methamphetamine (crystal meth), and Toradol (ketorolac). Hallucinogenic drugs and entheogen are not limited to LSD (acid), NBOMe (n-bomb), and dimethyltryptamine (DMT) [30]. Stimulants (as in cocaine) and hallucinogens act via increasing the levels of serotonin mainly by acting on SERT located centrally (CNS) [31]. In fact, these drugs that may lead to an overall increase in 5-hydroxytryptamine (serotonin) or a subsequent effect on 5-HT$_{2A}$ receptor will exert a mydriatic effect, as in the case of psychedelics [11, 31]. Other conditions leading to abnormally dilated pupil include *benign episodic unilateral mydriasis*, cranial nerves neuropathy, traumatic brain injury, and mydriatic agents used for ophthalmologic examination such as tropicamide [32]. Oxytocin, the *love hormone*, can induce mild to moderate mydriatic effect; oxytocin is related to intimate emotional and social interactions. Hence, it increases in bursts during sexual intercourse; Pitocin (oxytocin) is also medicinally used to induce uterine contraction to either facilitate or induce a normal vaginal delivery [33, 34].

Similar cases were reported in drug fora, particularly from abusers of psychedelic substances including both males and females. One of the threads included this comment "*My friend has one pupil increased in size and one decreased. Permanently... It happened to him after I made a cacao from weed and we tripped our balls. It looks funny*" [35, 36]. In fact, some psychedelic users reported that they were able to control the size of their pupillary apertures voluntarily; a male has commented "*I can change the size of my pupils while looking in the mirror*" [35, 36]. This is remarkable given the fact that iridial muscles are strictly controlled involuntarily by autonomic innervation [36]. Perhaps, some neuronal (or neurochemical) modulation exists in psychedelic (ab)users. Contrary to psychedelic users, users and misusers of opium and opioid substances experience a constricted (miotic) pupil, or even a pinpoint pupillary aperture [37]. Heroin, fentanyl, codeine, methadone, and morphine act via stimulation of the PNS [38]. The New Zealander patient presented in this manuscript admitted taking these substances (opioids) too; she has also confirmed that her pupils could still react with some degree of constriction. She commented saying "*I do take tramadol and codeine as well, but they do the opposite to the eyes.*"

Clinical examination, including a thorough neurological exam, failed to detect any abnormalities apart from the bilaterally dilated pupils. Furthermore, MRI of the regions of the craniocervical and thoracic region could not detect any pathology. It is likely that changes may exist at a cellular level that cannot be detected with the conventional methods, or at the centrally located nuclei in the midbrain and the hypothalamus. Functional MRI (fMRI) can be useful to detect these changes, but it was not available in the medical institute at which the patient was examined [39, 40]. Transcranial magnetic stimulation (TMS) might be of value in detecting lesions in the limbic system, temporal lobe, or the prefrontal cortex. However, TMS is not suitable to detect deep-seated lesions in the hypothalamus or the midbrain [41, 42].

This level-of-evidence of this manuscript is level-5 in accordance with the classification system imposed by the *Oxford Centre for Evidence-Based Medicine* (CEBM) [43, 44].

4. Conclusion

The case of the New Zealander female presented in this manuscript is one of the few cases documented in the body of literature. The patient had a frequent use of NPS, psychedelics, and other psychoactive chemicals including antidepressant medications. It can be inferred that the burden of (ab)use of hallucinogenic and other NPS chemicals is not to be underrated, particularly in the developed world, including Australasia. These substances can be abused as early as childhood leading to irreversible consequences including adverse pathophysiological changes of body systems, dependence syndrome, incidents of intoxications, fatalities, and sudden death. The magnitude of these hazards is obscure in relation to the developing countries, including the Middle East, Asia, Africa, and Latin America. In connection with the Middle East, more in-depth epidemiological investigations are mandatory to infer an estimate in relation to the spread of psychedelic (ab)use.

Acknowledgments

Appreciation and gratitude are due to the administration of *the Terence McKenna Page*, a private group located on the Facebook social communication medium; the group is dedicated for psychedelics users. The author would also like to acknowledge efforts of Dr. Mayasa Mohammed Al-Hyali, for her insightful remarks in relation to Introduction of this manuscript.

References

[1] I. Brew, "Novel psychoactive substances," *British Journal of General Practice*, vol. 66, no. 644, p. 125, 2016.

[2] P. Dargan and D. Wood, Eds., *Novel Psychoactive Substances: Classification, Pharmacology and Toxicology*, Academic Press, 2013.

[3] L. Orsolini, D. Papanti, R. Vecchiotti, A. Valchera, J. Corkery, and F. Schifano, "Novel psychoactive substances," *European Psychiatry*, vol. 33, pp. S59–S60, 2016.

[4] O. Corazza, F. Schifano, P. Simonato et al., "Phenomenon of new drugs on the internet: the case of ketamine derivative methoxetamine," *Human Psychopharmacol: Clinical and Experimental*, vol. 27, no. 2, pp. 145–149, 2012.

[5] O. Corazza, S. Assi, P. Simonato et al., "Promoting innovation and excellence to face the rapid diffusion of novel psychoactive substances in the EU: the outcomes of the ReDNet project," *Human Psychopharmacology: Clinical and Experimental*, vol. 28, no. 4, pp. 317–323, 2013.

[6] S. Fazel, P. Bains, and H. Doll, "Substance abuse and dependence in prisoners: A systematic review," *Addiction*, vol. 101, no. 2, pp. 181–191, 2006.

[7] M. D. Vaz, T. D. Raj, and K. D. Anura, *Guyton & Hall Textbook of Medical Physiology: A South Asian Edition*, Elsevier Health Sciences, 2014.

[8] R. R. Gainetdinov and M. G. Caron, "Monoamine transporters: from genes to behavior," *Annual Review of Pharmacology and Toxicology*, vol. 43, no. 1, pp. 261–284, 2003.

[9] R. B. Rothman and M. H. Baumann, "Monoamine transporters and psychostimulant drugs," *European Journal of Pharmacology*, vol. 479, no. 1-3, pp. 23–40, 2003.

[10] N. V. Cozzi, A. Gopalakrishnan, L. L. Anderson et al., "Dimethyltryptamine and other hallucinogenic tryptamines exhibit substrate behavior at the serotonin uptake transporter and the vesicle monoamine transporter," *Journal of Neural Transmission*, vol. 116, no. 12, pp. 1591–1599, 2009.

[11] M. E. Liechti, "Novel psychoactive substances (designer drugs): overview and pharmacology of modulators of monoamine signalling," *Swiss Medical Weekly*, vol. 145, 2015.

[12] N. Hohmann, G. Mikus, and D. Czock, "Effects and risks associated with novel psychoactive substances," *Deutsches Ärzteblatt International*, vol. 111, no. 9, pp. 139–147, 2014.

[13] S. Eilers, D. Q. Bach, R. Gaber et al., "Accuracy of self-report in assessing Fitzpatrick skin phototypes I through VI," *JAMA Dermatology*, vol. 149, no. 11, pp. 1289–1294, 2013.

[14] S. Majewski, C. Carneiro, E. Ibler et al., "Digital dermoscopy to determine skin melanin index as an objective indicator of skin pigmentation," *Journal of Surgical Dermatology*, vol. 1, no. 1, 2016.

[15] P. Richardson and W. E. Schulenburg, "Bilateral congenital mydriasis," *British Journal of Ophthalmology*, vol. 75, no. 10, pp. 632-633, 1992.

[16] A. Abbaspour, P. Khadiv Parsi, F. Khalighi-Sigaroodi, and R. Ghaffarzadegan, "Optimization of atropine extraction process from atropa belladonna by modified bubble column extractor with ultrasonic bath," *Iranian Journal of Chemistry and Chemical Engineering*, vol. 35, no. 4, pp. 49–60, 2016.

[17] K. Dimitrov, D. Metcheva, and L. Boyadzhiev, "Integrated processes of extraction and liquid membrane isolation of atropine from Atropa belladonna roots," *Separation and Purification Technology*, vol. 46, no. 1-2, pp. 41–45, 2005.

[18] P. Śramska, A. Maciejka, A. Topolewska, P. Stepnowski, and Ł. P. Haliński, "Isolation of atropine and scopolamine from plant material using liquid-liquid extraction and EXtrelut® columns," *Journal of Chromatography B*, vol. 1043, pp. 202–208, 2017.

[19] M. Wilkes, C. Y. Wright, J. L. Du Plessis, and A. Reeder, "Fitzpatrick skin type, individual typology angle, and melanin index in an African population: steps toward universally applicable skin photosensitivity assessments," *JAMA Dermatology*, vol. 151, no. 8, pp. 902-903, 2015.

[20] K. T. Patton, *Anatomy and physiology*, Elsevier Health Sciences, 2015.

[21] A. Presland and J. Price, "Ocular anatomy and physiology relevant to anaesthesia," *naesthesia & Intensive Care Medicine*, vol. 18, no. 1, pp. 27–32, 2017.

[22] C. Daluwatte, J. H. Miles, S. E. Christ, D. Q. Beversdorf, T. N. Takahashi, and G. Yao, "Atypical pupillary light reflex and heart rate variability in children with autism spectrum disorder," *Journal of Autism and Developmental Disorders*, vol. 43, no. 8, article no. 1741, pp. 1910–1925, 2013.

[23] P. Kaufman, L. Leonard, and A. Albert, *Adler's Physiology of the Eye*, Elsevier Health Sciences, 2011.

[24] C. J. K. Ellis, "The pupillary light reflex in normal subjects," *British Journal of Ophthalmology*, vol. 65, no. 11, pp. 754–759, 1981.

[25] P. H. Heller, F. Perry, D. L. Jewett, and J. D. Levine, "Autonomic components of the human pupillary light reflex," *Investigative Ophthalmology & Visual Science*, vol. 31, no. 1, pp. 156–162, 1990.

[26] J. A. Cahill and J. Ross, "Eye on children: Acute work-up for pediatric horner's syndrome. case presentation and review of the literature," *Journal of Emergency Medicine*, vol. 48, no. 1, pp. 58–62, 2015.

[27] W. F. Maloney, B. R. Younge, and N. J. Moyer, "Evaluation of the causes and accuracy of pharmacologic localization in Horner's syndrome," *American Journal of Ophthalmology*, vol. 90, no. 3, pp. 394–402, 1980.

[28] H. L. Van der Wiel and J. Van Gijn, "The diagnosis of Horner's syndrome. Use and limitations of the cocaine test," *Journal of the Neurological Sciences*, vol. 73, no. 3, pp. 311–316, 1986.

[29] R. J. Pandit and R. Taylor, "Mydriasis and glaucoma: Exploding the myth. A systematic review," *Diabetic Medicine*, vol. 17, no. 10, pp. 693–699, 2000.

[30] S. Beharry and S. Gibbons, "An overview of emerging and new psychoactive substances in the United Kingdom," *Forensic Science International*, vol. 267, pp. 25–34, 2016.

[31] B. E. Blough, A. Landavazo, A. M. Decker, J. S. Partilla, M. H. Baumann, and R. B. Rothman, "Interaction of psychoactive tryptamines with biogenic amine transporters and serotonin receptor subtypes," *Psychopharmacology*, vol. 231, no. 21, pp. 4135–4144, 2014.

[32] F. S. Bersani, O. Corazza, P. Simonato et al., "Drops of madness? Recreational misuse of tropicamide collyrium; early warning alerts from Russia and Italy," *General Hospital Psychiatry*, vol. 35, no. 5, pp. 571–573, 2013.

[33] B. Behnia, M. Heinrichs, W. Bergmann et al., "Differential effects of intranasal oxytocin on sexual experiences and partner interactions in couples," *Hormones and Behavior*, vol. 65, no. 3, pp. 308–318, 2014.

[34] C. S. Carter, "Oxytocin pathways and the evolution of human behavior," *Annual Review of Psychology*, vol. 65, pp. 17–39, 2014.

[35] Erowid.com. Erowid Experience Vaults (accessed 07 May 2017). https://erowid.org/experiences/.

[36] The Terence McKenna Page. The Terence McKenna Experience. (accessed 07 May 2017) https://www.facebook.com/groups/terencemckenna/.

[37] A. E. Neice, M. Behrends, M. P. Bokoch, K. M. Seligman, N. M. Conrad, and M. D. Larson, "Prediction of opioid analgesic efficacy by measurement of pupillary unrest," *Anesthesia and Analgesia*, vol. 124, no. 3, pp. 915–921, 2017.

[38] T. K. Nuckols, L. Anderson, I. Popescu et al., "Opioid prescribing: a systematic review and critical appraisal of guidelines for chronic pain," *Annals of Internal Medicine*, vol. 160, no. 1, pp. 38–47, 2014.

[39] K. Rubia, A. A. Alegria, A. I. Cubillo, A. B. Smith, M. J. Brammer, and J. Radua, "Effects of stimulants on brain function in attention-deficit/hyperactivity disorder: A systematic review and meta-analysis," *Biological Psychiatry*, vol. 76, no. 8, pp. 616–628, 2014.

[40] F. Mueller, C. Lenz, M. Steiner et al., "Neuroimaging in moderate MDMA use: a systematic review," *Neuroscience and Biobehavioral Reviews*, vol. 62, pp. 21–34, 2016.

[41] J. J. López-Ibor, M.-I. López-Ibor, and J. I. Pastrana, "Transcranial magnetic stimulation," *Current Opinion in Psychiatry*, vol. 21, no. 6, pp. 640–644, 2008.

[42] J. O'Shea and V. Walsh, "Transcranial magnetic stimulation," *Current Biology*, vol. 17, no. 6, pp. R196–R199, 2007.

[43] B. Phillips, C. Ball, D. Sackett, D. Badenoch, D. Straus, and B. Haynes, "Oxford Centre for Evidence-Based Medicine-Levels of Evidence (March 2009)," (accessed 6 January 2017). http://www.cebm.net/oxford-centre-evidence-based-medicine-levels-evidence-march-2009/.

[44] R. Smith and D. Rennie, "Evidence-based medicine—an oral history," *JAMA*, vol. 311, no. 4, pp. 365–367, 2014.

Emotional Lability as a Unique Presenting Sign of Suspected Chronic Traumatic Encephalopathy

Shauna H. Yuan[1] **and Sonya G. Wang**[2]

[1]Department of Neurosciences, University of California, San Diego, La Jolla, CA 92093, USA
[2]Department of Neurology, University of Minnesota, Minneapolis, MN 55455, USA

Correspondence should be addressed to Shauna H. Yuan; shyuan@ucsd.edu

Academic Editor: Samuel T. Gontkovsky

Chronic traumatic encephalopathy (CTE) is a neurodegenerative disease caused by head trauma. Diagnosis of this disease is difficult as reliable biomarkers have not been established and often this clinical entity is underappreciated with poor recognition of its clinical presentations (Lenihan and Jordan, 2015). The definitive diagnosis of CTE is determined by identification of neurofibrillary tangles in the perivascular space around the sulci in postmortem tissue (McKee et al., 2015). However, performing brain biopsies searching for neurofibrillary tangles is not a feasible option for early diagnosis. Thus, diagnosis of suspected CTE in the living has been based on clinical suspicion using proposed research criteria of clinical presentations. In addition, neuroimaging techniques have shown some promise in assisting diagnosis. Clinically, CTE is more commonly known to be associated with memory impairment and executive function disorder (Stern et al., 2013). However, here, we present two unique cases of prior professional football players where behavioral changes were the first identifying factors in clinical presentation and discuss possible neuroimaging options to help with CTE diagnosis. Because behavioral changes can be mistaken for other neuropsychological diseases, recognizing differing clinical constellations is critical to early diagnosis, early intervention, and improving patient care in suspected CTE.

1. Introduction

Chronic traumatic encephalopathy (CTE) has been associated with popular American contact sports, such as football, hockey, and soccer. The clinical presentation of CTE can be divided into two different groups. One group presents with changes in cognitive function, including memory and executive impairment. A second group presents with behavioral changes, including impulsivity and violent behavior prior to mood or cognitive decline [1]. This second group often can be misdiagnosed as having a psychiatric disorder and is not as easily recognized. Clinical diagnostic criteria for CTE have been proposed for research purposes but have yet to be widely disseminated for clinical purposes [1]. The utility of neuroimaging, such as MRI (magnetic resonance imaging) and PET (position emission tomography), has been evaluated to assist in early diagnosis [2]. This case report describes two unique presentations of behavioral changes as early signs of suspected CTE and provides further discussion regarding neuroimaging possibilities. This information is essential in helping to increase awareness of the differing clinical presentations of CTE.

The definitive diagnosis for CTE is neuropathological evidence of early perivascular tau deposition in the brain [3]. Tau is a microtubule binding protein, important for axonal transport. Abnormal phosphorylated tau deposition is also found in other types of neurodegenerative diseases, such as Alzheimer's disease [4]. In later stages of CTE, tau deposition appears in other regions of the brain [5, 6].

Without biomarkers, CTE continues to be a diagnostic dilemma [7]. The clinical presentation overlaps with psychiatric presentations such as depression and memory impairment. There are several proposed diagnostic criteria for research purposes [8–10] and these include history of repetitive head trauma and cognitive and/or behavioral impairment. Often symptoms associated with CTE may be ignored, and, therefore, raising awareness and recognizing the symptoms are critical. Below, we present two cases of professional

TABLE 1: Patient clinical information. Patient clinical information is compared.

	Patient A	Patient B
Age	39	41
Onset	mid-30s	30
History of concussion	yes	yes
Age of playing contact sports	5	13
Childhood/premorbid psychiatric history	no	no
Family history of Alzheimer's disease or other dementia	no	no

American football players to illustrate behavioral and memory changes suggesting early symptoms for suspected CTE. Included in their cases are background demographic data in Table 1.

2. Case Presentation

2.1. Patient A. Patient A was a 39-year-old right-handed former professional football player. He presented to Memory Disorders Clinic in a tertiary care hospital for evaluation of memory problems. He first developed mood problems with irritability, depression, and social withdrawal about the time he retired from professional football in his early 30s. He experienced significant mood swings, sometimes laughing uncontrollably, rocking, pacing, and grumbling. He also had suicidal ideations. Later, short-term memory problems started insidiously and gradually worsened into his mid-30s. He was quick to forget, constantly repeated questions, often forgot his appointments, and misplaced objects. He had difficulty with directions and relied on GPS to get around. He would forget to pay his bills, and thus management of the finances was taken over by his caregiver. He had difficulty performing at his job, for he could not remember the tasks. He also became frustrated easily and could not multitask.

Patient A started playing football at age of 5. He played football for total of 25 years. He experienced eight concussions, in which he lost consciousness in four of them. In addition, he experienced brief "bell rung," hitting his head and seeing stars, which occurred at least once if not more every time he played football. There is no family history of Alzheimer's disease.

His MOCA score was 20/30 and the CDR was 1. On the neuropsychological testing, patient exhibited significant deficit in multiple domains, including complex attention and executive and memory functioning (Table 2). Patient A's MRI brain was normal. Patient did not carry a psychiatric diagnosis previously. Diagnosis was major neurocognitive disorder, chronic traumatic encephalopathy, and major depressive disorder based on history and neuropsychological testing.

2.2. Patient B. Patient B was a 41-year-old right-handed ex-professional football player. He started feeling depressed at age of 30 and it gradually worsened over the years. He developed significant mood swings for three to four years where he cycled between feeling sad, crying, laughing, and becoming angry. He was not diagnosed or treated for mood problems, for he never sought medical help. He has lost interest in his hobbies and slowly reduced his daily activities to lying around at home.

Memory problems started at about age of 39. The memory problems had an insidious onset and gradual progression. Patient B had trouble recalling details of events. He needed to write things down; otherwise, they would not get done. He repeated questions several times a day.

His activities of daily living (ADLs), which are daily self-care activities, including eating, bathing, dressing toileting, transferring, and continence, were not entirely intact. He required reminders to take showers. Although he could dress himself, he required prompting to dress appropriately for the occasion. His instrumental ADLs (iADLs), which are activities requiring skills to successfully live independently, were affected. He was able to go shopping by himself; he could pick out the items and pay for them. His wife took over paying the bills completely, to ensure that bills were paid on time, because he forgot to pay certain bills. His driving was unaffected. He had not had any accidents and had not gotten lost. However, he used the GPS to help him get around. He continued to participate in doing household chores but typically needed assistance. For example, he could start the laundry but would forget to finish the laundry.

He started playing football since age of 13. He played 9-year professional football and 4-year college football. He played football for total of 18 years. He has had numerous events associated with seeing stars/seeing light/dazed for a few minutes during the season. He could not remember how many he had but reported having had quite a few. He did remember experiencing being knocked out four times and being escorted off the field.

His MOCA score was 23/30 and the CDR was 1. On the neuropsychological testing, patient exhibited significant deficit in multiple domains, including complex attention and executive functioning (Table 2). MRI was normal. His neuropsychological testing results and clinical history fulfilled the criteria of DSM V for major neurocognitive disorder, for he had deficits, which interfered with daily life in two different domains.

3. Discussion

This case report highlights an essential understanding of how CTE can develop in sports players as early as their 30s and can uniquely present with mood problems prior to memory and executive function problems.

These two cases show a similar history to other professional American sports players as both started playing football as children (Table 1). Both played in high school, college, and then professionally for approximately 10 years. Patient A started playing at an earlier age than patient B by 10 years. It is possible that patient A developed disease earlier than patient B for patient A started playing earlier. The number of years of exposure to the sport correlates with disease severity [11].

CTE is a tauopathy. NFT, tau-positive astrocytes, tau-positive cell processes that preferentially involve the cortical

TABLE 2: Neuropsychological testing results. Patient neuropsychological testing showing impaired memory and cognitive functions in multiple domains. *T* score of 50 is average. One standard deviation is 10 points. For example, one standard deviation below is 40.

Test	Patient A T score	Patient B T score
Complex attention		
WAIS IV digit span	30	47
WAIS IV arithmetic	37	43
WAIS IV letter number sequencing	37	
WAIS IV coding	27	53
WAIS IV symbol search	27	50
WAIS IV cancellation	30	37
DKEFS trails-visual scanning	30	50
DKEFS trails-number sequencing	27	50
DKEFS trails-letter sequencing	20	57
CATA commission errors		21
CPT omission errors		26
CPT commission errors		31
Speech sounds perception	43	40
Seashore rhythm	25	41
Visual-perceptual and motor/visual-motor functioning		
WAIS-IV block design	53	43
WAIS-IV visual puzzles	37	40
WAIS-IV matrix reasoning	50	63
DKEFS tower test	40	70
Executive functioning		
Verbal fluency (FAS)	32	53
Trails B	37	See TN/LS
Category test	38	36
WAIS-IV similarities	40	40
DKEFS trails number/letter switching	See Trails B	57
DKEFS letter fluency	37	53
DKEFS category fluency	37	50
DKEFS switching: total correct	43	37
DKEFS switching: accuracy	40	40
DKEFS color/word inhibition	20	37
DKEFS color/word inhibition switch	20	40
DKEFS word context test	40	53
Language functioning		
Boston naming test	N/A	N/A
Category fluency (animal naming)	37	53
DKEFS letter fluency	37	53
BDAE complex ideational material	n/a	N/A
DKEFS word context test	40	53
DKEFS category fluency	See above	53
Memory functioning		
WMS-IV logical memory I	23	40
WMS-IV logical memory II	23	33
WMS-IV verbal paired associates I	33	43
WMS-IV verbal paired associates II	23	47
WMS-IV visual reproduction I	37	43
WMS-IV visual reproduction II	27	50
WMS-IV designs I	43	N/A
WMS-IV designs II	40	N/A

sulci, medial temporal lobe, diencephalon, and brainstem are observed on brain autopsy. The tau pathology is characteristically perivascular, most pronounced at the sulcal depths, and preferentially involves the superficial cortical layers. These microscopic changes accumulate over time and help increase our understanding of its pathophysiology; however, at this time, these tau changes do not help clinicians in the diagnosis of the disease.

With regard to neuroimaging, both patients retained normal brain MRIs and thus relying on brain imaging may not be helpful in early diagnosis. CTE patients can develop cavum pellucidum with brain trauma; however, this is only in a small subgroup of patients with CTE [11]. More recently, PET imaging has been considered as a potentially useful neuroimaging modality for detecting CTE pathology. Already, a PET compound, PiB (Pittsburgh Compound B), has been developed that tracks amyloid deposition in Alzheimer's disease and helps in understanding amyloid-beta pathology after head trauma [12]. In the last two years, tau specific tracers for PET have been developed, THK5317, THK5351, AV1451, and PBB3. Due to the complexity and variability of different types of tau deposits in different diseases, these tracers will need to be evaluated for efficacy in diagnosing CTE and in understanding its pathology [13]. With future understanding of the tau specific PET tracers, the patients presented in this case report, may have further confirmatory data indicating a definitive diagnosis of CTE.

For now, these two patients fall into the clinical research diagnostic criteria of mood disorder prior to memory deficits for CTE [8–10]. Their age of onset (30s–40s) is also consistent with the behavioral symptoms presenting at a younger age compared to the age of presentation for cognitive symptoms [1]. Clinical features of CTE include impairments in mood (depression, suicidality, and irritability), behavior (explosivity, violence, and impulsivity), cognition (impaired memory, executive dysfunction, and diminished concentration), and motor functioning (parkinsonism, dysarthria, gait changes, and weakness). A longitudinal study of children in higher risk concussion sports and their development into professional sports players would be most beneficial in identifying and describing CTE. At this present time, CTE is often under-recognized or misdiagnosed. It is crucial for clinicians to be particularly aware of the varying presentations of CTE, especially when patients initially complain of emotional lability or behavioral symptoms.

References

[1] R. A. Stern, D. H. Daneshvar, C. M. Baugh et al., "Clinical presentation of chronic traumatic encephalopathy," *Neurology*, vol. 81, no. 13, pp. 1122–1129, 2013.

[2] P. Sparks, T. Lawrence, and S. Hinze, "Neuroimaging in the diagnosis of chronic traumatic encephalopathy," *Clinical Journal of Sport Medicine*, p. 1, 2017.

[3] A. C. McKee et al., "The first NINDS/NIBIB consensus meeting to define neuropathological criteria for the diagnosis of chronic traumatic encephalopathy," *Acta Neuropathol*, vol. 131, no. 1, pp. 75–86, 2016.

[4] D. M. Holtzman, J. C. Morris, and A. M. Goate, "Alzheimer's disease: the challenge of the second century," *Science Translational Medicine*, vol. 3, no. 77, p. 77sr1, 2011.

[5] A. C. McKee, T. D. Stein, P. T. Kiernan, and V. E. Alvarez, "The neuropathology of chronic traumatic encephalopathy," *Brain Pathology*, vol. 25, no. 3, pp. 350–364, 2015.

[6] J. Mez, D. H. Daneshvar, P. T. Kiernan et al., "Clinicopathological evaluation of chronic traumatic encephalopathy in players of american football," *Journal of the American Medical Association*, vol. 318, no. 4, pp. 360–370, 2017.

[7] M. W. Lenihan and B. D. Jordan, "The clinical presentation of chronic traumatic encephalopathy," *Current Neurology and Neuroscience Reports*, vol. 15, no. 5, 2015.

[8] J. Victoroff, "Traumatic encephalopathy: review and provisional research diagnostic criteria," *NeuroRehabilitation*, vol. 32, no. 2, pp. 211–224, 2013.

[9] P. H. Montenigro, C. M. Baugh, D. H. Daneshvar et al., "Clinical subtypes of chronic traumatic encephalopathy: literature review and proposed research diagnostic criteria for traumatic encephalopathy syndrome," *Alzheimer's Research & Therapy*, vol. 6, no. 5-8, article no. 68, 2014.

[10] B. D. Jordan, "The clinical spectrum of sport-related traumatic brain injury," *Nature Reviews Neurology*, vol. 9, no. 4, pp. 222–230, 2013.

[11] T. D. Stein, V. E. Alvarez, and A. C. McKee, "Concussion in chronic traumatic encephalopathy," *Current Pain and Headache Reports*, vol. 19, no. 10, p. 47, 2015.

[12] M. Sundman, P. M. Doraiswamy, and R. A. Morey, "Neuroimaging assessment of early and late neurobiological sequelae of traumatic brain injury: Implications for CTE," *Frontiers in Neuroscience*, vol. 9, article no. 334, 2015.

[13] L. Saint-Aubert, L. Lemoine, K. Chiotis, A. Leuzy, E. Rodriguez-Vieitez, and A. Nordberg, "Tau PET imaging: present and future directions," *Molecular Neurodegeneration*, vol. 12, no. 1, article no. 19, 2017.

Comorbid Normal Pressure Hydrocephalus with Parkinsonism: A Clinical Challenge and Call for Awareness

A. Cucca,[1] M. C. Biagioni,[1] K. Sharma,[1] J. Golomb,[2] R. M. Gilbert,[1] A. Di Rocco,[1] and J. E. Fleisher[3]

[1]*Department of Neurology, The Marlene & Paolo Fresco Institute for Parkinson's & Movement Disorders, New York University School of Medicine, NYU Langone Medical Center, New York, NY, USA*
[2]*Department of Neurosurgery, Adult Hydrocephalus Program, NYU School of Medicine, New York, NY, USA*
[3]*Department of Neurological Sciences, Rush University Medical Center, Chicago, IL, USA*

Correspondence should be addressed to A. Cucca; alberto.cucca@nyumc.org

Academic Editor: Pablo Mir

Idiopathic normal pressure hydrocephalus (iNPH) is the most common cause of hydrocephalus in adults. The diagnosis may be challenging, requiring collaborative efforts between different specialists. According to the International Society for Hydrocephalus and Cerebrospinal Fluid Disorders, iNPH should be considered in the differential of any unexplained gait failure with insidious onset. Recognizing iNPH can be even more difficult in the presence of comorbid neurologic disorders. Among these, idiopathic Parkinson's disease (PD) is one of the major neurologic causes of gait dysfunction in the elderly. Both conditions have their peak prevalence between the 6th and the 7th decade. Importantly, postural instability and gait dysfunction are core clinical features in both iNPH and PD. Therefore, diagnosing iNPH where diagnostic criteria of PD have been met represents an additional clinical challenge. Here, we report a patient with parkinsonism initially consistent with PD who subsequently displayed rapidly progressive postural instability and gait dysfunction leading to the diagnosis of concomitant iNPH. In the following sections, we will review the clinical features of iNPH, as well as the overlapping and discriminating features when degenerative parkinsonism is in the differential diagnosis. Understanding and recognizing the potential for concomitant disease are critical when treating both conditions.

1. Background

Idiopathic normal pressure hydrocephalus (iNPH) is a neurological condition clinically characterized by the triad of gait dysfunction, cognitive abnormalities, and urinary disorders [1]. iNPH is morphologically characterized by the expansion of the lateral and third cerebral ventricles in the absence of macroscopic obstructions to the CSF outflow. The pathogenesis of iNPH remains unknown; however CSF dynamics show two major abnormalities: a pulsatile increase in CSF pressure and an increased outflow resistance. Ventricular enlargement with near normalization of hydrostatic pressure takes place but the pathophysiology involved in these phenomena remains highly disputed [2]. Typically, iNPH shows an insidious onset without any specific prior event detectable on medical history. The progression is usually slow, spanning months or years. Gait dysfunction is usually the first reported abnormality and is characterized by reduced step height during the swing phase, reduced stride length and reduced velocity [3–5]. Equilibrium-related gait variables are particularly affected, including wide base, increased external rotation of the knees, and enlarged foot rotation angles [6]. Other frequent features include propulsion or retropulsion, festination, freezing of gait (FoG), and hesitancy of gait which may confer a "magnetic" character. Kinematic abnormalities of the lower limbs show a bilateral and symmetric distribution [7]. Dynamic balance during transitional movements, like standing or turning, is severely impaired. Cognitive symptoms of iNPH include impaired attention, short-term recall, and executive function that ultimately evolve into dementia [8]. In a recent observational study, up to 46% of patients with NPH were found to display depressive symptoms, and apathy is also common [9]. Bladder symptoms usually involve detrusor hyperactivity, manifesting as increased urinary urgency and frequency [10, 11]. According to the International Society for Hydrocephalus and Cerebrospinal Fluid Disorders guidelines, "probable NPH" is defined by the combination of gait dysfunction with insidious onset after age 40 without precipitating events, lasting at least 3–6 months in the absence of comorbidities which could fully explain the symptoms [12]. In clinical practice, the latter carries the most controversy. First, the age of these patients, usually between the 6th and the 7th decade of life, is associated with a high risk of comorbid factors potentially affecting walking, such as peripheral neuropathy, arthritis, or degenerative spine disease. Therefore it can be difficult to know whether the gait disorder is purely due to iNPH. For the same reason, a coexisting neurodegenerative condition like idiopathic Parkinson's disease (PD) or other parkinsonism must also be considered. Since each condition requires different treatments, recognizing coexisting PD and iNPH is essential.

2. Case Report

A 79-year-old right-handed female with lumbar spondylosis and chronic low back pain presented with a two-year, slowly progressive history of mild left hand resting tremor, stooped posture, generalized slowness, and fatigue. She reported a decline in her balance, though denied falls, and she was able to walk independently. She denied urinary symptoms, constipation, dysphagia, hypophonia, hyposmia, and symptoms of REM behavioral disorder. She denied cognitive or behavioral problems and denied previous exposure to neuroleptics, antiemetics, or head trauma. Her family history was noncontributory. Baseline examination revealed a pleasant woman with normal mental status who scored a 28/30 on the Montreal Cognitive Assessment (MoCA), with points missed for delayed recall. She displayed mild hypomimia with decreased blink rate. Myerson's sign was present, with no palmomental and no grasp reflex. Vertical saccades were slightly hypometric in both directions. There was a near-constant, low-frequency chin tremor. Her slow pill-rolling tremor of the left hand was unmasked by distraction and contralateral activation, and associated cogwheeling was appreciated in the ipsilateral wrist. There was slight rigidity affecting the left extremities and mild bilateral bradykinesia. Chair mobility was normal, and her gait notable for bilaterally diminished arm swing, affecting the left more than the right. Cadence, stride length, and ground clearance were slightly reduced. She had no FoG. She recovered from the pull test in 4 steps, yielding a UPDRS motor score of 21. The remainder of her physical examination was notable for bilateral, symmetrically reduced deep tendon reflexes in the lower limbs and a positive Romberg test. Electromyography and nerve conduction studies demonstrated a primarily sensory, large fiber peripheral neuropathy affecting both legs, with no evidence of radiculopathy, plexopathy, or myopathy. The patient was diagnosed with PD according to the United Kingdom Parkinson's Disease Society Brain Bank (UKPDSBB) criteria. She was started on rasagiline 1 mg once a day.

Six months later, she reported occasional detailed visual hallucinations with retained insight and progressive decline in her hand dexterity. Her physical examination was unchanged. A brain MRI revealed mild prominence of the ventricular system and cortical sulci along with multiple foci of periventricular, subcortical, and brainstem T2/FLAIR hyperintensities, consistent with chronic nonspecific microvascular changes (Figure 1). Rasagiline was discontinued due to a lack of efficacy and the potential contribution to hallucinations. Carbidopa-levodopa 25–100 mg was initiated and gradually titrated up to one full tablet TID. After 6 months, the patient reported improvements in stiffness, general slowness, and tremor. Her UPDRS motor score on levodopa improved by 19% and hallucinations completely resolved.

Over the following months, the patient experienced progressive gait deterioration with marked unsteadiness, particularly during transfers, with frequent falls and severe FoG. Near-falls began occurring daily, she was unable to walk unassisted when outdoors, and FoG episodes became disabling. She also reported increased urinary frequency, occasional urinary incontinence, mild forgetfulness affecting her short-term memory, and difficulties with word retrieval. Her mood significantly deteriorated, with increased apathy and pervasive sadness. On examination, her MoCA decreased to 22/30, with abnormal verbal recall, visuospatial function, executive function, and mental calculation. Her examination was notable for severe gait failure, with markedly decreased stride length and cadence, en bloc turns, freezing, and absent postural reflexes. Her gait failure was notably out of proportion to her otherwise stable appendicular signs. Carbidopa-levodopa was increased up to 1.5 tablets TID without benefit.

In considering the possibility of iNPH, we ordered a repeat brain MRI (Figure 1). The ventricular size was further increased and ventriculomegaly was out of proportion to sulcal enlargement. Confluent areas of T2 hyperintensity were detected in the periventricular white matter. On sagittal sections, a strong flow void was noted at the cerebral aqueduct (Figure 2). The patient underwent a large volume lumbar puncture (LP) with pre- and post-LP testing. Approximately 40 cc of clear CSF was withdrawn. Standard CSF analysis was unremarkable. Observation of gait after LP revealed improved velocity and uniformity of cadence relative to pre-LP baseline. There was a distinct improvement in the patient's ability to make 180° turns with no evidence of FoG. Video gait analysis was performed on a distance of 18 m with postprocessing of gait speed and stride length. Both parameters significantly improved compared to her pre-LP condition (Figure 3). Additionally, her post-LP neuropsychological assessment revealed significant improvement in Trail Making B (Table 1).

Given her response to LP, a ventricular-peritoneal (VP) shunt was placed without complications. Over the following weeks, she experienced a dramatic improvement in balance and walking. She was able to walk unassisted for long distances. Her functional independence, per the Schwab and England Activities of Daily Living scale, improved from 80% (doing most of daily chores takes twice as long) to

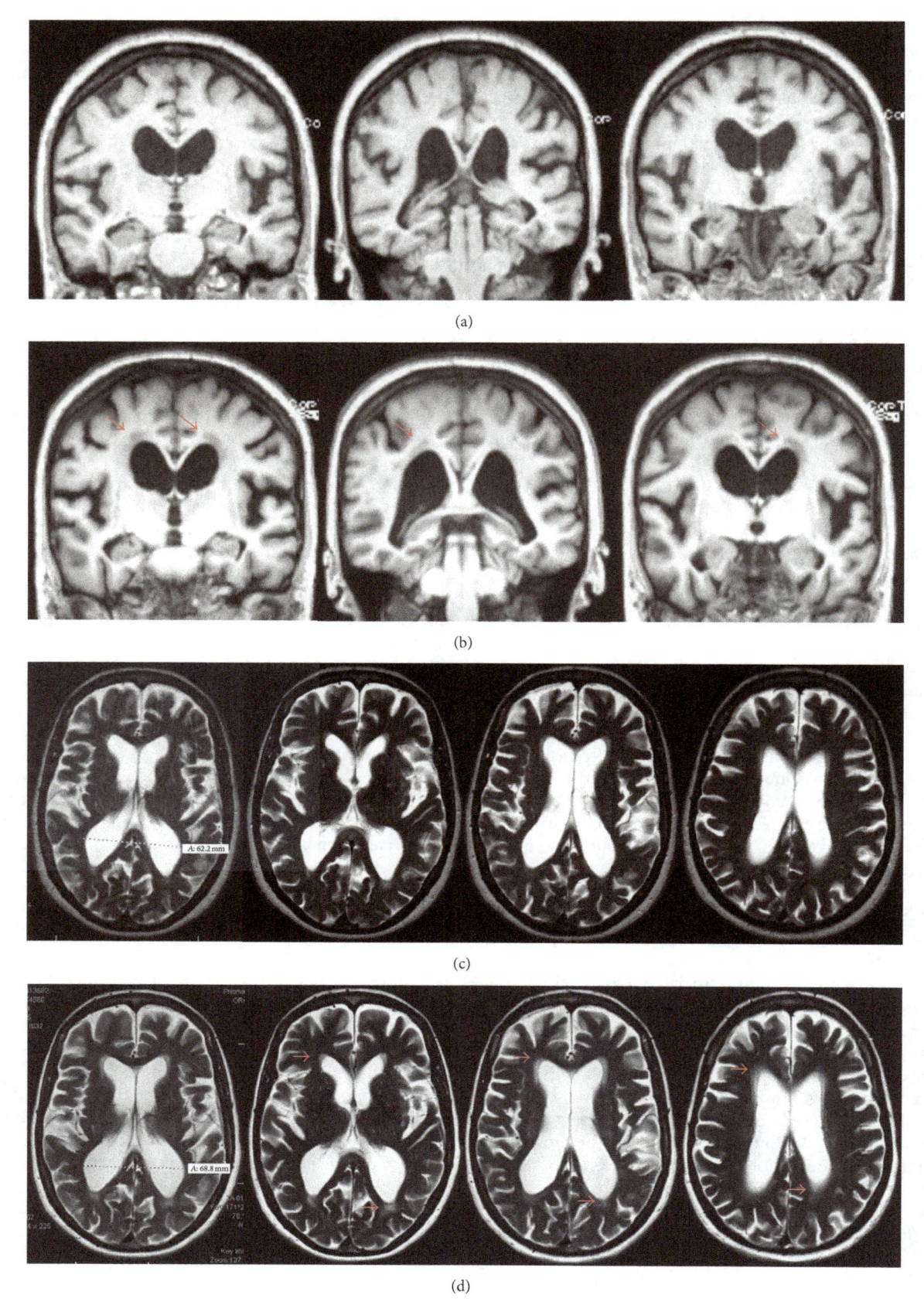

Figure 1: Brain MRI imaging. (a) Baseline coronal MPR sequences. (b) One-year follow-up coronal MPR sequences: periventricular white matter hypointensity (red arrows). Slight narrowing of cortical gyri on the vertex with enlarged Sylvian fissure. (c) Baseline Axial T2-weighted sequences. (d) One-year follow-up axial T2-weighted sequences: increased periventricular white matter hyperintensity (red arrows).

Table 1: Functional independence, neuropsychological assessment, and freezing of gait.

	Pre-LP	Post-LP	Postshunt	6 months after shunt
Schwab and England ADL	80%, completely independent in most chores; takes twice as long	80%, completely independent in most chores; takes twice as long	100%, completely independent; able to do all chores without slowness, difficulty, or impairment	100%, completely independent; able to do all chores without slowness, difficulty, or impairment
MoCA	22		25	26
Trail Making A	52.0 sec	36.4 sec	29.1 sec	39.1 sec
Trail Making B	93.3 sec	95.8 sec	71.8 sec	69.7 sec
UPDRS part II FoG	2 (occasional freezing when walking)		0 (none)	0 (none)

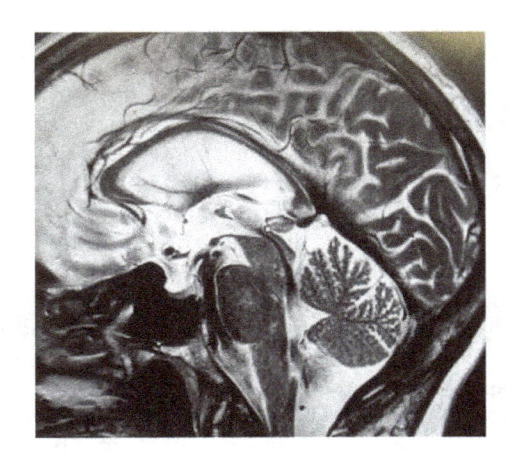

Figure 2: One-year follow-up brain MRI, sagittal T2 section. A strong flow void artifact is noted at the Sylvian aqueduct.

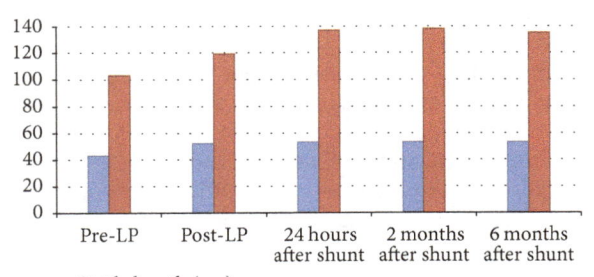

Figure 3: Video gait analysis at distance of 18 m.

100% (completely independent, able to do all chores without slowness, difficulty, or impairment). Falls, near-falls, and her bladder symptoms ceased. UPDRS part II FoG item improved from 2 to 0. On examination, walking speed, stride length, and heel strike significantly increased, with resolution of FoG. Her pull test normalized. Gait profile and neuropsychological assessment were repeated according to the same baseline procedures approximately two and six months after shunt placement (Figure 3 and Table 1). On both postshunt assessments, video analysis showed a significant and sustained improvement in stride length and mean gait velocity. Neuropsychological assessment revealed a significant improvement in all measured outcomes, and her MoCA improved by 3 points. Improvements in gait and balance were sustained over one year of follow-up. Appendicular symptoms including bradykinesia, stiffness, and resting tremor persisted but were well controlled without adjustments in the patient's dopaminergic regimen.

3. Discussion

Our patient presented with a two-year history of progressive slowness, fatigue, and mild asymmetric resting tremor. According to UKPDSBB, the clinical diagnosis of PD requires the presence of bradykinesia and at least one of the following: muscular rigidity, 4–6 Hz resting tremor, and postural instability. Baseline physical examination revealed the presence of all cardinal features included in the UKPDSBB criteria for PD, and our patient was diagnosed accordingly. In 2015, the International Movement Disorder Society (MDS) published revised PD diagnostic criteria [15]. The presence of "recurrent falls because of impaired balance within 3 years of onset" is among the red flags arguing against a diagnosis of clinically established PD. Notably, each red flag must be countered by at least one supportive diagnostic criterion, including a clear and dramatic response to dopaminergic therapy (a ≥30% improvement on clinical examination, for which our patient's 19% initial improvement did not qualify), unequivocal motor fluctuations, levodopa-induced dyskinesias, rest tremor of a limb, and either olfactory loss or cardiac sympathetic denervation. In our case, while she initially met the UKPDSBB criteria for PD, the patient's rapid progression of gait impairment and recurrent falls within 3 years are red flags arguing against idiopathic PD; her rest tremor constitutes one of the supportive criteria to argue *for* the PD diagnosis; however two supportive criteria are required to counterbalance these red flags. The concomitant presence of NPH may challenge the practical applicability of these criteria in the setting of comorbidities. Alternatively, this discrepancy may suggest that she has parkinsonism, but not idiopathic PD. It is likely that a longer follow-up period will provide meaningful observational data to either confirm or challenge the diagnosis of underlying PD.

Approximately 2.5 years after her PD diagnosis, our patient's gait and balance dramatically deteriorated, a far more rapid decline than expected for PD and disproportionate to her otherwise well-controlled parkinsonian symptoms. Optimization of dopaminergic therapy is considered the first line strategy to relieve FoG and improve gait function in PD; however this was ineffective [16]. Additionally, she reported the insidious onset of psychological, cognitive, and urologic symptoms. For all of the above reasons, we considered the possibility of NPH. From a clinical viewpoint, gait dysfunction is mandatory to diagnose iNPH. At least one more abnormality, namely, urinary symptoms or cognitive impairment, is required to support a probable diagnosis [17]. Radiologically, iNPH is characterized by a noncongenital, nonobstructive enlargement of ventricular size not attributable to cerebral atrophy, as indicated by an Evans index greater than 0.3. Supportive criteria include enlargement of the temporal horns of the lateral ventricles out of proportion to the degree of hippocampal atrophy; upbowing of the corpus callosum with callosal angle $\geq 40°$; and abnormal MRI signal intensity of the periventricular white matter [18]. Additionally, the Sylvian fissure is typically enlarged, particularly when compared to otherwise tight cortical sulci with crowding of the gyri at the vertex (the so-called "high convexity sign"). Long echo-time brain MRI sequences can detect the aqueduct flow void artifact due to hyperdynamic CSF flow. Our patient's MRIs were obtained at baseline and approximately one year later when iNPH was suspected. Although slice differences limit optimal comparability, a subtle high convexity sign was appreciable on her follow-up MRI, as was moderate ventriculomegaly, periventricular white matter changes, and a prominent flow void at the Sylvian aqueduct; however the imaging did not demonstrate disproportionately enlarged subarachnoid spaces or a grossly enlarged Sylvian fissure. Our patient underwent a large volume tap test, yielding a marked objective improvement in gait function. She was diagnosed with comorbid iNPH and successfully treated with VP shunt. Dramatic benefits in gait, neuropsychological domains, and clinical assessments were immediately observed and sustained over one-year follow-up.

Between 46 and 63% of patients with iNPH show some degree of benefit from large volume CSF subtraction [18, 19]. CSF tap test is regarded as an important test for the prediction of shunt effectiveness, with a sensitivity ranging from 70% to 80%, according to different observations [20, 21]. In the absence of a clear response to single tap test, a three day-long continuous lumbar drain can be considered to increase diagnostic accuracy. However, according to the international guidelines, a decision exclusively based on predictive tests exposes patients to a high risk of misdiagnosis. False negatives include those patients who, despite underlying iNPH, fail to significantly improve after the test, possibly due to a high degree of comorbidity or to irreversible progression of the disease following an extensive delay in diagnosis. False positives, conversely, may involve a placebo response inherent to any invasive medical procedure, particularly where the patient has expectations of benefit [22]. Hence, a positive response to a tap test should be regarded as a mere supportive criterion [23]. Shunt placement may still be considered in the absence of a clear response to predictive tests when a strong clinical suspicion remains, though the patient must be counseled appropriately and have clear expectations. CSF drainage is the only effective treatment and is generally configured between a lateral cerebral ventricle and the abdominal cavity (VP shunt). The guidelines of the American Academy of Neurology support the use of a shunt as effective therapy emphasizing that diagnostic delay is the major cause of poor therapeutic outcome [24].

4. Comorbid iNPH and Degenerative Parkinsonism: A Call for Awareness

The role of comorbidity in patients with iNPH must be considered according to International Society for Hydrocephalus and Cerebrospinal Fluid Disorder [25]. Identifying comorbidities in patients with iNPH is critical, allowing for optimization of the patient's care for each diagnosis, maximizing their clinical outcome. As recently observed by Broggi et al., given current demographic trends, the coexistence of iNPH and neurodegenerative diseases is expected to increase [26]. According to a Swedish population study, the prevalence of iNPH is approximately 200/100,000 in the range of age from 70 to 79 [13]. According to preliminary data from an ongoing prospective single-center study, approximately 45% of patients meeting the diagnostic criteria of probable iNPH show concurrent signs of parkinsonism [27]. Importantly, these patients display decreased striatal uptake on I123-ioflupane (DatScan) single-photon emission computed tomography (SPECT), consistent with an underlying degenerative parkinsonism. Recently, Odagiri et al. retrospectively analyzed 127 patients with definite iNPH [14]. Twenty-one of these patients reported parkinsonian symptoms including tremor, hypomimia, and stiffness and were referred for a metaiodobenzylguanidine SPECT to rule out an underlying alpha-synucleinopathy. One-third of this sample showed reduced cardiac uptake. Since iNPH does not cause cardiac sympathetic-adrenergic denervation, SPECT positivity has been interpreted as an actual comorbidity between iNPH and alpha-synucleinopathy. The possibility that cooccurrence of iNPH and PD may represent more than just a comorbidity but rather a discrete phenotype resulting from a common pathogenic substrate remains to be conclusively addressed.

Diagnosing both conditions in the same patient requires a willingness to critically review the established diagnosis, appreciate deviations from the usual course, and consider potential explanations. For example, an individual with levodopa-responsive parkinsonism who develops new, pervasive gait failure and subacute cognitive complaints might have concomitant iNPH. Conversely, a patient successfully shunted for iNPH who develops progressive, asymmetric parkinsonism should raise suspicion for degenerative parkinsonism. In Table 2, we compare the main clinical and epidemiological aspects of iNPH and PD to guide the diagnostic process and highlight key differences between these two conditions. Both PD and iNPH are considered among the most common gait disorders in elderly and both are "hypokinetic movement disorders," characterized by reduced speed, reduced stride length, and poor ground clearance along with an abnormal dynamic equilibrium manifesting as insufficient adaptation to sudden perturbations with increased risk of

TABLE 2: Comparing signs and symptoms of iNPH versus PD.

	iNPH	PD
Prevalence	2 cases/1000 in individuals > 70 years old [13]	10 cases/1,000 in individuals 70–79 years old [14]
Age at onset	Adults over the age of 60	Incidence peak between 70 and 79 years
Urinary disturbance	Common, nonspecific	Common, nonspecific
Cognitive dysfunction	Frontal, executive dysfunction	Frontal, executive dysfunction; global cognitive impairment usually denotes disease progression
Bradykinesia	62% of patients display bradykinesia affecting their lower limbs symmetrically; upper limbs are typically spared	Cardinal feature of the disease; upper limbs are usually affected early on in an asymmetric fashion
Rest tremor	Absent	Cardinal feature of the disease; observed in about 60% of patients
Rigidity	Rare	Cardinal feature of the disease; observed in about 60% of patients
Hallucinations	Absent	Usually manifesting with visual misperceptions and passage illusions with retained insight; florid hallucinations typically arise in advanced stages
Cortical deficits (aphasia, apraxia, agnosia)	Absent	Rare
Response to L-dopa	Absent, mild, or inconsistent	Excellent, sustained, supportive diagnostic criteria
Response to shunt placement	>60% of patients	Absent
MRI/CT	Ventriculomegaly	Noncontributory
Time course of gait failure	Early feature	If present early, regarded as a "red flag" for the diagnosis of disease
Gait velocity	Decreased	Decreased
Step length	Decreased	Decreased
Arm swing	Normal	Reduced or abolished
Freezing of gait	Early feature	Most commonly observed in the advanced stages
Responsiveness to cues	Absent or poor	Significant
Step height	Reduced	Reduced
Base	Wide	Narrow

falling [28–30]. FoG is frequently encountered in both disorders, defined as the episodic inability to generate effective stepping manifesting with the patient's feeling of having his feet glued to the floor [31]. Generally, most clinicians tend to favor the diagnosis of iNPH in the presence of a wide-based, prominently magnetic gait with relatively spared arm swing [32]. Conversely, PD is more likely to be considered when global bradykinesia, narrow gait base, reduced arm swing, responsiveness to cues, asymmetric rigidity, bradykinesia, resting tremor, or camptocormia are observed. However, most of the behavioral and cognitive abnormalities in PD—such as executive dysfunction, apathy, depression, and bradyphrenia—can overlap with those observed in patients with iNPH [33]. Parkinsonian signs—including bradykinesia and rigidity—are commonly observed in the lower limbs of patients with iNPH. It is also a common clinical experience that mixed hydrocephalic and parkinsonian gait features coexist, with various degrees of levodopa responsiveness.

In a recent review of 16 studies including 1256 iNPH patients, Espay et al. showed that shunt responsiveness, one of the cornerstones of iNPH diagnosis, declines dramatically over longer observational periods, challenging the current diagnostic construct [34]. In these patients, the frequent finding of associated neurodegenerative pathologies on postmortem examinations suggests that ventricular enlargement may signal subclinical parenchymal changes, therefore representing the only macroscopic sign of a neurodegenerative disorder. In the absence of known secondary causes of hydrocephalus, iNPH should therefore represent a diagnosis of exclusion and the possibility of an underlying neurodegenerative disease manifesting with hydrocephalic presentation must be carefully considered. For these patients, any interventional approach should be extensively discussed and proper counseling offered, highlighting the potential for short-lived benefits from shunting.

5. Conclusion

Here we reported a case of comorbid iNPH in a patient suffering from idiopathic PD. Both PD and iNPH represent prevalent, treatable conditions in the elderly. Despite the recent implementation of international guidelines, diagnostic accuracy of iNPH remains poor. Without appropriate recognition of iNPH symptoms, patients may be missing the possibility of improving their quality of life and functional independence. Suspecting iNPH in the setting of PD represents an additional diagnostic challenge and may reflect a radiographic and symptomatic expression of the underlying neurodegenerative disease, though further study is required. We hope to raise awareness about the potential overlap of these two conditions to optimize patient care.

References

[1] B. R. Nassar and C. F. Lippa, "Idiopathic Normal Pressure Hydrocephalus," *Gerontology and Geriatric Medicine*, vol. 2, p. 233372141664370, 2016.

[2] S. Qvarlander, B. Lundkvist, L.-O. D. Koskinen, J. Malm, and A. Eklund, "Pulsatility in CSF dynamics: Pathophysiology of idiopathic normal pressure hydrocephalus," *Journal of Neurology, Neurosurgery & Psychiatry*, vol. 84, no. 7, pp. 735–741, 2013.

[3] D. Shprecher, J. Schwalb, and R. Kurlan, "Normal pressure hydrocephalus: Diagnosis and treatment," *Current Neurology and Neuroscience Reports*, vol. 8, no. 5, pp. 371–376, 2008.

[4] M. A. Williams and J. Malm, "Diagnosis and treatment of idiopathic normal pressure hydrocephalus," *Continuum: Lifelong Learning in Neurology*, vol. 22, no. 2, pp. 579–599, 2016.

[5] J. G. Nutt, C. D. Marsden, and P. D. Thompson, "Human walking and higher-level gait disorders, particularly in the elderly," *Neurology*, vol. 43, no. 2, pp. 268–279, 1993.

[6] H. Stolze, J. P. Kuhtz-Buschbeck, H. Drücke, K. Jöhnk, M. Illert, and G. Deuschl, "Comparative analysis of the gait disorder of normal pressure hydrocephalus and Parkinson's disease," *Journal of Neurology, Neurosurgery & Psychiatry*, vol. 70, no. 3, pp. 289–297, 2001.

[7] E. Mori, "Gait disturbance in idiopathic normal pressure hydrocephalus," *Brain and Nerve*, vol. 60, no. 3, pp. 219–224, 2008.

[8] P. Hellstrom, M. Edsbagge, E. Blomsterwall et al., "Neuropsychological effects of shunt treatment in idiopathic normal pressure hydrocephalus," *Neurosurgery*, vol. 63, no. 3, pp. 527–535, 2008.

[9] H. Israelsson, P. Allard, A. Eklund, and J. Malm, "Symptoms of depression are common in patients with idiopathic normal pressure hydrocephalus: The INPH-CRasH study," *Neurosurgery*, vol. 78, no. 2, pp. 161–168, 2016.

[10] M. Kiefer and A. Unterberg, "The differential diagnosis and treatment of normal-pressure hydrocephalus," *Deutsches Arzteblatt International*, vol. 109, no. 1-2, pp. 15–25, 2012.

[11] S. Jonas and J. Brown, "Neurogenic bladder in normal pressure hydrocephalus," *Urology*, vol. 5, no. 1, pp. 44–50, 1975.

[12] H. C. Jones and P. M. Klinge, "Hydrocephalus 2008, 17-20th September, Hannover Germany: A conference report," *Cerebrospinal Fluid Research*, vol. 5, article no. 19, 2008.

[13] D. Jaraj, K. Rabiei, T. Marlow, C. Jensen, I. Skoog, and C. Wikkelsø, "Prevalence of idiopathic normal-pressure hydrocephalus," *Neurology*, vol. 82, no. 16, pp. 1449–1454, 2014.

[14] H. Odagiri, T. Baba, Y. Nishio et al., "Clinical characteristics of idiopathic normal pressure hydrocephalus with Lewy body diseases," *Journal of the Neurological Sciences*, vol. 359, no. 1-2, pp. 309–311, 2015.

[15] R. B. Postuma, D. Berg, M. Stern et al., "MDS clinical diagnostic criteria for Parkinson's disease," *Movement Disorders*, vol. 30, no. 12, pp. 1591–1601, 2015.

[16] A. Cucca, M. C. Biagioni, J. E. Fleisher et al., "Freezing of gait in Parkinson's disease: from pathophysiology to emerging therapies," *Neurodegenerative Disease Management*, vol. 6, no. 5, pp. 431–446, 2016.

[17] N. Relkin, A. Marmarou, P. Klinge, M. Bergsneider, and P. M. Black, "Diagnosing Idiopathic Normal-pressure Hydrocephalus," *Neurosurgery*, vol. 57, no. suppl_3, pp. S2-4–S2-16, 2005.

[18] N. Miskin, H. Patel, A. M. Franceschi et al., "Diagnosis of Normal-Pressure Hydrocephalus: Use of Traditional Measures in the Era of Volumetric MR Imaging," *Radiology*, p. 161216, 2017.

[19] P. Klinge, A. Marmarou, M. Bergsneider, N. Relkin, and P. M. L. Black, "INPH guidelines, part V: Outcome of shunting in idiopathic normal-pressure hydrocephalus and the value of outcome assessment in shunted patients," *Neurosurgery*, vol. 57, no. 3, pp. -40–S2, 2005.

[20] M. Ishikawa, M. Hashimoto, E. Mori, N. Kuwana, and H. Kazui, "The value of the cerebrospinal fluid tap test for predicting shunt effectiveness in idiopathic normal pressure hydrocephalus," *Fluids and Barriers of the CNS*, vol. 9, no. 1, article no. 1, 2012.

[21] R. Walchenbach, E. Geiger, R. T. W. M. Thomeer, and J. A. L. Vanneste, "The value of temporary external lumbar CSF drainage in predicting the outcome of shunting on normal pressure hydrocephalus," *Journal of Neurology, Neurosurgery & Psychiatry*, vol. 72, no. 4, pp. 503–506, 2002.

[22] T. Liu, "Route of placebo administration: Robust placebo effects in laboratory and clinical settings," *Neuroscience & Biobehavioral Reviews*, vol. 83, pp. 451–457, 2017.

[23] A. Marmarou, M. Bergsneider, P. Klinge, N. Relkin, and P. M. L. Black, "INPH guidelines, part III: The value of supplemental prognostic tests for the preoperative assessment of idiopathic normal-pressure hydrocephalus," *Neurosurgery*, vol. 57, no. 3, pp. -17–S2, 2005.

[24] J. J. Halperin, R. Kurlan, J. M. Schwalb, M. D. Cusimano, G. Gronseth, and D. Gloss, "Practice guideline: Idiopathic normal pressure hydrocephalus: Response to shunting and predictors of response," *Neurology*, vol. 85, no. 23, pp. 2063–2071, 2015.

[25] J. Malm, N. R. Graff-Radford, M. Ishikawa et al., "Influence of comorbidities in idiopathic normal pressure hydrocephalus - research and clinical care. A report of the ISHCSF task force on comorbidities in INPH," *Fluids and Barriers of the CNS*, vol. 10, no. 1, article no. 22, 2013.

[26] M. Broggi, L. Romito, V. Redaelli, and A. Franzini, "Normal pressure hydrocephalus and Parkinsonism: The essential teamwork between the neurosurgeon and the neurologist," *World Neurosurgery*, vol. 82, no. 6, pp. E837–E838, 2014.

[27] M. Broggi, V. Redaelli, G. Tringali et al., "Normal Pressure Hydrocephalus and Parkinsonism: Preliminary Data on Neurosurgical and Neurological Treatment," *World Neurosurgery*, vol. 90, pp. 348–356, 2016.

[28] T. Pringsheim, N. Jette, A. Frolkis, and T. D. L. Steeves, "The prevalence of Parkinson's disease: a systematic review and meta-analysis," *Movement Disorders*, vol. 29, no. 13, pp. 1583–1590, 2014.

[29] A. Fasano, M. Plotnik, F. Bove, and A. Berardelli, "The neurobiology of falls," *Neurological Sciences*, vol. 33, no. 6, pp. 1215–1223, 2012.

[30] J. Jankovic, "Gait Disorders," *Neurologic Clinics*, vol. 33, no. 1, pp. 249–268, 2015.

[31] N. Giladi and A. Nieuwboer, "Understanding and treating freezing of gait in Parkinsonism, proposed working definition, and setting the stage," *Movement Disorders*, vol. 23, no. 2, pp. S423–S425, 2008.

[32] J. K. Krauss, J. P. Regel, D. W. Droste, M. Orszagh, J. J. Borremans, and W. Vach, "Movement disorders in adult hydrocephalus," *Movement Disorders*, vol. 12, no. 1, pp. 53–60, 1997.

[33] M. Picascia, B. Minafra, R. Zangaglia et al., "Spectrum of cognitive disorders in idiopathic normal pressure hydrocephalus," *Functional Neurology*, vol. 31, no. 3, pp. 143–147, 2016.

[34] A. J. Espay, G. A. Da Prat, A. K. Dwivedi et al., "Deconstructing normal pressure hydrocephalus: Ventriculomegaly as early sign of neurodegeneration," *Annals of Neurology*, vol. 82, no. 4, pp. 503–513, 2017.

Acute, Nontraumatic Spontaneous Spinal Subdural Hematoma: A Case Report and Systematic Review of the Literature

Leigh A. Rettenmaier,[1] Marshall T. Holland,[2] and Taylor J. Abel[2]

[1] University of Iowa Carver College of Medicine, 375 Newton Rd, Iowa City, IA 52242, USA
[2] Department of Neurosurgery, University of Iowa, 200 Hawkins Drive, Iowa City, IA 52245, USA

Correspondence should be addressed to Marshall T. Holland; marshall-holland@uiowa.edu

Academic Editor: Shahid Nimjee

Spontaneous spinal subdural hematoma (sSDH) is a rare condition outright. Moreover, cases that occur spontaneously in the absence of an identifiable etiology are considerably less common and remain poorly understood. Here, we present the case of a 43-year-old man with spontaneous sSDH presenting with acute onset low back pain and paraplegia. Urgent magnetic resonance imaging identified a dorsal SDH from T8 to T11 with compression of the spinal cord. Emergent T8–T10 laminectomies with intradural exploration and hematoma evacuation were performed. However, despite prompt identification and appropriate action, the patient's recovery was modest and significant disability remained at discharge. This unique and unusual case demonstrates that spontaneous sSDH requires prompt surgical treatment to minimize associated morbidity and supports the association between the presence of severe neurological deficits upon initial presentation with less favorable outcomes. We performed a comprehensive systematic review of spontaneous sSDH of unknown etiology, which demonstrates that emergent surgical intervention is indicated for patients presenting with severe neurological deficits and the presence of these deficits is predictive of poor neurological outcome. Furthermore, conservative management should be considered in patients presenting with mild neurological deficits as spontaneous resolution followed by favorable neurological outcomes is often observed in these patients.

1. Introduction

Although spontaneous spinal subdural hematoma (sSDH) is a rare condition, it is associated with significant morbidity and mortality [1]. Exceedingly less common are spontaneous sSDHs occurring in the absence of an identifiable etiology. A nearly equivalent incidence between males and females has been described, but given the rarity of spontaneous sSDH the exact incidence remains unknown [2]. While spontaneous sSDHs are most frequently described in association with coagulopathies, iatrogenic causes, or arteriovenous malformations [1], the pathogenesis of spontaneous sSDH largely remains unclear. Rupture of the vasculature within the subarachnoid or subdural space has been proposed as a potential pathogenic mechanism in certain cases. While some suggest that the bleeding originates from subarachnoid vessels with concomitant rupture into the subdural space following an increase in intra-abdominal or intrathoracic pressure, others have proposed an alternative theory that the bleeding begins in the subdural space itself [3, 4]. Clinical presentation is typified by symptoms representative of spinal cord injury: motor, sensory, and autonomic dysfunction resulting from spinal cord compression [1]. Options for treatment include surgical decompression, percutaneous drainage, or management with conservative therapies alone. In this report, we present the case of a spontaneous sSDH presenting as acute onset lower back pain with paraplegia with no identifiable cause. Given the rarity of this condition, we review the available literature describing spontaneous idiopathic sSDH to elucidate the epidemiology, presentation, pathogenesis, diagnosis, treatment, and outcome of this rare condition.

2. Case Report

2.1. Presentation. A 43-year-old man presented to the emergency department with acute onset paraplegia and lower back

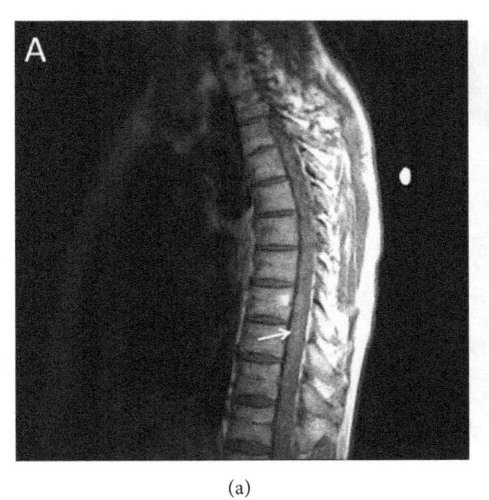

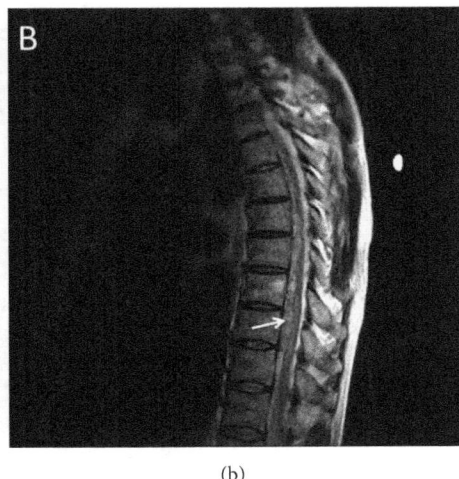

FIGURE 1: Preoperative MRI sagittal views T1 (a) and T2 (b) of the thoracic spine. White arrow indicates subdural hematoma.

pain that began in the absence of trauma. The patient reported feeling occasional paresthesia in his legs the preceding 2 months; however, the patient had not sought medical evaluation. The night prior to presentation, the patient reported moving quickly to avoid a bar fight that he was not involved in. Following this, he was able to proceed home without any noted difficulty. The following morning, the patient was able to walk, sit, and stand from the sitting position. However, after resting for a period of time, the patient experienced acute onset of unprovoked back pain and noted an inability to move his legs. This prompted emergent medical evaluation.

On examination, the patient was found to have grade 5/5 strength in his bilateral upper extremities and grade 0/5 strength throughout his bilateral lower extremities. He noted normal sensation in his upper extremities and slight decreased sensation in his lower extremities symmetrically. The patient had a postvoid residual of 1,500 cc. He had no history of recent surgical procedures and was not currently taking any prescription or over-the-counter medications.

Initial laboratory data revealed an elevated erythrocyte sedimentation rate of 68 (0–15), elevated C-reactive protein of 3 mg/dL (≤0.5), elevated WBC count of 17,300/μL (3.7–10.5), platelet count of 285,000/μL, partial thromboplastin time of 23 seconds (22–31), prothrombin time of 11 seconds (9–12), and an international normalized ratio of 1.1 (<4.0). Urine drug test was positive for amphetamines, benzodiazepine, and oxycodone.

Magnetic resonance imaging (MRI) with and without contrast of the spine was performed. T1- and T2-weighted images revealed an intradural, extramedullary heterogeneous subdural T2 signal and isointense T1 signal located ventral to the spinal cord spanning T8 to T11 causing displacement and compression of the thecal sac consistent with hyperacute or acute subdural hematoma. High T2 signal within the spinal cord at levels T10–T12 demonstrated the presence of spinal cord edema. (See Figure 1). Magnetic resonance angiography (MRA) of the thoracic spine revealed no evidence of arteriovenous malformation or arteriovenous fistula.

2.2. Operation. The patient was taken to the operating room emergently for T8–T10 laminectomies, with intradural exploration, and hematoma evacuation. Intraoperatively, a hematoma was visualized upon opening of the thecal sac and the hematoma was evacuated with gentle suction. Following evacuation, the spinal cord was visibly contused and swollen. Otherwise, inspection of the intradural space did not reveal any apparent abnormalities. Specifically, no evidence of abnormal vasculature or masses was observed. Hematoma fragments were collected and sent for histopathologic evaluation.

2.3. Postoperative Course and Histopathology. Postoperatively, the patient's initial strength was stable exhibiting grade 0/5 strength in bilateral lower extremities and grade 5/5 strength in bilateral upper extremities. Sensation was unchanged compared to preoperative evaluation. One-week following surgery, the patient's strength showed signs of improvement with grade 3/5 strength in right toe flexion. The patient's recovery was complicated by severe sepsis secondary to *Clostridium difficile* colitis. The patient was discharged on hospital day 25 to an acute rehabilitation facility. At discharge, the patient's examination remained unchanged with grade 3/5 strength in right toe flexion and otherwise 0/5 in all other lower extremity muscle groups and slightly diminished sensation in the bilateral lower extremities. Pathological samples taken at the time of surgery demonstrated acute hematoma with fragments of leptomeninges and meningothelial cells. There was no evidence of a vascular or neoplastic lesion.

Eight weeks following surgery, the patient continued to reside at an inpatient rehabilitation facility. His rehabilitation was complicated by development of a sacral wound requiring incision and drainage and placement of a wound vac. His lower extremity strength improved to consistent grade 2/5 throughout with reported rare ability to move his leg against gravity. His sensation remained stable with decreased (but present) sensation in the bilateral lower extremities. He had no bowel or bladder control using suppositories and self-catheterization techniques.

```
┌─────────────────────────────────┐
│ Databases (MEDLINE and Embase)  │
│ searched for "spinal," "subdural,"│
│ "hematoma," "spontaneous," and "acute" in│
│ various combination with Boolean operators│
│ "AND" and "OR" or as MESH terms │
└─────────────────────────────────┘
         │
         │        ┌────────────────────────────────────────────┐
         │───────▶│ Articles excluded if                       │
         │        │  (1) spinal SDH was precipitated by trauma or an│
         │        │      iatrogenic cause                      │
         │        │  (2) a coagulopathy is present             │
         │        │  (3) a known vascular abnormality was identified│
         │        │  (4) the spinal SDH was chronic            │
         │        │  (5) the patient was currently on an anticoagulant│
         │        │  (6) not in English                        │
         │        └────────────────────────────────────────────┘
         ▼
┌─────────────────────────────────┐
│ Relevant articles screened by   │
│ reviewing abstracts or full texts│
└─────────────────────────────────┘
         ▼
┌─────────────────────────────────┐
│ 38 papers (42 cases) selected   │
└─────────────────────────────────┘
```

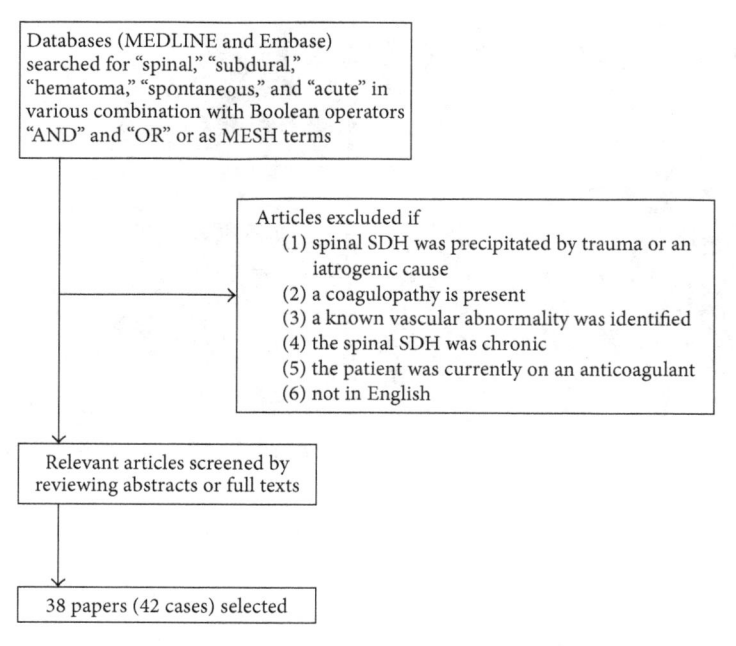

FIGURE 2: Flow chart detailing search strategy for review of literature.

2.4. Review of the Literature. A review of the English literature was conducted by searching Medline and Embase through November 2016. The terms "spinal subdural hematoma", "spontaneous spinal subdural hematoma" and "acute spinal subdural hematoma" were used. In a search of Medline, the MESH term "spinal subdural hematoma" returned 108 articles, "spontaneous" and "spinal subdural hematoma" yielded 28 articles, and "acute" and "spinal subdural hematoma" produced 25 articles. In a search of Embase, the terms "spinal hematoma", "spontaneous," and "subdural" generated 54 articles. The searches provided 215 papers, which were subsequently reviewed. Papers were excluded if the onset of the sSDH was precipitated by trauma or an iatrogenic cause, if a coagulopathy was present, if a known vascular abnormality was identified, if the sSDH was chronic, or if the patient was currently on an anticoagulant medication. After applying these restrictions, 38 papers were selected and 42 cases were included in the review of the literature (Table 1). Cases were indexed by patient age, gender, presenting symptoms, spinal level, additional medical conditions, treatment/surgical intervention, and patient outcome. Methods for the selection of articles are summarized in Figure 2.

3. Results

Forty-three patients with acute spontaneous sSDHs were identified in the review of the literature including the present case. Of the 43 patients, 18 were female, 24 were male, and 1 was unspecified. Patient age ranged from 27 years to 81 years with an average of 53.3 ($\pm$14) years. The predominant location of sSDHs was the thoracic spine. Of the 43 patients, 84% (36/43) demonstrated sSDHs spanning the thoracic spine, 23% (10/43) had cervical spine involvement, and 26% (11/43) demonstrated lumbosacral involvement. The location of the sSDH was limited to the cervical spine in only 2 of 43 patients, but 8 additional patients with cervical involvement had extension to the thoracic and/or lumbar regions. The extent of the sSDH ranged from a single level to up to 23 vertebral levels [22]. In 40% (17/43) of cases, the sSDH was limited to 4 or less levels, while 49% (21/43) involved 5 or more levels, and 11% (5/43) were unspecified.

In the review of the literature, back pain or interscapular pain was the most common presenting symptom with 63% (27/43) of patients reporting this as their initial symptom. Neck pain or stiffness was reported in 15% of patients (6/41), while headache was reported in 24% (10/41). Although cases with major bleeding risk factors, such as coagulopathy, were excluded from this study, several patients had additional underlying medical conditions (see Table 1). Of note, hypertension was most commonly encountered, being present in 16% (7/43) of patients identified in this review. Concurrent subarachnoid hemorrhage was described in 4 patients, while concurrent intracranial SDH was reported in 3 patients.

In most cases prior to 1991, myelography was the predominant diagnostic modality for sSDHs, whereas MRI was used in every subsequent case. Spinal angiography was performed in 21 of 43 cases in attempt to identify the source of bleeding. Given our inclusion criteria, no underlying vascular abnormalities were identified in any of the cases. Of the 43 patients, 20 patients (47%) underwent surgical decompression, 22 patients (51%) were managed with conservative therapies only, and 1 patient underwent lumbar puncture with percutaneous drainage of the sSDH. Of those patients managed with conservative therapies only, 86% (19/22) were reported to have either complete or good recovery, while the remaining 14% (3/22) experienced partial recovery. There were no reported cases of poor recovery with conservative therapy. Surgical intervention was employed in the treatment

TABLE 1: Summary of results from the literature review: Cases of spontaneous spinal subdural hematoma.

	Author and year	Age, years	Sex	Location	Presenting symptoms	Potential RFs	SAH	Treatment	Outcome
(1)	Ainslie, 1958 [5]	67	F	T8–T10	Back pain, paraparesis, bladder dysfunction	No	Yes	Laminectomy T8–T10	Complete recovery
(2)	Schaake and Schafer, 1970 [6]	74	M	NP	NP	NP	No	Surgery	Poor recovery
(3)	Anagnostopoulos and Gortvai, 1972 [7]	63	F	T8–T12	Back, arm, & abdominal pain, paraparesis, bladder dysfunction	No	No	Laminectomy T8–T12	Partial recovery
(4)	Reynolds and Turner, 1978 [8]	57	M	C4–C8	HA, hip pain, paraplegia, hypoesthesia, bowel dysfunction	No	No	Laminectomy C3–T1	Initial improvement then death (cardiopulmonary arrest)
(5)	Sakata and Kurihara, 1984 [9]	56	M	L2–S1	Back pain, paraparesis	Possible RA	No	Laminectomy L2–S1	Complete recovery
(6)	Swann et al., 1984 [10]	46	F	Thoraco-lumbar junction	HA, back pain w/ radiation to BLE, paraparesis	No	No	Percutaneous drainage	Complete recovery
(7)	Martinez et al., 1987 [11]	64	M	T5–T6	Paraparesis, hypoesthesia of BLE	No	No	Laminectomy T5–T6	Partial recovery
(8)	Mavroudakis et al., 1990 [12]	38	M	T1–T2	Interscapular pain w/ radiation to arm/nipple, paresthesia, HA, vomiting	No	Yes	Conservative	Complete recovery
(9)	Jacquet et al., 1991 [13]	51	M	T6–T8	Back pain, HA, fever, vomiting, slight opisthotonus	No	Yes	Laminectomy T5–T7	Complete recovery

TABLE 1: Continued.

	Author and year	Age, years	Sex	Location	Presenting symptoms	Potential RFs	SAH	Treatment	Outcome
(10)	Longatti et al., 1994 [14]	54	M	T5-L5	Back pain w/radiation to BLE & interscapular area, paraparesis, bladder dysfunction	HTN	No	Conservative	Complete recovery
(11)	Kang et al., 2000 [15, 16]	49	F	T5-L3	Back pain, paraparesis	No	No	Conservative	Complete recovery
(12)	Kuker et al., 2000 [16]	81	M	Mid T spine	Back pain, paraparesis bladder dysfunction	No	No	Surgery	Complete recovery
(13)	Kuker et al., 2000 [16]	56	F	Thoracolumbar	Paraparesis, bladder dysfunction	No	No	Surgery	Good recovery
(14)	Kirsch et al., 2000 [17]	42	M	Craniocervical junction	Paraplegia, bladder dysfunction	Suicide attempt with natural gas	No	Laminectomy T2–T5	No recovery
(15)	Kirsch et al., 2000 [17]	34	M	T1-T4	Midscapular pain, BLE paresthesia	No	No	Conservative	Complete recovery
(16)	Boukobza et al., 2001 [18]	74	M	T6-L4	Back pain, mild motor deficit in R LE	HTN	No	Conservative	Complete recovery
(17)	Maeda et al., 2001 [19]	29	F	T1-T4	HA, nausea, neck pain, paraplegia	No	No	Conservative	Partial recovery
(18)	Yamada et al., 2003 [20]	38	F	T1-T7	Interscapular pain, dysesthesia in BLE, bladder dysfunction, motor deficits in BLE	Postpartum, HTN	No	Conservative	Complete recovery

TABLE 1: Continued.

	Author and year	Age, years	Sex	Location	Presenting symptoms	Potential RFs	SAH	Treatment	Outcome
(19)	Thiex et al., 2005 [21]	78	M	T4–T11	Paraplegia, bladder dysfunction	No	No	R-sided hemilaminectomy; T5–T11	Death (due to another cause/not SDH)
(20)	Braun et al., 2007 [22]	76	F	Cervicothoracic	Back pain w/radiation to arms	No	No	Conservative	Complete recovery
(21)	Braun et al., 2007 [22]	72	F	Cervical t0 lumbar	Neck, pain, tetraparesis	No	No	Conservative	Complete recovery
(22)	Kyriakides et al., 2007 [23]	44	M	T2–T6	Back pain, paraplegia, bladder/bowel dysfunction	No	Yes	Laminectomy	Partial recovery
(23)	Kim et al., 2008 [24]	48	F	T1–T4	Paraplegia, bladder dysfunction	Fibromuscular dysplasia	No	Laminectomy T1–T4	No recovery
(24)	Montano et al., 2008 [25]	54	F	T6–T8	Back pain, bladder/bowel dysfunction, paraesthesia, hypoesthesia	Polycystic kidney disease	No	Surgery	Complete recovery
(25)	Ozdemir et al., 2008 [26]	50	M	T4–T8	Interscapular pain, paraparesis, hypoesthesia	No	No	Laminectomy T4–T6	Complete recovery
(26)	Al et al., 2009 [27]	57	M		HA, back pain, paraplegia, bladder/bowel dysfunction	No	No	Conservative	Complete recovery
(27)	Oh et al., 2009 [28]	59	F	C3–C6	Neck pain, L-sided hemiparesis	HTN, hyperlipidemia	No	Conservative	Complete recovery

TABLE 1: Continued.

	Author and year	Age, years	Sex	Location	Presenting symptoms	Potential RFs	SAH	Treatment	Outcome
(28)	Yang et al., 2009 [29]	35	F	L3-S1	HA, back pain, paraparesis	Concurrent intracranial SDH	No	Laminectomy	Complete recovery
(29)	Kakitsubata et al., 2010 [3]	66	M	T11-T12	HA, back pain, L LE pain	No	Yes	Conservative	Complete recovery
(30)	Nardone et al., 2010 [30]	37	M	C4-T4	HA, neck stiffness, cervical radicular pain, paraparesis, hypoesthesia	No	No	Conservative	Complete recovery
(31)	Liu et al., 2010 [31]	41	M	Mid T spine	Back pain, paraparesis, bladder dysfunction	Rhabdomyolysis, amphetamine abuse	No	Laminectomy T10-L1	Complete recovery
(32)	Nagashima et al., 2010 [32]	66	M	L1-S1	Leg pain, paraparesis, hypoesthesia, bowel dysfunction	Concurrent intracranial SDH, RA, HTN	No	Conservative	Complete recovery
(33)	Chung et al., 2011 [33]	45	F	T5-T11	Back pain, paraparesis, bladder dysfunction	HTN, DM	No	Conservative	Good recovery
(34)	Song et al., 2011 [34]	57	M	C1-T3	Neck & shoulder pain, paraparesis	Chronic renal failure, HTN	No	Conservative	Complete recovery
(35)	Yang et al., 2011 [35]	55	F	C2-T6	Paraplegia, hypoesthesia	HTN, DM	No	Conservative	Good recovery
(36)	Yang et al., 2011 [35]	38	M	C6-T5	HA, back pain, cold sweating, dizziness, vertigo, chest pain, hypoesthesia	No	No	Conservative	Good recovery

TABLE 1: Continued.

	Author and year	Age, years	Sex	Location	Presenting symptoms	Potential RFs	SAH	Treatment	Outcome
(37)	Cave and Sharobeem, 2013 [36]	65	M	T12	Back pain, paraplegia	No	No	Conservative	Partial recovery
(38)	Chung et al., 2014 [37]	66	F	C7–T4	HA, neck stiffness	No	No	Conservative	Complete recovery
(39)	Lin and Layman, 2014 [38]	70	M	L4–S1	Back pain, BLE weakness	HTN, hyperlipidemia, cancer, concurrent intracranial SDH	No	Conservative	Partial recovery
(40)	Oh and Eun, 2015 [39]	27	M	T5–T9	Back pain, paraparesis, hypoesthesia, bowel dysfunction, erectile dysfunction	No	No	Conservative	Good recovery
(41)	Visocchi et al., 2015 [40]	45	F	T1–T10	Back pain, paraplegia, anesthesia, bladder & bowel dysfunction	HIV+, HCV+, history of drug abuse	No	Laminectomy T1–T10	Partial recovery
(42)	Zhu et al., 2015 [41]	45	F	T9	Paraplegia, hypoesthesia	No	No	Laminectomy T8–T10	Partial recovery
(43)	Current case, 2017	43	M	T8–T11	Back pain, paraplegia	Drug abuse	No	Laminectomy T8–T10	Poor recovery

BLE: bilateral lower extremity; NP: data not provided; RA: rheumatoid arthritis; HTN: hypertension: L: left; DM: diabetes mellitus; SDH: subdural hematoma.

of 20 patients: 45% (9/20) experienced complete or good recovery, 25% (5/20) experienced partial recovery, 20% (4/20) experienced poor or no recovery, and there were 2 patient deaths (1 death was attributed to an unrelated factor). Of the 43 patients, 12 either presented with complete paraplegia or progressed to complete paraplegia shortly after presentation. Of these 12 patients, 8 underwent surgical intervention while the remaining 4 were managed conservatively. Outcomes for patients who underwent surgical decompression included partial recovery (3/8), poor or no recovery (3/8), or death (2/8), although 1 death was attributed to an unrelated factor. Patients presenting with complete paraplegia who were managed conservatively experienced complete or good recovery (50%; 2/4) or partial recovery (50%; 2/4).

4. Discussion

4.1. Epidemiology. Few publications exist addressing the exact prevalence of spontaneous sSDH; however, it appears to be quite rare. Domenicucci et al. presented a series of 106 cases of nontraumatic acute sSDH; this series reported near equal distribution of males and females with rates of 49% and 51%, respectively [2]. The average age in this series was 47.5 years (rang: 0.5–87 years). Similarly, Pereira et al. described a slight female predominance (1.25 female/1.0 male) in a series of 151 patients with nontraumatic spontaneous acute sSDH [1].

Spontaneous sSDH is most often associated with disorders related to impaired hemostatic mechanisms or following minor injury from iatrogenic causes. In a review of 151 patients with nontraumatic spontaneous acute sSDH, 46% of patients were either treated with anticoagulation therapy or harbored a coagulopathy attributable to a hematologic disorder [1]. In a separate review of 106 cases of nontraumatic acute sSDH, a large proportion of the cases were associated with either bleeding disorders or purely iatrogenic causes, representing 54% and 14% of the cases, respectively [2]. Bleeding disorders were mainly noted as those that impair the hemostatic mechanism including leukemia, hemophilia, thrombocytopenia, cryoglobulinemia, hemorrhagic diathesis, and polycythemia. Although less common, cases of spontaneous sSDH have been reported in the following conditions: ankylosing spondylitis [17, 42], systemic lupus erythematosus [43], fibromuscular dysplasia [24], cystic fibrosis [44], polycystic kidney disease [25], chronic renal failure [34], rhabdomyolysis [31], rheumatoid arthritis [32], pregnancy [45], and eclampsia [46]. Although an underlying coagulopathy, anticoagulant therapy, or an iatrogenic cause can be implicated in most cases of spontaneous sSDH, a significant proportion of patients have no readily identifiable cause; thus further investigation of these cases is warranted.

4.2. Presentation. Spontaneous sSDH often presents as acute severe back pain with radicular signs. It is frequently accompanied by sensory, motor, and autonomic dysfunction including erectile dysfunction and urinary retention [1, 14, 20, 39]. Domenicucci et al. reported the most common presenting symptoms to be motor deficits (57% of patients), spinal pain (45% of patients), radicular pain (22% of patients), and paresthesia [2]. Patients may also complain of headache and sphincter dysfunction. The severity of these deficits varies greatly from the presence of only pain without motor or sensory deficits to those of complete quadriplegia [2, 3]. Less common presentations include symptoms of central cord syndrome [12], hemiparesis [28], and initially only headache with neck stiffness [30, 37]. The present case represents a more severe instance with complete paraplegia on initial presentation. What typifies this pathology from an otherwise less worrisome diagnosis is an acute neurological change in the setting of no readily identifiable cause.

4.3. Pathogenesis. The pathogenesis of sSDHs is unclear as the bridging veins often implicated in the development of intracranial SDHs are not abundant within the spinal canal [47]. Some have suggested the bleeding in sSDHs results from rupture of vessels within the subarachnoid space following a rapid increase in intrathoracic or intra-abdominal pressure [4]. Any bleeding that originates from the vascular subarachnoid space would be subject to dilution by cerebrospinal fluid, thus preventing hematoma formation within the subarachnoid space. If bleeding within the subarachnoid space becomes sufficiently profuse, it may rupture into the subdural space [48]. Consistent with these propositions, cases in which spinal subarachnoid hemorrhage and SDHs coexist have been reported [3, 12, 23]. Alternatively, rupture of small extra-arachnoid vessels lying along the dural surface may be the source of bleeding in sSDHs [3]. Ultimately, it is difficult to determine whether the source of bleeding originates from within the subarachnoid or subdural space.

Although our patient denied intravenous drug use, a history of drug abuse cannot be excluded, especially considering the positive urine drug test for amphetamines. Two cases of spontaneous sSDH in association with amphetamines have previously been reported [31, 40]. Amphetamine use has been associated with both intracranial hemorrhage and cerebral vasculitis [49]. Although a direct causal link cannot be made, amphetamine use may have contributed to the development of sSDH in the present case considering the absence of other definitive contributing factors and the suggested mechanisms relating amphetamine use to vascular pathologies.

4.4. Diagnosis. MRI is considered the gold standard in the evaluation of sSDHs as it is capable of visualizing spinal hematomas as well as other spinal cord pathologies. The appearance of the sSDH on MR imaging is dependent on its duration and oxygenation and has been previously described [22]. Prior literature has shown that contrast-enhanced time-resolved MR angiography was 88% sensitive, 90% specific and had a positive predictive value of 88%, and negative predictive value of 90% for detection of spinal dural arterial venous fistulas [50]. Digital subtraction spinal angiography is considered the gold standard for identifying vascular abnormalities and is frequently used in evaluation of the bleeding source [40]. However, Braun et al. suggest performing spinal angiography when clinical suspicion of vascular malformation exists based on MRI findings [22]. In the present case, MRA demonstrated no vascular malformations; the patient had a poor and declining neurological examination requiring emergent surgical intervention, and no evidence of a malformation was noted intraoperatively. Given all these factors, clinical observation rather than a follow-up spinal digital subtraction angiograph was elected.

4.5. Treatment and Outcomes. Three treatment options exist in the management of sSDH: surgical evacuation, conservative medical management, and percutaneous drainage. If only mild deficits are present, conservative management is reasonable. However, in the face of clinical deterioration or severe motor/sensory deficits, surgical evacuation is advised [23]. Percutaneous drainage may be considered in cases where the hematoma is located dorsally and there is absence of coagulopathy [10, 15]. The current patient underwent urgent surgical decompression in light of the severe neurological deficits on initial presentation. Results from the literature review reveal that a greater proportion of patients experience complete or good neurological recovery when managed with conservative therapies alone (86%) versus those who underwent surgical interventions (47%). However, patients presenting with severe neurological deficits are more likely to receive surgical interventions, therefore introducing bias in favor of conservative management. In patients presenting with severe neurological deficits, urgent surgical decompression is indicated. Although when only modest neurological deficits are present, conservative therapies may be considered over surgical intervention.

The mortality rates in patients with spontaneous nontraumatic sSDH has decreased in recent years and is currently reported to be 1.3%. However, the associated morbidity, including serious neurologic deficits, is substantially higher and is reported to be 28% [1]. Pereira et al. examined factors that predict outcome in patients with spontaneous nontraumatic sSDH. Neurologic status at presentation was the strongest predictor of good outcomes; only 34% of patients with preexisting neurologic deficits had favorable outcomes compared to 83% of patients devoid of neurologic deficits at initial presentation. In the present case, the patient initially presented with severe neurologic dysfunction. Despite urgent surgical decompression, the patient has experienced limited recovery and persistent paraparesis. Other factors identified as predictive of favorable outcome include absence of coagulopathy, lumbar puncture, or other associated diseases. This may suggest outcomes in idiopathic cases will be more favorable as, by definition, they lack coagulopathies and iatrogenic factors. While the presence of subarachnoid hemorrhage has been implicated in theories regarding the etiology of spontaneous sSDH, the presence of subarachnoid hemorrhage was not found to be associated with outcome. Surgery was also not found to be associated with a more favorable outcome; however, Pereira et al. note a potential bias as patients in better clinical condition are less likely to receive surgical interventions.

5. Conclusion

Although rare, spontaneous sSDH should be considered in patients presenting with progressive motor, sensory, and autonomic deficits in addition to other intraspinal hematomas and inflammatory lesions. Although more common in patients with coagulopathies or following iatrogenic causes, sSDH can occur in the absence of an obvious underlying cause. The present case is illustrative of the substantial morbidity associated with the condition despite rapid diagnosis and surgical intervention. Due to the significant morbidity associated with the spontaneous sSDH, special consideration should be given to this diagnosis in patients with suggestive symptoms. Furthermore, surgical intervention is recommended in patients presenting with severe neurological deficits, although presence of these deficits is predictive of less favorable outcome. Conservative management should be strongly considered in patients with minor deficits as a large proportion of patients treated in this manner achieve favorable neurological recovery.

References

[1] B. J. Pereira, A. N. de Almeida, V. M. Muio, J. G. de Oliveira, C. V. de Holanda, and N. C. Fonseca, "Predictors of Outcome in Nontraumatic Spontaneous Acute Spinal Subdural Hematoma: Case Report and Literature Review," *World Neurosurgery*, vol. 89, pp. 574–577.e7, 2016.

[2] M. Domenicucci, A. Ramieri, P. Ciappetta, and R. Delfini, "Nontraumatic acute spinal subdural hematoma: report of five cases and review of the literature," *Journal of Neurosurgery*, pp. 65–73, 1999.

[3] Y. Kakitsubata, S. J. Theodorou, D. J. Theodorou et al., "Spontaneous spinal subarachnoid hemorrhage associated with subdural hematoma at different spinal levels," *Emergency Radiology*, vol. 17, no. 1, pp. 69–72, 2010.

[4] J. P. Rader, "Chronic subdural hematoma of the spinal cord: report of a case," *The New England Journal of Medicine*, vol. 253, pp. 374–376, 1955.

[5] J. P. Ainslie, "Paraplegia due to spontaneous extradural or subdural haemorrhage," *British Journal of Surgery*, vol. 45, no. 193, pp. 565–567, 1958.

[6] T. Schaake and E. R. Schafer, "Spontaneous haemorrhage in the spinal canal.," *Journal of Neurology, Neurosurgery & Psychiatry*, vol. 33, no. 5, pp. 715-716, 1970.

[7] D. I. Anagnostopoulos and P. Gortvai, "Spontaneous Spinal Subdural Haematoma," *British Medical Journal*, vol. 1, no. 5791, p. 30, 1972.

[8] A. F. Reynolds and P. T. Turner, "Spinal subdural hematoma," *Rocky Mountain Medical Journal*, vol. 75, no. 4, pp. 199-200, 1978.

[9] T. Sakata and A. Kurihara, "Spontaneous spinal subdural hematoma. A case report," *The Spine Journal*, vol. 9, no. 3, pp. 324–326, 1984.

[10] K. W. Swann, C. K. Chung, and H. J. Kim, "Spontaneous spinal subdural hematoma with spontaneous resolution," *Spinal Cord*, vol. 38, no. 3, pp. 192–196, 1984.

[11] R. Martinez, J. Vaquero, and F. Gilsanz, "Spontaneous spinal subdural hematoma. Case report," *Journal of Neurosurgical Sciences*, vol. 31, no. 3, pp. 157-158, 1987.

[12] N. Mavroudakis, M. Levivier, and G. Rodesch, "Central cord syndrome due to a spontaneously regressive spinal subdural hematoma," *Neurology*, vol. 40, no. 8, pp. 1306-1308, 1990.

[13] G. Jacquet, J. Godard, M. Orabi, S. Sönmez, and R. Steimlé, "Spinal subdural hematoma," *Zentralblatt Fur Neurochirurgie*, vol. 52, no. 3, pp. 131-135, 1991.

[14] P. L. Longatti, P. Freschi, M. Moro, G. Trincia, and A. Carteri, "Spontaneous spinal subdural hematoma," *Journal of Neurosurgical Sciences*, vol. 38, no. 3, pp. 197-199, 1994.

[15] H.-S. Kang, C.-K. Chung, and H. J. Kim, "Spontaneous spinal subdural hematoma with spontaneous resolution," *Spinal Cord*, vol. 38, no. 3, pp. 192-196, 2000.

[16] W. Kuker, R. Thiex, S. Friese et al., "Spinal subdural and epidural haematomas: diagnostic and therapeutic aspects in acute and subacute cases," *Acta Neurochir (Wien)*, vol. 142, no. 7, pp. 777-785, 2000.

[17] E. C. Kirsch, M. S. Khangure, D. Holthouse, and W. McAuliffe, "Acute spontaneous spinal subdural haematoma: MRI features," *Neuroradiology*, vol. 42, no. 8, pp. 586-590, 2000.

[18] M. Boukobza, D. Haddar, M. Boissonet, and J. J. Merland, "Spinal subdural haematoma: a study of three cases," *Clinical Radiology*, vol. 56, pp. 475-480, 2001.

[19] M. Maeda, J. Mochida, E. Toh, K. Nishimura, and T. Nomura, "Nonsurgical treatment of an upper thoracic spinal subdural hemorrhage," *Spinal Cord*, vol. 39, no. 12, pp. 657-661, 2001.

[20] K. Yamada, T. Nakahara, K. Yamamato, T. Muranaka, and Y. Ushio, "Nontraumatic spinal subdural haematoma occurring in a postpartum period," *Acta Neurochir (Wien)*, vol. 145, no. 2, pp. 151-155, 2003.

[21] R. Thiex, A. Thron, J. M. Gilsbach, and V. Rohde, "Functional outcome after surgical treatment of spontaneous and nonspontaneous spinal subdural hematomas," *Journal of Neurosurgery: Spine*, vol. 3, no. 1, pp. 12-16, 2005.

[22] P. Braun, K. Kazmi, P. Nogués-Meléndez, F. Mas-Estellés, and F. Aparici-Robles, "MRI findings in spinal subdural and epidural hematomas," *European Journal of Radiology*, vol. 64, no. 1, pp. 119-125, 2007.

[23] A. E. Kyriakides, R. K. Lalam, and W. S. El Masry, "Acute spontaneous spinal subdural hematoma presenting as paraplegia: A rare case," *The Spine Journal*, vol. 32, no. 21, pp. E619-E622, 2007.

[24] S. D. Kim, J. O. Park, S. H. Kim, Y. H. Lee, D. J. Lim, and J. Y. Park, "Spontaneous thoracic spinal subdural hematoma associated with fibromuscular dysplasia," *Journal of Neurosurgery: Spine*, vol. 8, no. 5, pp. 478-481, 2008.

[25] N. Montano, C. G. Nucci, F. Doglietto et al., "Teaching NeuroImage: Spontaneous idiopathic spinal subdural hematoma," *Neurology*, vol. 71, no. 10, p. e27, 2008.

[26] O. Ozdemir, T. Calisaneller, E. Yildirim, H. Caner, and N. Altinors, "Acute spontaneous spinal subdural hematoma in a patient with bilateral incarcerated inguinal hernia," *Joint Bone Spine*, vol. 75, no. 3, pp. 345-347, 2008.

[27] B. Al, C. Yildirim, S. Zengin, S. Genc, I. Erkutlu, and A. Mete, "Acute spontaneous spinal subdural haematoma presenting as paraplegia and complete recovery with non-operative treatment," *BMJ Case Reports*, 2009.

[28] S. H. Oh, I. Han, Y. Koo, and O. Kim, "Acute Spinal Subdural Hematoma Presenting with Spontaneously Resolving Hemiplegia," *Journal of Korean Neurosurgical Society*, vol. 45, no. 6, p. 390, 2009.

[29] M. S. Yang, Y. W. Tung, T. H. Yang et al., "Spontaneous spinal and intracranial subdural hematoma," *Journal of the Formosan Medical Association*, vol. 108, no. 3, pp. 258-261, 2009.

[30] R. Nardone, A. Kunz, J. Kraus et al., "Spontaneous subdural spinal haematoma presenting as occipital headache: a case report," *Acta Neurologica Belgica*, vol. 110, no. 3, pp. 268-269, 2010.

[31] C. Liu, C. Cheng, and D. Cho, "Rhabdomyolysis Accompanied by Spontaneous Spinal Subdural and Subarachnoid Hematoma Related to Amphetamine Abuse," *The Spine Journal*, vol. 35, no. 2, pp. E71-E73, 2010.

[32] H. Nagashima, A. Tanida, I. Hayashi et al., "Spinal subdural haematoma concurrent with cranial subdural haematoma: Report of two cases and review of literature," *British Journal of Neurosurgery*, vol. 24, no. 5, pp. 537-541, 2010.

[33] T. T. Chung, H. Cheng-Ta, L. Ming-Ying, and J. Da-Tong, "Spontaneous spinal subdural hematoma: A rare case report and review of the literature," *Journal of Medical Sciences*, vol. 31, no. 4, pp. 181-183, 2011.

[34] T. J. Song, Lee J. B., Choi Y. C., Lee K. Y., and Kim W. J., "Treatment of spontaneous cervical spinal subdural hematoma with methylprednisolone pulse therapy," *Yonsei Medical Journal*, vol. 52, no. 1, pp. 692-694, 2011.

[35] N.-R. Yang, S. J. Kim, Y. J. Cho, and D. S. Cho, "Spontaneous resolution of nontraumatic acute spinal subdural hematoma," *Journal of Korean Neurosurgical Society*, vol. 50, no. 3, pp. 268-270, 2011.

[36] J. J. Cave and K. M. Sharobeem, "A rare case of spontaneous spinal subdural haematoma that developed after using an electric drill," *Cerebrovascular Disease*, vol. 35, p. 349, 2013.

[37] J. Chung, I. S. Park, S. Hwang, and J. Han, "Acute Spontaneous Spinal Subdural Hematoma with Vague Symptoms," *Journal of Korean Neurosurgical Society*, vol. 56, no. 3, pp. 269-271, 2014.

[38] J. C. Lin and K. Layman, "Spontaneous spinal subdural hematoma of intracranial origin presenting as back pain," *Journal of Emergency Medicine*, vol. 47, no. 5, pp. 552-556, 2014.

[39] Y. M. Oh and J. P. Eun, "Idiopathic spontaneous spinal subdural hematoma causing transient paraparesis: Case report with a review of the literature," *Neurosurgery Quarterly*, vol. 25, no. 4, pp. 484-487, 2015.

[40] M. Visocchi, G. La Rocca, F. Signorelli, R. Roselli, Z. Jun, and A. Spallone, "10 Levels thoracic no-intrumented laminectomy for huge spontaneous spinal subdural hematoma removal. report of the first case and literature review," *International Journal of Surgery Case Reports*, pp. 57-62, 2015.

[41] Y. J. Zhu, D. Q. Peng, F. Shen, and L. L. Wang, "Spontaneous thoracic ventral spinal subdural hematoma mimicking a tumoral lesion: a case report," *Journal of Medical Case Reports*, vol. 9, no. 132, 2015.

[42] J. Sokoloff, M. N. Coel, and R. J. Ignelzi, "Spinal subdural hematoma," *Radiology*, vol. 120, no. 1, p. 116, 1976.

[43] K. Hirano, M. Tada, N. Sasahira et al., "Incidence of malignancies in patients with IgG4-related disease," *Internal Medicine*, vol. 53, no. 3, pp. 171-176, 2014.

[44] D. Zochodne, G. Hinton, R. Del Maestro et al., "Intradural spinal hematoma in an infant with cystic fibrosis," *Pediatric Neurology*, vol. 2, no. 5, pp. 311-313, 1986.

[45] S. Pujol and R. Torrielli, "Neurological accidents after epidural anesthesia in obstetrics," *Cahiers D'Anesthesiologie*, vol. 44, no. 4, pp. 341-345, 1996.

[46] T. T. Lao, S. H. Halpern, D. MacDonald, and C. Huh, "Spinal subdural haematoma in a parturient after attempted epidural anaesthesia," *Canadian Journal of Anesthesia*, vol. 40, no. 4, pp. 340-345, 1993.

[47] R. N. Edelson, N. L. Chernik, J. B. Posner et al., "Spinal Subdural Hematomas Complicating Lumbar Puncture," *JAMA Neurology*, vol. 31, no. 2, pp. 134–137, 1974.

[48] N. Russell and B. Benoit, "Spinal subdural hematoma a review," *World Neurosurgery*, vol. 20, no. 2, pp. 133–137, 1983.

[49] N. Buxton and N. S. McConachie, "Amphetamine abuse and intracranial haemorrhage," *Journal of the Royal Society of Medicine*, vol. 93, no. 9, pp. 472–477, 2016.

[50] A. M. Saindane, S. R. Boddu, F. C. Tong, S. Dehkharghani, and J. E. Dion, "Contrast-enhanced time-resolved mra for pre-angiographic evaluation of suspected spinal dural arterial venous fistulas," *Journal of NeuroInterventional Surgery*, vol. 7, no. 2, pp. 135–140, 2015.

Familial Hemiplegic Migraine with Severe Attacks: A New Report with *ATP1A2* Mutation

E. Martínez,[1] R. Moreno,[2] L. López-Mesonero,[1] I. Vidriales,[2] M. Ruiz,[1] A. L. Guerrero,[1] and J. J. Tellería[3]

[1]Neurology Department, Hospital Clínico Universitario, Valladolid, Spain
[2]Clinical Analysis Department, Hospital Clínico Universitario, Valladolid, Spain
[3]IBGM, University of Valladolid, Valladolid, Spain

Correspondence should be addressed to A. L. Guerrero; gueneurol@gmail.com

Academic Editor: Mathias Toft

Introduction. Familial hemiplegic migraine (FHM) is a rare disorder characterized by migraine attacks with motor weakness during the aura phase. Mutations in CACNA1A, ATP1A2, SCN1A, and PRRT2 genes have been described. *Methods.* To describe a mutation in ATP1A2 gene in a FHM case with especially severe and prolonged symptomatology. *Results.* 22-year-old woman was admitted due to migraine-type headache and sudden onset of right-sided weakness and aphasia; she had similar episodes in her childhood. Her mother was diagnosed with hemiplegic migraine without genetic confirmation. She presented with fever, decreased consciousness, left gaze preference, mixed aphasia, right facial palsy, right hemiplegia, and left crural paresis. Computed tomography (CT) showed no lesion and CT perfusion study evidenced oligohemia in left hemisphere. A normal brain magnetic resonance (MR) was obtained. Impaired consciousness and dysphasia began to improve three days after admission and mild dysphasia and right hemiparesis lasted for 10 days. No recurrences were reported during a follow-up of two years. We identified a variant in heterozygous state in ATP1A2 gene (p.Thr364Met), pathogenic according to different prediction algorithms (SIFT, PolyPhen2, MutationTaster, and Condel). *Conclusion.* Prolonged and severe attacks with diffuse hypoperfusion in a FHM seemed to be specially related to ATP1A2 mutations, and p.T364M should be considered.

1. Introduction

Familial hemiplegic migraine (FHM) is an uncommon type of migraine with aura including motor weakness with at least one first- or second-degree relative affected [1]. FHM is considered a monogenic disorder with autosomal dominant inheritance pattern. Though there may be other loci to be identified, FHM is subdivided into three types: FHM1 with mutations in *CACNA1A* gene on chromosome 19, FHM2 in *ATP1A2* gene on chromosome 1, and FHM3 in which mutations in *SCN1A* gene on chromosome 2 have been identified [1]. These genes are implicated not only in ion channel but also in other molecules as synaptosomal associated protein. Moreover, there are typical cases that do not have a mutation in one of the main genes described, suggesting that other genes are still to be identified [2].

The clinical spectrum of this disorder varies from moderate headache accompanied by motor weakness to coma, with description of cases associated with permanent ataxia, epileptic seizures, mental retardation, and chronic progressive cerebellar atrophy [2].

We describe a mutation in *ATP1A2* gene in a case of FHM with especially severe attacks.

2. Case Report

A 22-year-old Caucasian woman was admitted due to a clinical picture of right-sided weakness and aphasia accompanied by a migraine-type headache (throbbing pain on the left side, with nausea and photophobia) initiated when she woke up. She had previously suffered similar clinical episodes 7 years before and during her childhood. Her mother presented with

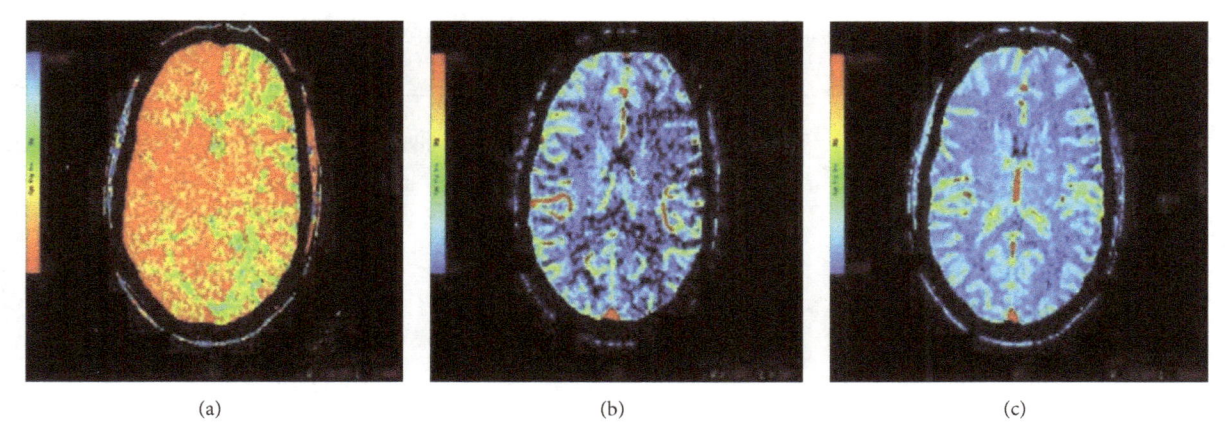

FIGURE 1: Perfusion computed tomography. TC revealed increased mean transit time (a) and diminished cerebral blood flow (b) with preserved cerebral volume (c). These changes were observed throughout the entire left cerebral hemisphere not confined to a particular vascular territory including the territory of anterior, middle, and posterior cerebral arteries (PCA).

multiple episodes of migraine with motor weakness. Our patient was adopted during early childhood and did not have a relationship with her family; so, a more accurate description on her mother's clinical picture was not available. She has no brothers or sisters.

In the anamnesis of possible triggers, she reported that, ten days before admission, she had suffered a mild head trauma during a traffic collision (she did not call for medical care for this reason). At admission, clinical exam showed a left gaze preference, predominantly nonfluent aphasia, and right facial palsy with right hemiplegia.

Urgent unenhanced CT was normal, but perfusion CT revealed increased mean transit time (MTT) and diminished cerebral blood flow (CBF) throughout the entire left cerebral hemisphere not confined to a particular vascular territory including the territory of anterior (ACA), middle (MCA), and posterior cerebral arteries (PCA) (Figure 1). Cerebral blood volume (CBV) was normal. Findings were consistent with hypoperfusion throughout all the left cerebral hemisphere. Cerebrovascular study was completed with an angiography TC and carotid ultrasound with no alterations. Transcranial Duplex revealed a generalized acceleration in both middle cerebral arteries with absence of arterial occlusion. A diffusion-weighted brain magnetic resonance imaging (DWB-MRI) was performed 3 days after clinical onset and it showed no restricted diffusion on the region of perfusion abnormality with normal signal intensity of the brain parenchyma.

On the second day, aphasia worsened, and somnolence and body temperature of 38° appeared. A lumbar puncture was performed without pleocytosis nor hyperproteinorrachia. Cerebrospinal fluid (CSF) microbiological studies and serum extensive biochemical, hematological, or immunological determinations were carried out with normal results. An electroencephalogram (EEG) recording showed diffuse delta activity.

The patient was empirically treated with acetylsalicylic acid and acyclovir during the first days. The clinical picture evolved favorably but in a slow way; fever and diminished level of consciousness disappeared on day 4, and motor deficit and dysphasia resolved, respectively, 6 and 8 days after onset. No recurrence of neurological symptoms was observed during a follow-up of 2 years.

As usual in our protocols for FHM studies, we carried out exome sequencing and subsequently analyzed the coding sequences of *SCN1A*, *CACNA1A*, *ATP1A2*, *NOTCH3*, and *PRRT2* genes in order to identify potential pathogenic mutations. DNA was extracted from peripheral blood according to standard protocols. DNA quality was determined by continuous reading of optical density with the Nanodrop equipment. Its integrity was checked by electrophoresis and SYBR Green II staining. After checking the quality, we proceeded to the capture and massive sequencing of human gene exons by using the SureSelect Human All Exon Kit 51 Mb (Agilent®) assay and Hiseq2000 (Illumina®) sequencer with a 30x mean coverage depth. The bioinformatic analysis allowed us to identify single nucleotide variants and small insertions and deletions relative to the reference genome [25]. Once obtained, the exonic sequences were aligned against the human genome reference, and we proceeded to the selective detection of all possible variants in candidate genes. Variants reported with frequencies over 1% in dbSNP, 1000 Genomes, and Exome Variant Server were excluded and the results were analyzed assuming a dominant model of inheritance according to the model expected for the disease and the indicated genes.

We identified a heterozygous variant within *ATP1A2* gene. This variant has not been reported in more than 6500 control individuals [26]. Sequence analysis revealed C>T transition (missense mutation) in position 160098515 of chromosome 1. This variation in *ATP1A2* gene produces Thr to Met amino acid substitution at position 364 of the coded protein (p.T364M).

The substituted amino acid is strongly conserved, since it is present in homologous proteins in all recorded mammals, reptiles, and fishes. Several in silico tests strongly suggest that Thr to Met substitution should strongly affect the *ATP1A2* function: PolyPhen shows a damaging score of 1.000

TABLE 1: Mutations described in *ATP1A2* gene related to FHM.

Mutation	Phenotypic characteristics
D718N [1]	Long-lasting hemiplegic migraine, seizures, and mental retardation
P979L [1]	Recurrent coma, seizures, mental retardation, and interictal mild cerebellar signs
R689Q [2]	Benign familial infantile convulsions
K794Q [2]	Spectrum between alternating hemiplegia of childhood (AHC) and FHM
A1033G, T345A [3]	Coma
E700K [2]	FHM
R593W and V628M [4]	FHM
M731T and T376M [5]	Pure FHM
A606T, N717K, R1002Q [6]	Severe hemiplegia
T415M [7]	Dysphasia and drowsiness and attacks triggered by mild head injury
V362E [8]	Mood alterations, classified as a borderline personality
P796S [8]	Mild mental impairment, in addition to hemiplegic migraine
D999H [8, 9]	Seizures
G900R [8]	Coma, high fever, and status epilepticus
G301R [10, 11]	FHM with interictal cerebellar symptoms
R548C [12]	Epilepsy
G855R [13]	Febrile seizures
G902L [14]	Fever, coma, and cortical edema in MR
V338A, Q927P [11]	Coma
G715R [15]	Aphasia, coma, and brain edema
R548H [16]	Hemiplegic migraine associated with basilar migraine
M731T [17]	Psychotic aura symptoms
p.T364M [18]	Prolonged hemiplegia, aphasia, somnolence, and fever in a child
R1007W [19]	Drowsiness with myoclonic seizures
S220L, R908Q [20]	Coma and aphasia
M731T [21]	Psychotic aura
R908Q [22]	FHM with prolonged aura
p.A348p [23]	Large family and severe and long-lasting attacks with coma and fever
c.G571A [24]	Neurosensorial hearing loss

and reports that Thr is always conserved in this position when compared with the homologous gene of 43 species; MutationTaster software test gives a probability of disease causing over 0.9999 and reports that this mutation has not been reported in 1000G or in ExAC databases; and, finally, SITF test gives a PROVEAN score of −5.166 (variants with scores under −2.5 are considered deleterious).

No further potential pathogenic mutations were found within *ATP1A2* or in the remaining candidate genes studied. The variant was validated by Sanger sequencing.

3. Discussion

FHM is a clinically heterogeneous disorder, with attacks varying from mild hemiparesis to severe long-lasting hemiplegia. Rare disturbances of consciousness (sometimes including coma), confusion, fever, and cerebrospinal fluid pleocytosis may occur [2].

There are more than 60 different missense mutations in *ATP1A2* gene. Other heterozygous mutations in *ATP1A2* gene have been reported in FHM patients [3–6, 9, 18]. We present a table with the mutations described in the literature from 2003 to 2016 and their main phenotypic characteristics (Table 1). Some of the mutations produce long-lasting attacks of hemiplegic migraine, but they are related to other neurological pathologies such as seizures and mental retardation [1], coma, and fever [23]. The case we present had no other neurological diseases apart from FHM.

To understand the relationship of the ATP1A2 gene with seizures, migraine, and coma, it is important to understand the pathophysiology of the mutations in ATP1A2 gene. This gene is on chromosome 1q23 and encodes α-2 subunit of Na^+/K^+ ATPase plasma membrane enzyme, which consumes ATP to actively transport Na^+ out of the cell and K^+ into the cell [9]. Na^+/K^+ ATPase protein is composed of three heteromeric subunits (α, β, and γ), and α is the catalytic one, which is composed of two subunits. The α-2 subunit is expressed in central nervous tissue, particularly astrocytes and pyramidal cells in the hippocampus. This α-2 subunit is composed of N-terminal region containing 4 membrane-spanning domains (M1–M4) and C-terminal region containing 6 membrane-spanning domains (M5–M10), which are linked by a large intracellular loop. This large M4-M5 loop contains critical functional sites and undergoes major conformational changes during the enzymatic cycle. Most of the *ATP1A2* gene mutations causing FHM2 are located within this loop [9]. In fact, the described mutation affects the M4-M5 loop. In silico software predicts severe conformational changes within this domain on the mutated protein. Moreover, Thr amino acid is highly conserved underlining its key role in this location of ATP1A2 protein. This variation in *ATP1A2* gene produces Thr to Met amino acid substitution at position 364 of the coded protein (p.T364M), leading to the dysfunction of the gene.

As Na^+/K^+ ATPase exchanges intracellular Na^+ for extracellular K^+, loss of Na^+/K^+ ATPase function results in raised extracellular K^+, which facilitates cortical spreading depression, the mechanism postulated to cause migraine aura. This ATPase dysfunction also results in raised intracellular Na^+, which will increase intracellular Ca^{2+} levels as a result of a decrease in Na^+/Ca^{2+} exchange. This raised intracellular Ca^{2+} also facilitates the cortical spreading depression [9] with the consequent hypoperfusion as we have shown in Figure 1. These biochemical alterations are capable of producing prolonged functional impairment but without causing lesion on neuroimaging (MRI).

The mutation present in our patient was previously described in an eight-year-old female who presented with prolonged attacks including hemiplegia, aphasia, lethargy, and fever [18]. As in our case, cerebrospinal fluid was unremarkable, and electroencephalogram showed diffuse slowing. Hypoperfusion was not shown in perfusion CT as in our patient.

4. Conclusion

In conclusion, prolonged and severe attacks with diffuse hypoperfusion in a FHM seemed to be specially related to *ATP1A2* mutations, and p.T364M mutation should be considered.

Competing Interests

The authors declare that they have no competing interests.

References

[1] Headache Classification Committee of the International Headache Society (IHS), "The International Classification of Headache Disorders, 3rd edition (beta version)," *Cephalalgia*, vol. 33, no. 9, pp. 629–808, 2013.

[2] M. J. M. Van Den Maagdenberg, G. M. Terwindt, J. Haan, R. R. Frants, and M. D. Ferrari, "Genetics of headaches," *Handbook of Clinical Neurology*, vol. 97, pp. 85–97, 2010.

[3] K. J. Swoboda, E. Kanavakis, A. Xaidara et al., "Alternating hemiplegia of childhood or familial hemiplegic migraine?: a novel *ATP1A2* mutation," *Annals of Neurology*, vol. 55, no. 6, pp. 884–887, 2004.

[4] M.-J. Castro, A. H. Stam, C. Lemos et al., "Recurrent *ATP1A2* mutations in Portuguese families with familial hemiplegic migraine," *Journal of Human Genetics*, vol. 52, no. 12, pp. 990–998, 2007.

[5] J. C. Jen, A. Klein, E. Boltshauser et al., "Prolonged hemiplegic episodes in children due to mutations in *ATP1A2*," *Journal of Neurology, Neurosurgery and Psychiatry*, vol. 78, no. 5, pp. 523–526, 2007.

[6] M.-J. Castro, B. Nunes, B. de Vries et al., "Two novel functional mutations in the Na^+,K^+-ATPase α2-subunit *ATP1A2* gene in patients with familial hemiplegic migraine and associated neurological phenotypes," *Clinical Genetics*, vol. 73, no. 1, pp. 37–43, 2008.

[7] K. R. J. Vanmolkot, A. H. Stam, A. Raman et al., "First case of compound heterozygosity in Na,K-ATPase gene ATP1A2 in familial hemiplegic migraine," *European Journal of Human Genetics*, vol. 15, no. 8, pp. 884–888, 2007.

[8] L. Deprez, S. Weckhuysen, K. Peeters et al., "Epilepsy as part of the phenotype associated with *ATP1A2* mutations," *Epilepsia*, vol. 49, no. 3, pp. 500–508, 2008.

[9] D. M. Fernandez, C. K. Hand, B. J. Sweeney, and N. A. Parfrey, "A novel *ATP1A2* gene mutation in an Irish familial hemiplegic migraine kindred," *Headache*, vol. 48, no. 1, pp. 101–108, 2008.

[10] M. Spadaro, S. Ursu, F. Lehmann-Horn et al., "A G301R Na+/K+-ATPase mutation causes familial hemiplegic migraine type 2 with cerebellar signs," *Neurogenetics*, vol. 5, no. 3, pp. 177–185, 2004.

[11] F. Riant, A. Ducros, C. Ploton, C. Barbance, C. Depienne, and E. Tournier-Lasserve, "De novo mutations in *ATP1A2* and *CACNA1A* are frequent in early-onset sporadic hemiplegic migraine," *Neurology*, vol. 75, no. 11, pp. 967–972, 2010.

[12] A. Lebas, L. Guyant-Maréchal, D. Hannequin, F. Riant, E. Tournier-Lasserve, and D. Parain, "Severe attacks of familial hemiplegic migraine, childhood epilepsy and *ATP1A2* mutation," *Cephalalgia*, vol. 28, no. 7, pp. 774–777, 2008.

[13] B. De Vries, A. H. Stam, M. Kirkpatrick et al., "Familial hemiplegic migraine is associated with febrile seizures in an FHM2 family with a novel de novo *ATP1A2* mutation," *Epilepsia*, vol. 50, no. 11, pp. 2503–2504, 2009.

[14] J. P. Dreier, K. Jurkat-Rott, G. G. Petzold et al., "Opening of the blood-brain barrier preceding cortical edema in a severe attack of FHM type II," *Neurology*, vol. 64, no. 12, pp. 2145–2147, 2005.

[15] S. De Sanctis, G. S. Grieco, L. Breda et al., "Prolonged sporadic hemiplegic migraine associated with a novel de novo missense *ATP1A2* gene mutation," *Headache*, vol. 51, no. 3, pp. 447–450, 2011.

[16] P. Bøttger, S. Glerup, B. Gesslein et al., "Glutamate-system defects behind psychiatric manifestations in a familial hemiplegic migraine type 2 disease-mutation mouse model," *Scientific Reports*, vol. 6, Article ID 22047, 2016.

[17] A. Ambrosini, M. D'Onofrio, G. S. Grieco et al., "Familial basilar migraine associated with a new mutation in the ATP1A2 gene," *Neurology*, vol. 65, no. 11, pp. 1826–1828, 2005.

[18] I. Toldo, D. Cecchin, S. Sartori et al., "Multimodal neuroimaging in a child with sporadic hemiplegic migraine: a contribution to understanding pathogenesis," *Cephalalgia*, vol. 31, no. 6, pp. 751–756, 2011.

[19] T. Pisano, S. Spiller, D. Mei et al., "Functional characterization of a novel C-terminal *ATP1A2* mutation causing hemiplegic migraine and epilepsy," *Cephalalgia*, vol. 33, no. 16, pp. 1302–1310, 2013.

[20] C. Roth, T. Freilinger, G. Kirovski et al., "Clinical spectrum in three families with familial hemiplegic migraine type 2 including a novel mutation in the *ATP1A2* gene," *Cephalalgia*, vol. 34, no. 3, pp. 183–190, 2014.

[21] J. Barros, A. Mendes, I. Matos, and J. Pereira-Monteiro, "Psychotic aura symptoms in familial hemiplegic migraine type 2 (ATP1A2)," *Journal of Headache and Pain*, vol. 13, no. 7, pp. 581–585, 2012.

[22] J. U. Blicher, A. Tietze, M. J. Donahue, S. A. Smith, and L. Ostergaard, "Perfusion and pH MRI in familial hemiplegic migraine with prolonged aura," *Cephalalgia*, vol. 36, no. 3, pp. 279–283, 2016.

[23] N. Pelzer, D. Blom, A. Stam et al., "Recurrent coma and fever in familial hemiplegic migraine type 2. A prospective 15-year follow-up of a large family with a novel *ATP1A2* mutation," *Cephalalgia*, 2016.

[24] S.-K. Oh, J.-I. Baek, K. M. Weigand et al., "A missense variant of the *ATP1A2* gene is associated with a novel phenotype of progressive sensorineural hearing loss associated with migraine," *European Journal of Human Genetics*, vol. 23, no. 5, pp. 639–645, 2015.

[25] "Human reference genome, 19th version (Genome Reference Consortium GRCh37)," https://genome.ucsc.edu/FAQ/FAQreleases.html.

[26] OMIM # 602481, http://omim.org/entry/602481.

Ketamine Infusion Used to Successfully Control Refractory Status Epilepticus in a Pregnant Patient

Murad Talahma [iD], Vivek Sabharwal, Yana Bukovskaya, and Fawad Khan

Department of Neurocritical Care, Ochsner Health System, New Orleans, LA, USA

Correspondence should be addressed to Murad Talahma; mmmtalahma@gmail.com

Academic Editor: Chin-Chang Huang

The management of SE during pregnancy is especially challenging to the treating physician. While antiepileptic medications might cause teratogenicity, SE can have significant morbidity and mortality on both the mother and the developing fetus. This case report demonstrated the successful use of ketamine infusion in the management of RSE in pregnancy without affecting the immediate outcome of pregnancy. The fetus survived this complicated ICU stay and outpatient follow-up was generally uncomplicated. The pregnancy was ended with a delivery of a normal female newborn.

1. Introduction

Worldwide, an estimated half million women of childbearing age have been diagnosed with epilepsy [1]. The management of seizures during pregnancy poses the challenge of striking a balance between the risks of complications from seizures in the mother and the possible teratogenic effects of antiepileptic drugs (AEDs) on the developing fetus. Ketamine is an N-methyl-D-aspartate (NMDA) receptor antagonist that has been used with increasing frequency in the management of refractory and super-refractory status epilepticus (SE); however, to our knowledge, its successful use in pregnancy has never been reported. We present a case in which ketamine was used to manage refractory SE in a pregnant patient without affecting the outcome of the pregnancy.

2. Case Report

The patient is a 37-year-old female with a history of epilepsy secondary to astrocytoma that had been surgically resected and followed with radiation and chemotherapy a year prior to the current presentation. Her seizure semiology ranged from focal seizures to generalized tonic-clonic seizures. Her outpatient AEDs included levetiracetam (LEV), valproic acid (VPA), and zonisamide (ZNS). Ten days prior to her presentation, she discovered that she was pregnant and decided to self-discontinue her VPA. She experienced a significant increase in her seizure frequency, for which she was admitted to our neurocritical care unit (NCCU). Initially her home doses of LEV and ZNS were increased from 1500 mg bid to 2000 mg bid and from 200 mg bid to 300 mg bid, respectively. The patient's blood levels of LEV and ZNS on admission were 23 ug/mL and 29 mcg/mL, respectively, which are within therapeutic ranges.

On day 2 of her hospitalization, she was started on daily prenatal vitamins in addition to 4 mg folic acid. Transvaginal ultrasound showed a single intrauterine pregnancy corresponding with a 6-week, 6-day gestation by crown rump length.

The patient continued to have intermittent seizures involving both sides of the face with associated confusion. She was placed on continuous electroencephalogram (EEG) monitoring that showed right hemisphere focal SE. Her seizures continued at a rate of multiple episodes per hour, and she failed to respond to a total of 10 mg of lorazepam administered in 2 mg doses; thus the decision was made to intubate and start anesthetic agents. Continuous propofol infusion was initiated without a bolus dose at a rate of 30 mcg/kg/min and titrated to 45 mcg/kg/min; however, further up titrations were not tolerated because of dose

Table 1: "The timeline of different antiepileptic medications during ICU stay".

Therapy in ICU [Day 1-Day 15]			
Anesthetics			
		Dose Range	Therapeutic Monitoring
Ketamine	Day 3-9	50 -150 mcg/kg/min	N/A
Propofol	Day 3-5	10-40 mcg/kg/min	N/A
Maintenance AEDs			
		Total Daily Dose	
Levetiracetam	Day 1-15	3000mg-9000mg	18.4-88.9 ug/mL
Lacosamide	Day 2-15	400 mg-500 mg	
Oxcarbazepine	Day 4-15	600 mg-800 mg	5-10 mcg/mL
Zonisamide	Day 7-15	600 mg	11-29 mcg/mL
Ancillary Therapy			
Pyridoxine	Day 3-15	50 mg	3 ug/L
Magnesium Sulfate Infusion	Day 3-7	Maintain serum Mg 3-3.5	3.1-3.8 mg/dL
IV Methylprednisolone	Day 4-6	1000 mg	N/A

related hypotension. She received a bolus of 80 mg ketamine intravenously (IV) and was started on a continuous ketamine infusion at a rate of 100 mcg/kg/min. Additionally, a continuous infusion of magnesium sulfate was initiated. Her EEG continued to show right focal SE presenting with both clinical and subclinical seizures; thus the ketamine infusion rate was increased to 150 mcg/kg/min. Nine hours after the initiation of ketamine, the seizures stopped both clinically and electrographically. Twenty-four hours later, propofol was discontinued. Twenty-four hours after propofol was stopped, the seizure suppression continued, so the ketamine infusion was gradually decreased to 75 mcg/kg/min while continuing her maintenance AED regimen, which included LEV 3000 mg q8h, ZNS 300 mg bid, oxcarbazepine 300 mg bid, and lacosamide 200 mg bid. On day 7 of ketamine, the infusion rate was decreased to 50 mcg/kg/min for 6 hours, then to 30 mcg/kg/min, and subsequently discontinued. The patient remained seizure-free both clinically and electrographically (Table 1).

She remained intubated for a total of 8 days and was successfully extubated. She remained on EEG monitoring for 3 additional days which showed no seizures. After 2 weeks in the NCCU, she was transitioned to a regular floor. On day 18 of her hospitalization, ZNS was discontinued. She remained in the hospital for an additional 5 days, experienced no clinical seizures, and was subsequently discharged home.

Multiple ultrasounds after discharge showed a normal fetus, appropriate to gestational age, and normal amniotic fluids. Fetal echocardiogram showed no evidence of cardiac anomalies. The patient was admitted for elective caesarean section at 37 weeks and 5 days' gestation and delivered a single viable female. The baby scored 9 on both the 1-minute and 5-minute Apgar scores. The patient and the newborn were discharged 4 days postoperatively in stable condition. At the most recent follow-up visit 38 weeks after the birth of the baby discharge she denied any further episodes of status epilepticus. She reported no cognitive deficits or mood changes. Her baby was brought to the clinic and was notably healthy while achieving all normal developmental milestones.

3. Discussion

The definition of SE has evolved over the years, starting with the initial definition in 1993 by the Epilepsy Foundation of America that required repetitive seizures for 30 minutes; however, the time was subsequently reduced to 20, then 10, and most recently 5 minutes [2]. When SE fails to respond to 2 AEDs, it is referred to as refractory SE. When seizure activity continues for 24 hours or more after initiation of anesthetic treatment, it is considered super-refractory SE [3]. An estimated 31%-43% of patients with SE will develop refractory SE [4] and 10%-15% will develop super-refractory SE [3]. Both refractory and super-refractory SE carry a significantly higher mortality and morbidity than SE, and their management poses a significant challenge, particularly given the absence of strong evidence or consensus in the literature to guide management.

The relationship between pregnancy and seizures is complicated, given the physiological changes of pregnancy on seizure control and AED requirements. Seizures are not only harmful to the mother, but hypoxia and acidosis resulting from convulsive seizures can have a harmful effect on the developing fetus as well. Although most women with epilepsy will be seizure-free during pregnancy, approximately one-third will have an increase in their seizure frequency [5], and the timing of the seizures is evenly distributed among trimesters [6]. The frequency of SE in pregnancy ranges from 0% to 1.3% compared to 1.6% in the general epilepsy population [1]. Compliance with AEDs might be a major factor in the control of seizures during pregnancy, but other factors such as hormonal changes, changes in protein binding that affect the volume of distribution of AEDs, and the change in renal clearance and intestinal absorption of AEDs may affect seizure control and management during pregnancy.

One of the primary factors in the development of both refractory and super-refractory SE is the unique changes in the neuroreceptors at the synapses and blood brain barrier. As seizures continue, the GABA A receptors move to the inner side of the membrane, while the NMDA receptors move in the opposite direction [2]. These changes explain the development of pharmacoresistance to the AEDs, such as benzodiazepines and propofol, that work on GABA receptors as the seizure activity continues. The finding that NMDA receptors are upregulated during SE increased interest in using agents such as ketamine that block NMDA receptors. The neurocritical care community has been reluctant to use ketamine to treat SE patients because of reports in the literature from the 1960s and 1970s that showed the potential for ketamine to increase the intracranial pressure in neurologically ill patients; however those reports have been contradicted by more recent data from patients with both traumatic and nontraumatic brain injury [7].

Conflicting data about the safety of ketamine has been published. While early studies showed that ketamine can be neuroprotective [8], others showed that ketamine can cause cerebral atrophy [9]. Similar conflicting results have been reported in animal studies. In one study of rats with traumatic brain injury, ketamine was associated with neuronal apoptosis [7], while others showed that ketamine can prevent learning impairment when administered immediately after the onset of SE [10].

Ketamine use in the management of SE provides a promising choice given its unique mechanism of action on the NMDA receptors, availability, fast onset of action, and generally benign side effect profile. Some of the side effects of ketamine include hallucinations, arrhythmia, and hypersalivation. The sympathetic properties of ketamine might be helpful if hypotension is a concern, but ketamine should be used with caution or avoided in patients with coronary artery disease or severe hypertension.

Reports about the use of ketamine during pregnancy in the literature are primarily cases of anesthesia for caesarian section, with some reports of recreational use of the drug during pregnancy. Some animal studies have shown teratogenic effects of ketamine. Ketamine crossed the placenta rapidly and equilibrated between the maternal and fetal circulation when studied in pregnant ewes [11]. The litter pregnant rats that received ketamine in their second trimester had memory impairment, as well as depression-like and anxiety-like behavioral disorder [12]. A report of an infant's late exposure to recreational ketamine showed some association with intrauterine growth retardation, remarkable hypotonia, and poor reflexes [13].

To our knowledge, this is the first case report in the literature of ketamine use for refractory SE during pregnancy. Our patient experienced resolution of RSE with the use of intravenous infusion of ketamine. She remained on ketamine infusion for a total of 7 days. No acute adverse effects were noted. She reported no long-term adverse effects after discharge from the hospital. No complications occurred during the caesarean Section. At 9 months the baby was healthy and achieved all development milestones.

4. Conclusion

The management of SE during pregnancy is especially challenging to the treating physician. While antiepileptic medications might cause teratogenicity, SE can have significant morbidity and mortality on both the mother and the developing fetus. This case report demonstrated the successful use of ketamine infusion in the management of RSE in pregnancy without affecting the immediate outcome of pregnancy. The fetus survived this complicated ICU stay and outpatient follow-up was generally uncomplicated. The pregnancy was ended with a delivery of a normal female newborn.

References

[1] C. L. Harden, J. Hopp, T. Y. Ting et al., "Practice Parameter update: Management issues for women with epilepsy–Focus on pregnancy (an evidence-based review): Obstetrical complications and change in seizure frequency: Report of the Quality Standards Subcommittee and Therapeutics and Technology Assessment Subcommittee of the American Academy of Neurology and American Epilepsy Society," *Neurology*, vol. 73, no. 2, pp. 126–132, 2009.

[2] C. G. Wasterlain and J. W. Y. Chen, "Mechanistic and pharmacologic aspects of status epilepticus and its treatment with new antiepileptic drugs," *Epilepsia*, vol. 49, supplement 9, pp. 63–73, 2008.

[3] S. Shorvon and M. Ferlisi, "Erratum: The outcome of therapies in refractory and super-refractory convulsive status epilepticus and recommendations for therapy (Brain (2012) 135 (2314-2328) DOI: 10.1093/brain/aws091)," *Brain*, vol. 136, no. 7, p. 2326, 2013.

[4] S. A. Mayer, J. Claassen, J. Lokin, F. Mendelsohn, L. J. Dennis, and B. F. Fitzsimmons, "Refractory status epilepticus: frequency, risk factors, and impact on outcome," *JAMA Neurology*, vol. 59, no. 2, pp. 205–210, 2002.

[5] R. L. Beach and P. W. Kaplan, "Chapter 15 Seizures in Pregnancy," in *Epilepsy in Women - The Scientific Basis for Clinical Management*, vol. 83 of *International Review of Neurobiology*, pp. 259–271, Elsevier, 2008.

[6] T. Tomson, "Seizure control and treatment in pregnancy: Observations from the EURAP epilepsy pregnancy registry," *Neurology*, vol. 66, no. 3, pp. 354–360, 2006.

[7] F. A. Zeiler, "Early Use of the NMDA Receptor Antagonist Ketamine in Refractory and Superrefractory Status Epilepticus," *Critical Care Research and Practice*, vol. 2015, Article ID 831260, 5 pages, 2015.

[8] D. G. Fujikawa, "The temporal evolution of neuronal damage from pilocarpine-induced status epilepticus," *Brain Research*, vol. 725, no. 1, pp. 11–22, 1996.

[9] E. E. Ubogu, S. M. Sagar, A. J. Lerner, B. N. Maddux, J. I. Suarez, and M. A. Werz, "Ketamine for refractory status epilepticus : A case of possible ketamine-induced neurotoxicity," *Epilepsy & Behavior*, vol. 4, no. 1, pp. 70–75, 2003.

[10] L. S. Stewart and M. A. Persinger, "Ketamine Prevents Learning Impairment When Administered Immediately after Status

Epilepticus Onset," *Epilepsy & Behavior*, vol. 2, no. 6, pp. 585–591, 2001.

[11] G. C. Musk, J. D. Netto, G. L. Maker, and R. D. Trengove, "Transplacental transfer of medetomidine and ketamine in pregnant ewes," *Laboratory Animals*, vol. 46, no. 1, pp. 46–50, 2012.

[12] T. Zhao, Y. Li, W. Wei, S. Savage, L. Zhou, and D. Ma, "Ketamine administered to pregnant rats in the second trimester causes long-lasting behavioral disorders in offspring," *Neurobiology of Disease*, vol. 68, pp. 145–155, 2014.

[13] P. Su, Y. Chang, and J. Chen, "Infant With In Utero Ketamine Exposure: Quantitative Measurement of Residual Dosage in Hair," *Pediatrics and Neonatology*, vol. 51, no. 5, pp. 279–284, 2010.

Bilateral Ganglion Cysts of the Ligamentum Flavum in the Cervical Spine Causing a Progressive Cervical Radiculomyelopathy and Literature Review

Juneki Kim,[1] Jin-gyu Choi,[1] and Byung-chul Son[1,2]

[1]*Department of Neurosurgery, Seoul St. Mary's Hospital, College of Medicine, The Catholic University of Korea, Seoul, Republic of Korea*
[2]*Catholic Neuroscience Institute, College of Medicine, The Catholic University of Korea, Seoul, Republic of Korea*

Correspondence should be addressed to Byung-chul Son; sbc@catholic.ac.kr

Academic Editor: Abbass Amirjamshidi

Here we report a unique case of bilateral ganglion cysts originating from the ligamentum flavum in the cervical spine. Degenerative cysts of the ligamentum flavum are rare lesions, and most had been reported in the lumbar spine. Its occurrence in the cervical spine is extremely rare: only eight have been reported. A 66-year-old male patient presented with progressive paraparesis, pain, and paresthesia in his bilateral T1 dermatomes that had lasted for three weeks. Magnetic resonance imaging of the cervical spine demonstrated a well-demarcated cystic lesion in the bilateral dorsolateral aspects of the C7/T1 segment and significant compression of the cervical cord. All case reports of ganglion cysts of the cervical ligamentum flavum including the present one showed characteristic symptoms and signs of myelopathy such as paraparesis or quadriparesis associated with varying degrees of paresthesia or pain in the upper extremities. Ganglion cysts of the cervical ligamentum flavum are considered a cause of cervical radiculomyelopathy due to cervical intraspinal cystic lesions. Bilateral occurrence and associated subluxation of the involved cervical segments again support the degenerative pathogenesis of ganglion cysts of the ligamentum flavum in the cervical spine.

1. Introduction

Ganglion cysts of the ligamentum flavum are uncommon degenerative spinal lesions that are mostly encountered in the lumbar spine [1–6]. Cervical localization is rare and may cause severe myelopathy [7]. These cysts accompany degenerative changes of the spine and can be differentiated from synovial and other degenerative spinal cysts based on location and histopathological features [7]. To our knowledge, only five cases have been reported, and all were associated with myelopathy [7–11]. Here, we report a case of bilateral ganglion cyst of the ligamentum flavum in the cervical spine that presented with gradual paraparesis along with bilateral cervical radicular pain.

2. Case Presentation

A 66-year-old male patient, usually in good health, presented progressive paraparesis of three weeks' duration. Three months prior to admission, he had worked hard for four to five hours a day for three months. He developed posterior neck pain and was treated several times with acupuncture. Three weeks earlier, the left leg had lost strength, and his right leg began to flex within a week. Eventually, he could not stand by himself due to the gradual progression of the paraparesis; he also felt paresthesia and pain on his bilateral medial upper arm. No urinary incontinence developed. He was admitted to a hospital and had magnetic resonance imaging (MRI) of the cervical spine and was referred for further evaluation.

Neurologic examination showed paraparesis and ataxia. Decreased motor strength, mainly of the quadriceps and adductors, was noted in his lower extremities, 4/5 on his right side and 3/5 on the left. He had more pronounced deep tendon reflex in his left patellar than in his right one. His upper extremities showed no weakness, but he had pain associated with paresthesia and hypesthesia in bilateral C8

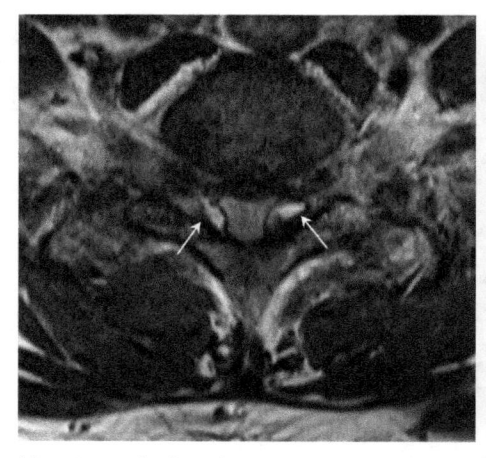

(a) A T2-weighted, axial MRI image showing bilateral ganglion cysts (arrows) of the ligamentum flavum at C7/T1. The rim of the cyst shows low signal intensity connected to the low signal intensity in the ligamentum flavum, and the cyst's contents were heterogenous, with both high and low signals on the left side

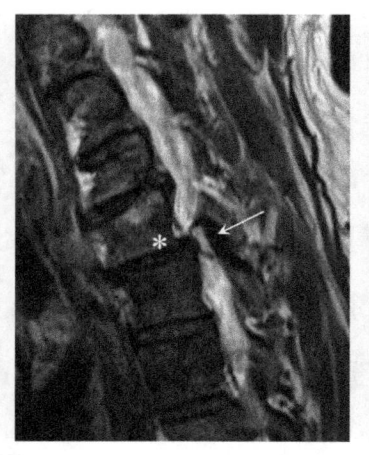

(b) A T2-weighted, sagittal MRI image showing the ganglion cyst (arrow) of the ligamentum flavum at C7/T1. Note the mild anterior subluxation of C7 to T1 (asterisk)

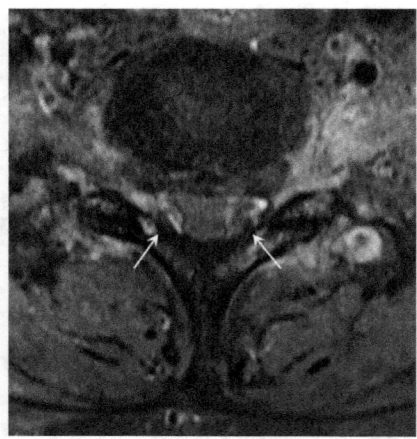

(c) An axial T1-weighted, enhanced MRI image showing variable, contrast enhancement of the cyst wall (arrows)

FIGURE 1: Magnetic resonance imaging (MRI) findings of bilateral ganglion cysts of the ligamentum flavum at C7/T1.

dermatomes. We observed no urinary difficulty. MRI of the cervical spine revealed bilateral extradural cystic masses that compromised the dural sac at the level of C7/T1 (Figure 1). The lesion was isointense in T1-weighted images and showed a hyperintense core with a peripheral hypodense ring in T2-weighted images. The wall of the cyst showed strong enhancement with gadolinium. We observed mild subluxation of C7 over T1 in the sagittal T2-weighted MRI and found prominent degenerative osteoarthritic changes in the bone scan. Considering the progressive neurologic deficits, we planned surgical treatment.

After a laminectomy of C7 and small medial facetectomy of C7/T1, we removed a hypertrophied ligamentum flavum and exposed the underlying dura. We found a fibrotic, extradural cyst on the internal aspect of the ligamentum flavum (Figure 2) that was embedded within the inner aspect of the ligamentum flavum with no connection with the facet joint or dura mater. When we violated the cyst wall, we found thick, mucous fluid. The cyst wall adhered densely to the underlying, lateral margin of the dura, and we carefully dissected the adhesion under microscopy. After we completely removed the bilateral cysts of the ligamentum flavum and the adjacent hypertrophied ligamentum flavum, we found the dura and the bilateral C8 root to be decompressed.

The postoperative course was uneventful. Immediately after the operation, the patient's severe pain and paresthesia of the bilateral medial upper arm corresponding to the T1 dermatome were alleviated. Although he experienced immediate functional improvement in both legs, the weakness in both legs improved only slowly over the six months following the operation. There was no weakness or sensory deficit in his arms and legs at the one-year postoperative follow-up and no neck pain or radiological instability.

3. Discussion

3.1. Pathogenesis of Ganglion Cysts of the Ligamentum Flavum in the Cervical Spine. Intraspinal degenerative cysts are rare and usually located in the lumbar spine [1–6]. Because the joint capsule is often considered to be the origin of these lesions, they are called juxtafacet cysts to indicate both synovial and ganglion cysts [12, 13]. Owing to their similar locations and cystic contents, the terms "spinal synovial cyst" and "spinal ganglion cyst" have been used interchangeably [6]. Initially, the suggested difference between synovial and ganglion cysts was that the former often contain clear and serous fluid whereas the latter contain gelatinous, highly viscous fluid [12]. However, differentiation between them is only possible with pathological findings [6]. Synovial cysts are lined with pseudostratified columnar cells, whereas ganglion cysts have no synovial cell lining and no communication with the joint cavity [6, 9, 10, 13, 14]. In the present case, the cysts did not communicate with the facet joint but were instead imbedded in the ligamentum flavum intraoperatively, and we found no synovial lining on microscopic examination. Therefore, we made the diagnosis of ganglion cyst.

It has been suggested that ganglion cysts are caused by myxoid degeneration and cystic softening of the connective tissue of the joint capsule or tendon sheath as a result of degenerative process or trauma [7]. The pathogenesis of degeneration of the ligamentum flavum is still unclear, but it can be considered in the context of degenerative change [7]. Aging and repeated microtrauma due to spinal motion lead to degenerative changes including loss of elastic fibers, thickening with chondrocyte proliferation and calcifications, and formation of collagen fibers [6]. Loss of elasticity predisposes the ligamentum flavum to mechanical stress injury, resulting in scar remodeling and ganglion cyst formation [6]. The

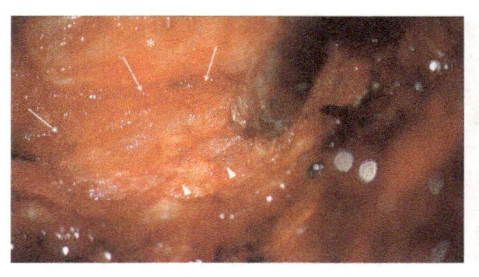

(a) An intraoperative photograph showing the outer wall of ganglion cyst (arrows) at the right side of C7/T1. The ligamentum flavum was bulged with the cyst, and the lateral margin of the dura (asterisk) was compressed. The cut edge of the facet (arrowheads)

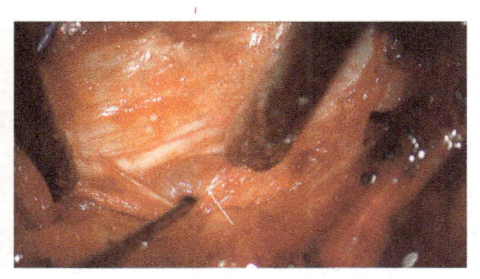

(b) After the outer wall of the ligamentum flavum cyst was cleared, a degenerated cystic portion was found (arrow). The underlying dura (asterisk) was dissected and decompressed

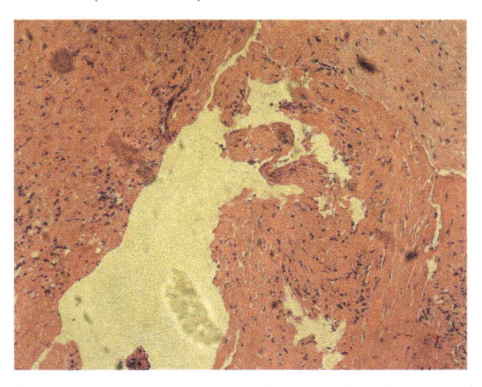

(c) A histologic specimen showing the absence of synovial cell lining of the inner cystic wall (×40, H & E stain)

FIGURE 2: Intraoperative photograph showing the ganglion cyst of the ligamentum flavum.

current case is unique because of the bilateral occurrence of the ligamentum flavum ganglion cyst and associated mild subluxation. We think that bilateral occurrence and associated subluxation further support the pathogenesis of degenerative changes involving the ligamentum flavum. Indeed, in the literature, all of the case reports involved people over age 60 (Table 1).

3.2. Symptoms, Diagnosis, and Treatment of Ganglion Cysts in the Cervical Ligamentum Flavum.

Symptoms and signs of myelopathy with or without cervical radiculopathy association are the most common presenting symptoms in symptomatic ganglion cysts of the ligamentum flavum in the cervical spine. In our review of the literature regarding theses cysts, six of seven reported cases (86%), including the current case, showed paraparesis or quadriparesis owing to their location within the narrow cervical spinal canal. Most symptoms and signs of myelopathy are gradual and insidious (Table 1). However, an occurrence of sudden Brown-Sequard syndrome within three hours due to a ganglion cyst of the cervical ligamentum flavum has been reported [10]. Although the symptomatic cervical ligamentum flavum ganglion cysts in the literature have been small (8 to 15 mm in diameter), all reported cases showed characteristic symptoms and signs of myelopathy: gait disturbance and paraparesis [15–17].

MRI is the imaging study of choice in the diagnosis of ganglion cysts in the cervical spine, although histopathologic examination is needed for definitive diagnosis [7]. The MRI findings of the ganglion cysts are characteristic; the cyst contents are hypointense on T1-weighted images and hyperintense on T2-weighted images [6, 7, 9, 10, 14]. The peripheral rims of the cysts are hypointense on T2-weighted images with gadolinium enhancement. The treatment for symptomatic ganglion cysts of the ligamentum flavum in the cervical spine is surgery. All reported cases of ganglion cervical spine cysts caused serious neurologic deficits, and surgical treatment universally resulted in neurologic improvement.

Surgical excision of ganglion cysts of the cervical spine with posterior laminectomy appears to be a straightforward for decompressing the spinal cord, removing the ganglion cysts, addressing the connection to the facet joint, and taking histologic specimens for definitive diagnosis. All case reports regarding symptomatic ganglion cysts of the cervical ligamentum flavum adopted surgical excision via laminectomy, and the prognosis of surgical treatment is favorable. Although some degree of adhesion between the dura and the ganglion cyst was always mentioned, no surgical morbidity or neurologic compromise was reported. Gradual recovery of the symptoms and signs of radiculomyelopathy appear to occur within 6 to 12 months postoperatively.

TABLE 1: Summary of the reported cases of ganglion cysts of the ligamentum flavum in the cervical spine.

Author/year	Number of cases	Age/sex	Presenting symptom/signs	Location	Diagnostic modality	Treatment	Prognosis follow-up period	Associated condition
Takano et al., 1992	1	72/m	Spastic paraparesis, 1 yr bilat. C6 paresthesia	C3/4, lt	MRI, OR, histology connection (−)	C3–6 laminectomy	Rapid recovery unknown F-U	
Yamamoto et al., 2001	2	81/m	Progr. paraparesis, 1 mo neck pain, bilat. arm leg paresthesia	C3/4, lt	MRI, OR, histology connection (−)	Laminectomy C3–7 laminoplasty	Improved, 2 mos	
		65/m	Spastic quadriparesis rt arm pain	C3/4, rt	MRI, M-CT connection (−)	Laminectomy C3–7 laminoplasty	Improved, 2 mos	
Shima et al., 2002	1	66/m	Paraparesis and numbness	C7/T1, rt	MRI, OR, histology connection (−)	Laminoplasty C3–6	Complete recovery, 9 mos	
Chenng et al., 2006	1	58/m	Sudden Brown-Sequard synd. lt-sided hemiparesis rt-sided hemianalgesia below T4	C6/7, lt	MRI, OR, histology connection (+)	Laminectomy C6-7	Complete recovery, 4 mos	CRF
Yahara et al., 2009	1	63/f	Myelopathy below C5, bilat. hand paresthesia	C4/5, lt	MRI, OR, histology connection (−)	Laminectomy C4/5 instrumentation, fusion	Complete recovery, 1 yr	RA 15 yrs C4/5 instability
Muzii et al., 2010	1	60/m	Progr. paraparesis, 1 yr ataxia, hyperreflexia	C4/5 midline	MRI, OR, histology connection (−)	C4/5 laminectomy	Complete recovery, 1 yr mild spastic gait	
Brotis et al., 2012	1	82/f	Progr. quadriparesis, 3 mos bilat. arm paresthesia, neck pain	C3/4, lt	MRI, OR, histology connection (−)	Laminectomy C3	Complete recovery, 6 mos	HBP, DM hypothyroidism
Current case, 2017	1	66/m	Paraparesis, 3-week bilat. T1 paresthesia, pain	C7/T1, bilat.	MRI, OR, histology connection (−)	Laminectomy C7	Complete recovery, 12 mos	C7/T1 subluxation

Bilat.: bilateral, CRF: chronic renal failure, DM: diabetes mellitus, HBP: hypertension, lt: left, mos: months, OR: operation, progr.: progressive, RA: rheumatoid arthritis, and rt: right. Connection (−)/(+): presence/absence of communication to the facet joint.

4. Conclusions

We here report a very rare case of bilateral ganglion cysts of the cervical ligamentum flavum that presented with progressive myelopathy and radiculopathy. The characteristic bilateral occurrence and associated cervical subluxation at the involved segment supported the degenerative pathophysiology in the cyst.

References

[1] A. F. Abdullah, R. W. Chambers, and D. P. Daut, "Lumbar nerve root compression by synovial cysts of the ligamentum flavum. Report of four cases," *Journal of Neurosurgery*, vol. 60, no. 3, pp. 617–620, 1984.

[2] J. K. Baker and G. W. Hanson, "Cyst of the ligamentum flavum," *Spine*, vol. 19, no. 9, pp. 1092–1094, 1994.

[3] C. B. Bärlocher and R. W. Seiler, "Vertebral erosion and a ligamentum flavum cyst," *Journal of Neurosurgery: Spine*, vol. 93, no. 2, pp. 335-335, 2000.

[4] J. Haase, "Extradural cyst of ligamentum flavum l4 - A case," *Acta Orthopaedica*, vol. 43, no. 1, pp. 32–38, 1972.

[5] H. Terada, Y. Yokoyama, N. Kamata, T. Hozumi, and T. Kondo, "Cyst of the ligamentum flavum," *Neuroradiology*, vol. 43, no. 1, pp. 49–51, 2001.

[6] A. Yamamoto, I. Nishiura, H. Handa, and A. Kondo, "Ganglion cyst in the ligamentum flavum of the cervical spine causing myelopathy: report of two cases," *Surgical Neurology*, vol. 56, no. 6, pp. 390–395, 2001.

[7] V. F. Muzii, P. Tanganelli, G. Signori, and A. Zalaffi, "Ganglion cyst of the ligamentum flavum: a rare cause of cervical spinal cord compression. A case report," *Journal of Neurology, Neurosurgery and Psychiatry*, vol. 81, no. 8, pp. 940-941, 2010.

[8] A. G. Brotis, E. Z. Kapsalaki, E. K. Papadopoulos, and K. N. Fountas, "A cervical ligamentum flavum cyst in an 82-year-old woman presenting with spinal cord compression: a case report and review of the literature," *Journal of Medical Case Reports*, vol. 6, article no. 92, 2012.

[9] Y. Takano, T. Homma, H. Okumura, and H. E. Takahashi, "Ganglion cyst occurring in the ligamentum flavum of the cervical spine: a case report," *Spine*, vol. 17, no. 12, pp. 1531–1533, 1992.

[10] W. Y. Chenng, C. C. Shen, and M. C. Wen, "Ganglion cyst of the cervical spine representing with Brown-Sequard syndrome," *Journal of Clinical Neuroscience*, vol. 95, supplement 1, pp. 193-142, 2006.

[11] L. F. Chen, C. C. Lui, M. H. Cheng, and J. W. Lin, "Ganglion cyst in the ligamentum flavum of the cervicothoracic junction," *Journal of the Formosan Medical Association*, vol. 95, pp. 490–492, 1996.

[12] C. C. Kao, S. S. Winkler, and J. H. Turner, "Synovial cyst of spinal facet. Case report," *Journal of Neurosurgery*, vol. 41, no. 3, pp. 372–376, 1974.

[13] O. Hatem, G. Bedou, C. Négre, J. L. Bertrand, and J. Camo, "Intraspinal cervical degenerative cyst. report of three cases," *Journal of Neurosurgery*, vol. 95, no. 1, pp. 139–142, 2001.

[14] M. A. Stoodley, N. R. Jones, and G. Scott, "Cervical and thoracic juxtafacet cysts causing neurologic deficits," *Spine*, vol. 25, no. 8, pp. 970–973, 2000.

[15] P. Fransen, G. P. Pizzolato, P. Otten, A. Reverdin, R. Lagier, and N. De Tribolet, "Synovial cyst and degeneration of the transverse ligament: an unusual cause of high cervical myelopathy. case report," *Journal of Neurosurgery*, vol. 86, no. 6, pp. 1027–1030, 1997.

[16] Y. Shima, S. L. G. Rothman, K. Yasura, and S. Takahashi, "Degenerative intraspinal cyst of the cervical spine: case report and literature review.," *Spine*, vol. 27, no. 1, pp. E18–22, 2002.

[17] Y. Yahara, Y. Kawaguchi, S. Seki, Y. Abe, T. Oya, and T. Kimura, "Ligamentum flavum cyst of the cervical spine associated with rheumatoid arthritis," *Journal of Orthopaedic Science*, vol. 14, no. 2, pp. 215–218, 2009.

Differential Effects of Awake Glioma Surgery in "Critical" Language Areas on Cognition: 4 Case Studies

Djaina Satoer,[1] Elke De Witte,[2] Marion Smits,[3] Roelien Bastiaanse,[4] Arnaud Vincent,[1] Peter Mariën,[2,5] and Evy Visch-Brink[1,6]

[1]Department of Neurosurgery, Erasmus MC University Medical Center, Rotterdam, Netherlands
[2]Department of Clinical and Experimental Neurolinguistics, Free University of Brussels, Brussels, Belgium
[3]Department of Radiology, Erasmus MC University Medical Center, Rotterdam, Netherlands
[4]Center for Language and Cognition Groningen (CLCG), University of Groningen, Groningen, Netherlands
[5]Department of Neurology and Memory Clinic, ZNA Middelheim, Antwerp, Belgium
[6]Department of Neurology, Erasmus MC University Medical Center, Rotterdam, Netherlands

Correspondence should be addressed to Djaina Satoer; d.satoer@erasmusmc.nl

Academic Editor: Abbass Amirjamshidi

Awake surgery with electrocorticosubcortical stimulation is the golden standard treatment for gliomas in eloquent areas. Preoperatively, mostly mild cognitive disturbances are observed with postoperative deterioration. We describe pre- and postoperative profiles of 4 patients (P1–P4) with gliomas in "critical" language areas ("Broca," "Wernicke," and the arcuate fasciculus) undergoing awake surgery to get insight into the underlying mechanism of neuroplasticity. Neuropsychological examination was carried out preoperatively (at T1) and postoperatively (at T2, T3). At T1, cognition of P1 was intact and remained stable. P2 had impairments in all cognitive domains at T1 with further deterioration at T2 and T3. At T1, P3 had impairments in memory and executive functions followed by stable recovery. P4 was intact at T1, followed by a decline in a language test at T2 and recovery at T3. Intraoperatively, in all patients language positive sites were identified. Patients with gliomas in "critical" language areas do not necessarily present cognitive disturbances. Surgery can either improve or deteriorate (existing) cognitive impairments. Several factors may underlie the plastic potential of the brain, for example, corticosubcortical networks and tumor histopathology. Our findings illustrate the complexity of the underlying mechanism of neural plasticity and provide further support for a "hodotopical" viewpoint.

1. Introduction

Awake surgery is considered the golden standard treatment for low-grade gliomas (LGG) in eloquent regions to optimize tumor resection while preserving neurological and cognitive functions and hence quality of life [1, 2]. However, deficits in cognitive functions, that is, language, memory, attentional, and executive functions, occur in the (pre- and) postoperative phase of awake glioma surgery [3–5].

Eloquent regions typically include the left dominant perisylvian brain regions. DES has provided evidence for a "hodotopical" (i.e., dynamic) view of the organization of brain functions as opposed to a "topological" viewpoint (i.e., static organization of brain functions) [6–8]. Language functions are "classically" represented in cortical areas such as Broca's and Wernicke's area and in the subcortical tracts that connect different eloquent cortical regions. LGGs typically invade functional subcortical white matter tracts. However, due to the relative slow growth rate (i.e., 4 mm a year) of LGG, neural plasticity can be facilitated [9, 10]. This may be the reason that, instead of moderate to severe language problems, typically mild language disorders are observed in this patient group [11]. Despite intense intraoperative monitoring, brain tumor surgery resection may induce or aggravate the existing cognitive deficits. For a long time, complete recovery within 3 months was claimed to take place, but Satoer et al. [5].

found that cognitive recovery can continue until up to at least 1 year postoperatively. A recent review of cognition in glioma patients showed various pre- and postoperative cognitive profiles with deficits in various domains at different time-moments [12]. These findings point towards differential postoperative recovery courses of cognitive functions. Apart from individual variability in functional organization and language lateralization, other factors accounting for the potential of neuroplasticity are under debate. Tumor related characteristics (e.g., tumor volume, grade) may interfere with the course of cognitive recovery [13, 14]. Anticonvulsants and adjuvant therapy (radio- and chemotherapy) as well as the degree of seizures (frequency) may have impact on the functional cerebral network in brain tumor patients [15]. In this article, we describe 4 patients with a brain tumor in dominant perisylvian language areas in proximity of the arcuate fasciculus with differential pre- and postoperative cognitive profiles illustrating the diversity of neural plasticity processes.

2. Materials and Methods

2.1. Case Reports. This is a follow-up study of 4 patients that we selected based on tumor localization in perisylvian language areas. The patients (P1, P2, P3, and P4) were diagnosed with a glioma in the language dominant left hemisphere as identified with fMRI (see structural MRI scans for tumor localization in Figure 1 and resection cavity in Figure 2). The demographic and clinical characteristics of the patients are shown in Table 1. The tumor was in proximity to the posterior temporoparietal language regions "Wernicke" in patients P1, P2, and P4. In P4, the tumor extended frontally towards the frontal language region of "Broca" as well. In P3, the tumor was located in the frontal and insular gyrus, in proximity or possibly with minimal involvement of the inferior frontal gyrus, that is, "Broca," but not the posterior temporoparietal regions. Tumor locations in all patients were in the vicinity of the arcuate fasciculus (AF).

2.2. Procedure: Operation, Neuroimaging, and Pathological Findings. Between July 2011 and June 2013, patients were treated with awake brain surgery given the tumor location in or near presumed critical language regions. Electrical stimulation was carried out at cortical and subcortical level with a bipolar electrode. Object naming and repetition tasks were administered during stimulation, whereas more extensive language testing was conducted using the Dutch Linguistic Intraoperative Protocol (DuLIP) with spontaneous speech monitoring during resection [16].

Localization of the tumor was determined by a neuroradiologist using 3D T1-weighted images and 2D T2-weighted images. The pre- and postoperative tumor volume was calculated by manual delineation of 3-dimensional deviant signal intensity on T2-weighted MR images using Osirix version 4.1.2. (http://www.osirix-viewer.com/). Postoperative MRI scans were assessed at 6 months after surgery. The extent of the resection was calculated as the fraction (%) of the difference between the preoperative and postoperative volume divided by the preoperative volume. The histological type of the tumor (astrocytoma, oligodendroglioma, and oligoastrocytoma) and the World Health Organization (WHO) grade (2007) were determined by a neuropathologist, from tissue obtained during the tumor resection.

2.3. Neuropsychological Assessment. Pre- and postoperatively, we administered an extensive neuropsychological test-protocol (Table 2). *Language* tests are as follows: Boston Naming Test (BNT) or object naming (DuLIP), action naming, category and letter fluency, and Aachen Aphasia Test (AAT) subtests: repetition, writing to dictation, reading aloud, and Token Test. *Memory* tests are as follows: 15-word test (imprinting, recall); digit span. *Attentional and executive functions* tests are as follows: design fluency, Trail Making Tests A and B, and Stroop Color Word Tests I–III. Based on the normative data, z-scores were computed to compare performance of the patients to healthy controls. A clinical impairment is reflected by a z-score between -1.5 and -2; a pathological impairment is reflected by a z-score of ≥ -2. Postoperatively, P1 and P2 were tested at 6 weeks and 6 months and P3 and P4 at 3 months and 1 year. The study was approved by the Ethical Committee of Erasmus MC Rotterdam and University of Brussels. All patients gave written informed consent.

3. Results

Tumor volume ranged from $1.46\,\text{cm}^3$ to $108\,\text{cm}^3$. Pathological examination of tumor tissue obtained during resection revealed a LGG (WHO grade II) in P1 and P3 and a HGG in P2 (WHO grade IV) and in P4 (WHO grade III). The extent of resection (EoR) ranged from 58 to 89%. P1, P2, and P4 underwent postoperative radiotherapy (33 fraction doses of 1.8 Gy). All patients used anticonvulsants pre- and postoperatively (see Table 2).

3.1. Neuropsychological Assessment: Pre-, Intra-, and Postoperative Course (See Table 3)

3.1.1. P1: Low-Grade Glioma in "Wernicke's" Area and Near AF. Preoperatively, the cognitive functions of P1 were intact ($z \geq -1.5$). During operation, speech arrest occurred after stimulation at the precentral gyrus (primary motor cortex) at the level of the mouth. Postoperatively, at 6 weeks a clinical deficit in a memory test was observed (15 WT imprinting; $z = -1.60$) which recovered at 6 months. No other cognitive deficits were observed ($z \geq -1.5$).

3.1.2. P2: High-Grade Glioma in "Wernicke's" Area Near AF. Preoperatively, P2 had clinically or pathologically significant impairments in language (letter fluency; $z = -1.90$, AAT Token Test; $z = -5.35$), and attention and executive deficits (TMT B: $z = -1.60$, TMT BA: $z = -1.90$, Stroop I: $z = -2.00$, Stroop II: $z = -2.20$, and Stroop III: $z = -1.90$). During surgery cortical stimulation in the posterior superior temporal gyrus/angular gyrus triggered speech arrest. During stimulation of the AF, phonemic paraphasia occurred; these increased during resection near the AF, at which point resection was terminated. At 6 weeks postoperatively new deficits were found in language (object naming: $z = -6.28$,

TABLE 1: Demographic and clinical characteristics. Y = years, Hem. Dom. = hemispheric dominance, M = male, L = left, R = right, AF = arcuate fasciculus, O = oligodendroglioma, GBM = glioblastoma, AO = anaplastic oligodendroglioma, EoR = extent of resection, and AED = antiepileptic drugs.

Case	Gender	Age (y)	Education (y)	Handedness	Onset symptoms	Hem. Dom.	Cortical area	Subcortical area	WHO grade (2007)	Histology	EoR (%)	AED	Adjuvant therapy
P1	M	45	15	L	Seizure	L	Temporoparietal ("Wernicke")	AF	II (low)	O	58.34	Yes	Radio
P2	M	63	12	R	Language problems	L	Temporoparietal ("Wernicke")	AF	IV (high)	GBM	88.68	Yes	Radio
P3	M	41	16	R	Seizure	L	Frontal and insular ("Broca")	AF	II (low)	O	52.73	Yes	No
P4	M	33	15	R	Seizure	L	Temporoparietal and frontal ("Wernicke" and "Broca")	AF	III (high)	AO	81.48	Yes	Radio

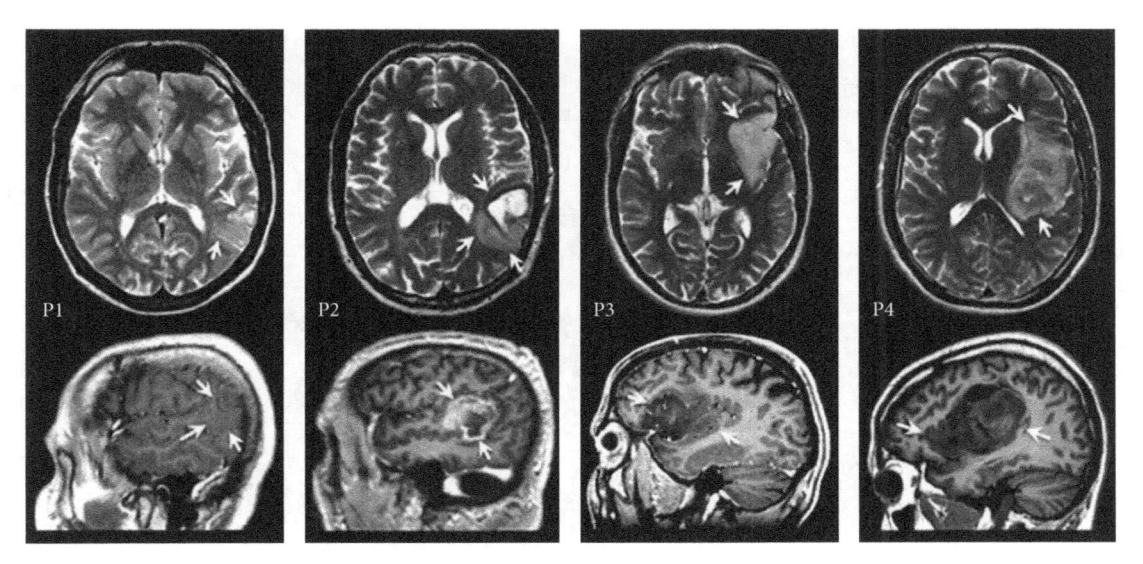

FIGURE 1: Preoperative MRI scans axial T2 weighted and sagittal T1 weighted (contrast-enhanced in P1 and in P3) sections depicting tumor localization (arrows).

TABLE 2: Neuropsychological assessment.

	Cognitive abilities and description of task
Language tests	
AAT [17]	
Repetition	Repeating phonemes, words, and sentences
Writing to dictation	Writing words and sentences on dictation
Reading out loud	Reading aloud words and sentences
Token Test	Comprehension of, pointing to, and manipulating geometric forms
Boston Naming Test [18]	Naming 60 pictures, presented in order of word frequency and word difficulty
Category fluency	Flexibility of verbal semantic thought: categories (e.g., animals) (within 1 min)
Letter fluency	Flexibility of verbal phonological thought: letters D, A, and T (within 1 min)
DuLIP [16]	
Syntactic fluency	Flexibility of verbal grammatical thought, producing verbs (within 1 min)
Object naming[1]	Word finding: naming objects
Action naming	Word finding, grammar: naming actions
Memory tests	
Digit span for/backward [19]	Verbal learning of digits: repeating the list of digits forward/backward
15-word test [19]	Verbal learning of words
Learning	Immediate recall: learning a list of 15 words, immediate recall for 5 times
Recall	Delayed recall: learning a list of 15 words, 1 delayed recall
Recognition	Delayed recognition: 1 delayed recognition out of 30 words
Attentional & executive tests	
Trail Making Test (TMT) [19]	
Trail Making Test A	Visuomotor speed, attention: connecting numbers in ascending order
Trail Making Test B	Divided attention/mental flexibility: connecting alternating numbers and letters
Stroop Color Word Test [19]	
Stroop I	Mental speed, selective attention: reading color words
Stroop II	Mental speed, selective attention: naming colors
Stroop III	Mental speed, selective attention: naming colors of printed words denoting another color
Design fluency [20]	Nonverbal fluency, attention, motor speed, visuoperceptual and constructional abilities

[1] Flanders: object naming from DuLIP, the Netherlands: Boston Naming Test.

TABLE 3: Pre- and postoperative neuropsychological test-scores P1–P4 (a–d). w = weeks, m = months, and y = years. **Pathological (severe) impairment: z-score ≤ -2 (marked with bold). *Clinical (mild) impairment: z-score ≤ -1.5 (marked with italic).

(a)

	P1		
	Preoperative results	Postoperative results (6 w)	Postoperative results (6 m)
Language			
Object naming (DuLIP)	0.13	0.63	0.63
Action naming (DuLIP)	0.76	0.76	0.76
Category fluency	0.10	−1.00	0.45
Letter fluency	1.10	−0.10	0.50
AAT Token Test	0.83	0.83	0.83
Memory			
15 WT imprinting	−0.10	*−1.60**	0.10
15 WT recall	−0.60	−0.60	−0.20
Digit span	0.67	0.33	1.00
Attention/executive functions			
Design fluency productivity	2.05	1.41	2.33
Design fluency flexibility	1.28	0.58	0.67
Design fluency strategy	1.08	2.05	1.28
TMTA	1.10	1.20	1.60
TMTB	1.40	1.70	2.10
TMTBA	0.90	1.20	1.40
Stroop I	−0.30	−0.40	−0.20
Stroop II	1.50	1.20	1.80
Stroop III	1.60	2.40	1.90
Stroop interference	1.00	2.30	1.20

(b)

	P2		
	Preoperative results	Postoperative results (6 w)	Postoperative results (6 m)
Language			
Object naming (DuLIP)	−0.64	**−6.28**	**−4.40**
Action naming (DuLIP)	−0.80	**−2.94**	−1.37
Category fluency	−1.20	**−2.50**	**−2.30**
Letter fluency	*−1.90*	**−2.70**	**−2.40**
AAT Token Test	**−5.35**	**−10.81**	**−5.35**
Memory			
15 WT imprinting	−0.64	**−3.90**	**−3.50**
15 WT recall	−0.80	**−3.10**	**−2.70**
Digit span	−1.20	**−3.00**	**−3.00**
Attention/executive functions			
Design fluency productivity	0.13	*−1.88*	**−2.05**
Design fluency flexibility	−0.25	−1.13	0.00
Design fluency strategy	0.84	−0.47	0.25
TMTA	0.20	**−4.10**	*−1.50*
TMTB	*−1.60*	**−4.30**	**−3.40**
TMTBA	*−1.90*	**−2.70**	**−3.10**
Stroop I	**−2.00**	**−5.40**	**−5.00**
Stroop II	**−2.20**	**−4.40**	**−5.10**

(b) Continued.

	P2		
	Preoperative results	Postoperative results (6 w)	Postoperative results (6 m)
Stroop III	−1.90*	**−3.40****	**−3.40****
Stroop interference	−0.60	−1.20	−0.30

(c)

	P3		
	Preoperative results	Postoperative results (3 m)	Postoperative results (1 y)
Language			
Boston Naming Test	−0.60	−0.27	−1.27
Category fluency	1.10	1.57	−0.46
Letter fluency	0.00	0.54	1.08
AAT Token Test	−0.10	−0.83	−0.83
AAT repetition	1.39	0.83	0.83
AAT reading aloud	0.54	0.54	0.54
AAT writing to dictation	0.54	0.54	0.54
Memory			
15 WT imprinting	−1.40	−0.40	0.40
15 WT recall	−1.60*	−0.50	1.00
Attention/executive functions			
TMTA	0.50	1.10	1.00
TMTB	**−2.40****	0.30	−0.20
TMTBA	**−3.00****	−0.40	−0.90
Stroop I	0.60	0.60	1.10
Stroop II	−0.30	−0.30	0.70
Stroop III	0.70	0.10	1.10
Stroop interference	1.10	0.30	0.80

(d)

	P4		
	Preoperative results	Postoperative results (3 m)	Postoperative results (1 y)
Language			
Boston Naming Test	−0.21	−0.74	0.05
Category fluency	0.75	−1.16	0.73
Letter fluency	−1.08	−1.26	−1.44
AAT Token Test	−0.47	0.99	−0.10
AAT repetition	0.28	**−4.17****	−1.39
AAT reading aloud	−0.49	−0.49	0.54
AAT writing to dictation	0.27	−0.27	0.00
Memory			
15 WT imprinting	−1.30	1.50	−0.10
15 WT recall	−0.70	0.00	0.40
Attention/executive functions			
TMTA	0.70	0.00	0.90
TMTB	−0.60	−1.40	0.00
TMTBA	−1.10	−1.60*	−0.60
Stroop I	0.80	−0.90	−0.30
Stroop II	1.10	0.00	−0.50
Stroop III	1.20	−0.50	−0.30
Stroop interference	0.60	−0.70	0.00

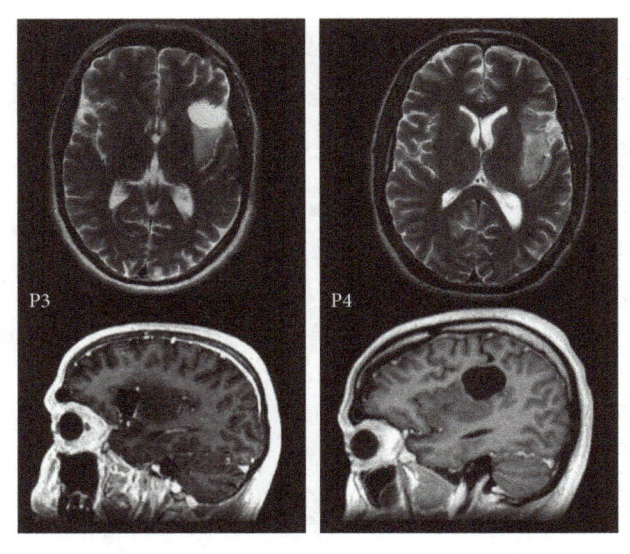

FIGURE 2: Postoperative MRI scans axial T2 weighted and sagittal T1 weighted P3 and P4.

action naming: $z = -2.94$, and category fluency: $z = -2.50$), in memory (15 WT imprinting: $z = -3.90$, 15 WT recall: $z = -3.10$, and digit span: $z = -3.00$), and in attention and executive functions (design fluency: productivity: $z = -1.88$, TMT A: $z = -4.10$). There was an increase of the preoperative deficits in language (letter fluency: $z = -2.70$, AAT Token Test: $z = -10.81$) and in attention and executive functions (TMT B: $z = -4.30$, TMT BA: $z = -2.70$, Stroop I: $z = -5.40$, Stroop II: $z = -4.40$, and Stroop III: $z = -3.40$). At 6 months postoperatively, improvement was observed in 1 subtest within the language domain (action naming: $z = -1.37$) and in the attention and executive functions (TMT A: $z = -1.50$), but further deterioration was found in another subtest (design fluency: productivity: $z = -2.05$).

3.1.3. P3: Low-Grade Glioma in "Broca's" Area and Near AF. Preoperatively P3 was clinically impaired in memory (15 WT recall: $z = -1.60$) and had selective pathological impairments in executive functioning (TMT B: $z = -2.40$, TMT BA: $z = -3.00$). During surgery speech arrest occurred with stimulation of the inferior frontal gyrus, below the motor cortex, and the parietal lobe (see Figure 3). Phonemic paraphasia and neologisms were elicited at the temporoparietal junction. At the subcortical level near the AF also phonemic paraphasia was elicited. At the motor cortex, stimulation triggered dysarthria and contraction of the tongue. At the end of resection, perseverations occurred at which point resection was terminated (see Figure 4). Postoperatively at 3 months, the patient had recovered from the observed preoperative impairments in memory (15 WT recall: $z = -0.50$) and executive functioning (TMT B: $z = 0.30$, TMT BA: $z = -0.40$), which remained stable during the follow-up of 1 year (15 WT: $z = 1.00$, TMT B: $z = -0.20$, and TMT BA: $z = -0.90$). No other impairments were present.

3.1.4. P4: High-Grade Glioma in "Wernicke's" Area with Extension to "Broca's" Area and Near AF. Preoperatively, P4 had no

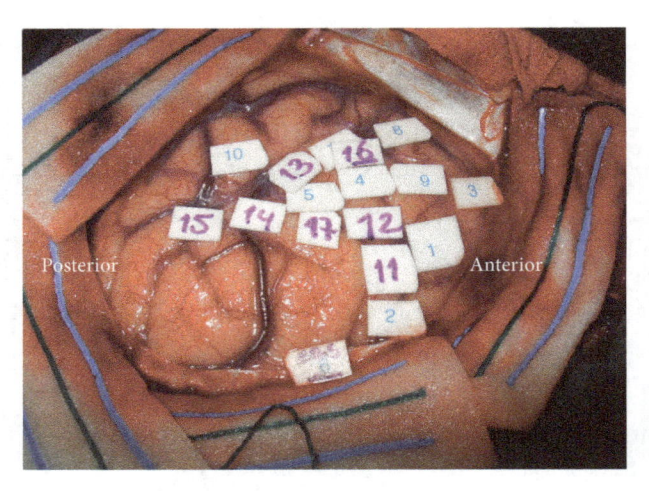

FIGURE 3: Intraoperative mapping P3. Cortical positive sites: speech arrest (1, 5, 7-9, and 13-14), dysarthria (2-4), neologism (10, 15), phonemic paraphasia (10, 15), and contraction of tongue (11-12, 16-17).

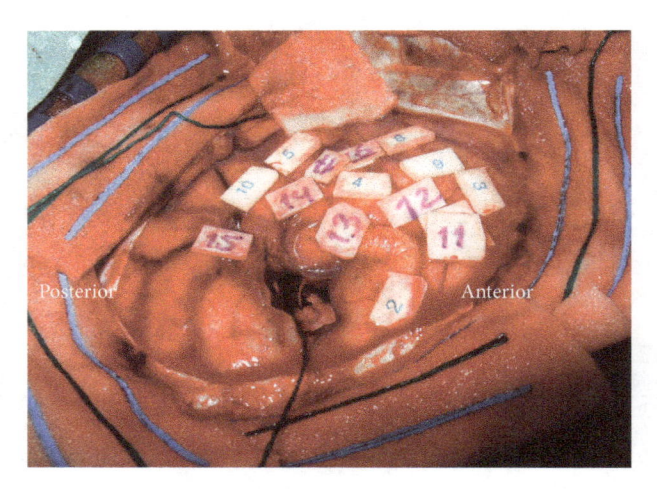

FIGURE 4: Resection cavity P3.

cognitive disorders. During surgery speech arrest was found when the inferior frontal gyrus was stimulated, below the motor cortex and in the temporal lobe. Phonemic paraphasia was elicited in the parietal lobe. Resection was terminated when perseverations occurred. At 3 months postoperatively, P4 developed a deficit in language (AAT repetition: $z = -4.17$) which had recovered at 1 year ($z = -1.39$) and in attention and executive functions (TMT BA: $z = -1.60$) which also recovered at 1 year ($z = -0.60$).

4. Discussion

A detailed examination of cognitive functions was conducted in 4 patients with brain tumors in or near "classical" language areas Broca, Wernicke, and the AF before and after awake surgery. Given the tumor localization it is remarkable that only in one patient (P2) a language disorder was present preoperatively. Our study revealed mixed cognitive profiles at pre- and postoperative time-points. Two patients (P1 and

P4) showed relatively intact cognitive performance, which may be explained by neural plasticity (i.e., reorganization of functions). By contrast, the other two cases (P2 and P3) demonstrated impairments in several cognitive domains pre- and/or postoperatively. These different findings are in line with a "dynamic" or "hodotopical" brain as opposed to a "static" or "topological" viewpoint [6]. Several factors may be related to the plastic potential of the brain such as different corticosubcortical networks (localization), tumor grade (low versus high), tumor volume, EoR, and the use of anticonvulsants and/or adjuvant therapy with irradiation.

P1 with a tumor in Wernicke's area appeared to have intact cognition, apart from a temporary clinical memory deficit at 6 weeks postoperatively. Intact cognition after glioma surgery in Wernicke's area has been reported previously [21]. By contrast, a multicognitive disturbed profile at pre- and postoperative level was found in P2 who had a very similar tumor localization. This implies that the "classical" language area Wernicke can also be related to other cognitive functions or that cognitive functions are disturbed when language is impaired (partly) in line with the model proposed by Coello et al. [22]. However, it is not possible to make strong assumptions about the interdependency of deficits in different cognitive domains. In P2, a simultaneous decline of language, memory, and executive functions at T2 illustrates this phenomenon where both verbal and nonverbal tasks deteriorated (verbal fluency and design fluency). Surprisingly, P3 with a tumor near Broca's area did not suffer from preoperative language deficits probably due to functional reorganization. Instead, impairments in the domains of memory and executive functions were observed which recovered within 3 months. P4 with a large tumor extending to Broca's and Wernicke's area had generally intact language performance, again in contrast with the "classical" language model, apart from a temporary decline on a repetition task at 3 months after surgery. Recently, the sensitivity of a repetition task was demonstrated in the intraoperative stimulation setting especially in or near the AF [23]. In all our patients the tumor was also located in or near the AF. Surgery in this area can cause a decline in phonological language performance [24]. A variety of pre- and postoperative cognitive disturbances in our patients demonstrate that this subcortical tract (AF) is not only associated with phonology. This has previously been observed in patients with lesions with a different etiology [25]. Hence, preservation of AF during surgery appears to be mandatory for the surveillance of (further) cognitive decline. Despite the detection of intraoperative language positive sites in all patients, different postoperative cognitive outcomes were observed. Tumor resection in proximity of a language positive site, but also preoperative language deficits, can be a risk factor for postoperative aphasia [26].

Apart from localization and the intraoperative procedure, the differential pre- and postoperative cognitive profiles in our patients could be attributed to tumor related factors, such as tumor grade. Noll et al. [27] found that patients with grade IV gliomas present with poorer preoperative cognitive performance (verbal learning, processing speed, executive functioning, and language) than patients with lower-grade gliomas (II, III). These differences were not related to tumor size, seizure status, and anticonvulsants or steroid use which points to evidence of a so-called "lesion momentum": faster growing tumors may be associated with more severe cognitive impairments. Our results are partly consistent with this line of reasoning. P2 with a high-grade glioma showed a preoperative disturbed cognitive profile (deficits in language, memory, and attention/executive functioning). Preserved cognitive functions in P1 were possibly facilitated by the slow growth rate of a low-grade tumor allowing "typical" functional reorganization (i.e., 4 mm p/y), that is, preoperative cognitive plasticity. A faster growth rate of a high-grade tumor, as in P2, could have more aggressively affected these preoperative cognitive functions. However, results in P3 and P4 do not concur with this hypothesis: P3 with a LGG presented disturbances of memory, attention, and executive functions whereas P4 with a HGG demonstrated overall intact cognitive performance. It is possible in this case (P4) that, due to fast tumor growth, mainly suppression of functional areas occurs, whereas the integrity of white matter bundles associated with function remains intact. Herbet et al. [28] showed via a probabilistic atlas that reorganization at subcortical level, in proximity to white matter tracts, could be less optimal than at cortical level. In addition, Trinh et al. [29] demonstrated that a subcortical injury was an independent predictor for longer-term neurological impairments underlining the importance of preservation of subcortical tracts. It may also be possible that genetic tumor mutation is associated with cognition: IDH1-mutant wild-type (isocitrate dehydrogenase), more aggressive than IDH1-mutant tumors, appeared to be associated with more severe cognitive impairments possibly hindering neuroplasticity [30].

Another intervening factor influencing preoperative cognitive performance could be tumor volume. Habets et al. [13] found that larger brain tumors in the left hemisphere were associated with poorer executive functioning. This explanation may hold for P2 who has a relatively large preoperative tumor volume and is suffering from more serious cognitive deficits compared to P1 with a smaller tumor and intact cognition. However, P3 and P4 showed the reversed pattern, with P4 having a larger tumor with intact cognitive performance and P3 with a smaller tumor and deficits.

EoR may have played a role as P2 and P4 underwent a more extensive tumor resection than P1 and P3. However, a recent follow-up study did not reveal a relation between EoR and cognitive decline [5]. Currently, there is only evidence that a more extensive resection is associated with longer survival in both LGG and HGG patients [31]. In addition, in all patients resection was conducted according to individual subcortical functional boundaries.

In general, (stimulation-induced) seizures and the use of anticonvulsants can be a risk factor for deficits in cognitive performance [32]. Deficits in information processing, attention, and executive functions were found to be related to the use of anticonvulsants in long-term glioma survivors (at least 1 year after diagnosis) in the absence of seizures [33]. In our patients, the use of medication may have added to cognitive defects or postoperative decline. However, all patients took anticonvulsants both before and after surgery, which makes it hard to draw any firm conclusions. Apart from antiepileptic drugs, radiotherapy may also have had negative effects on cognitive performance [34]. P1, P2, and P4 were treated with radiotherapy, of whom P2 and P4, but not P1, showed postoperative cognitive deterioration during the administration of irradiation. In addition, in all patients a "safe" fraction dose of maximally 2 Gy per session was administered, which is known to be associated with relative stable cognition for several years after irradiation [35].

Finally, some other factors should be taken into account when interpreting our results. Handedness may have interfered with the results, as P1 was left-handed as opposed to P2–P4. Language organization in left-handed people is not always consistent and can be represented in a more widespread network than in right-handed people [36]. However, all patients had tumors in the language dominant hemisphere as attested with fMRI. The detection of crossed cerebellar activation may add to the identification of language lateralization in (left-handed) brain tumor patients [37]. From these 4 cases, it is clear that cognitive functions cannot be related to a certain location in the brain. Unfortunately, we do not know when and until which period improvement of specific cognitive functions exactly takes place. Follow-up measurements were not administered at similar time-points in all patients, namely, 6 weeks or 3 months for early and 6 months or 1 year for late follow-up. However, a recent outcome study found that the postoperative interval of 3 and 6 months is crucial for language improvement, whereas recovery of the executive functions appeared to take longer than 6 months [38]. Evidently, larger subgroups with patients with a comparable brain tumor localization and, for instance, tumor grade need to be analyzed to investigate the different courses that underlie functional neural plasticity. No postoperative fMRI and diffusion tensor imaging studies were available; therefore, it is difficult to account for reorganization at both the structural and functional level.

Patients with brain tumors in "classical" language areas do not necessarily present language (or other cognitive) disturbances. Surgery can either improve or deteriorate (existing) cognitive (impairments) functions. The findings of these case studies provide therefore further support for neural plasticity within a "hodotopical" framework. It remains uncertain to which extent and which factors, such as localization, tumor grade, volume, EoR, and/or adjuvant therapy, contribute to neural plasticity. Hence, an extensive examination of cognitive functions with larger (sub)groups taking into account localization, tumor, and treatment related factors will elucidate prognostic factors of the plastic potential of the brain.

References

[1] P. C. De Witt Hamer, S. G. Robles, A. H. Zwinderman, H. Duffau, and M. S. Berger, "Impact of intraoperative stimulation brain mapping on glioma surgery outcome: A meta-analysis," *Journal of Clinical Oncology*, vol. 30, no. 20, pp. 2559–2565, 2012.

[2] H. Duffau, "Surgery of low-grade gliomas: towards a 'functional neurooncolngy'," *Current Opinion in Oncology*, vol. 21, no. 6, pp. 543–549, 2009.

[3] A. Talacchi, B. Santini, S. Savazzi, and M. Gerosa, "Cognitive effects of tumour and surgical treatment in glioma patients," *Journal of Neuro-Oncology*, vol. 103, no. 3, pp. 541–549, 2011.

[4] C. Papagno, A. Casarotti, A. Comi, M. Gallucci, M. Riva, and L. Bello, "Measuring clinical outcomes in neuro-oncology. A battery to evaluate low-grade gliomas (LGG)," *Journal of Neuro-Oncology*, vol. 108, no. 2, pp. 269–275, 2012.

[5] D. Satoer, E. Visch-Brink, M. Smits et al., "Long-term evaluation of cognition after glioma surgery in eloquent areas," *Journal of Neuro-Oncology*, vol. 116, no. 1, pp. 153–160, 2014.

[6] H. Duffau, "The huge plastic potential of adult brain and the role of connectomics: new insights provided by serial mappings in glioma surgery," *Cortex*, vol. 58, pp. 325–337, 2014.

[7] M. C. Tate, G. Herbet, S. Moritz-Gasser, J. E. Tate, and H. Duffau, "Probabilistic map of critical functional regions of the human cerebral cortex: Broca's area revisited," *Brain*, vol. 137, part 10, pp. 2773–2782, 2014.

[8] A. Bizzi, S. Nava, F. Ferrè et al., "Aphasia induced by gliomas growing in the ventrolateral frontal region: Assessment with diffusion MR tractography, functional MR imaging and neuropsychology," *Cortex*, vol. 48, no. 2, pp. 255–272, 2012.

[9] E. Mandonnet, J.-Y. Delattre, M.-L. Tanguy et al., "Continuous growth of mean tumor diameter in a subset of grade II gliomas," *Annals of Neurology*, vol. 53, no. 4, pp. 524–528, 2003.

[10] M. Desmurget, F. Bonnetblanc, and H. Duffau, "Contrasting acute and slow-growing lesions: a new door to brain plasticity," *Brain*, vol. 130, no. 4, pp. 898–914, 2007.

[11] D. Satoer, A. Vincent, M. Smits, C. Dirven, and E. Visch-Brink, "Spontaneous speech of patients with gliomas in eloquent areas before and early after surgery," *Acta Neurochirurgica*, vol. 155, no. 4, pp. 685–692, 2013.

[12] D. Satoer, E. Visch-Brink, C. Dirven, and A. Vincent, "Glioma surgery in eloquent areas: can we preserve cognition?" *Acta Neurochirurgica*, vol. 158, no. 1, pp. 35–50, 2016.

[13] E. J. J. Habets, A. Kloet, R. Walchenbach, C. J. Vecht, M. Klein, and M. J. B. Taphoorn, "Tumour and surgery effects on cognitive functioning in high-grade glioma patients," *Acta Neurochirurgica*, vol. 156, no. 8, pp. 1451–1459, 2014.

[14] E. C. Miotto, A. S. Junior, C. C. Silva et al., "Cognitive impairments in patients with low grade gliomas and high grade gliomas," *Arquivos de Neuro-Psiquiatria*, vol. 69, no. 4, pp. 596–601, 2011.

[15] J. J. Heimans and M. J. B. Taphoorn, "Impact of brain tumour treatment on quality of life," *Journal of Neurology*, vol. 249, no. 8, pp. 955–960, 2002.

[16] E. De Witte, D. Satoer, E. Robert et al., "The Dutch linguistic intraoperative protocol: a valid linguistic approach to awake brain surgery," *Brain and Language*, vol. 140, pp. 35–48, 2015.

[17] S. Graetz, P. De Bleser, and K. Willmes, *Akense Afasie Test*, Lisse: Swets & Zeitlinger, Dutch edition edition, 1991.

[18] E. Kaplan, H. Goodglass, and S. Weintraub, *Boston Naming Test*, Lippincott, Williams and Wilkins, Philadelphia-Tokyo, 2001.

[19] M. D. Lezak, *Neuropsychological Assessment*, Oxford University Press, New York, 2004.

[20] S. Goebel, R. Fischer, R. Ferstl, and H. M. Mehdorn, "Normative data and psychometric properties for qualitative and quantitative scoring criteria of the Five-point Test," *Clinical Neuropsychologist*, vol. 23, no. 4, pp. 675–690, 2009.

[21] S. Sarubbo, F. Latini, E. Sette et al., "Is the resection of gliomas in Wernicke's area reliable? Wernicke's area resection," *Acta Neurochirurgica*, vol. 154, no. 9, pp. 1653–1662, 2012.

[22] A. F. Coello, S. Moritz-Gasser, J. Martino, M. Martinoni, R. Matsuda, and H. Duffau, "Selection of intraoperative tasks for awake mapping based on relationships between tumor location and functional networks: A review," *Journal of Neurosurgery*, vol. 119, no. 6, pp. 1380–1394, 2013.

[23] J. Sierpowska, A. Gabarros, A. Fernandez-Coello et al., "Words are not enough: nonword repetition as an indicator of arcuate fasciculus integrity during brain tumor resection," *Journal of Neurosurgery*, pp. 1–11, 2016.

[24] S. Sarubbo, A. De Benedictis, S. Merler et al., "Towards a functional atlas of human white matter," *Human Brain Mapping*, vol. 36, no. 8, pp. 3117–3136, 2015.

[25] A. M. Rauschecker, G. K. Deutsch, M. Ben-Shachar, A. Schwartzman, L. M. Perry, and R. F. Dougherty, "Reading impairment in a patient with missing arcuate fasciculus," *Neuropsychologia*, vol. 47, no. 1, pp. 180–194, 2009.

[26] J. Ilmberger, M. Ruge, F.-W. Kreth, J. Briegel, H.-J. Reulen, and J.-C. Tonn, "Intraoperative mapping of language functions: A longitudinal neurolinguistic analysis - Clinical article," *Journal of Neurosurgery*, vol. 109, no. 4, pp. 583–592, 2008.

[27] K. R. Noll, C. Sullaway, M. Ziu, J. S. Weinberg, and J. S. Wefel, "Relationships between tumor grade and neurocognitive functioning in patients with glioma of the left temporal lobe prior to surgical resection," *Neuro-Oncology*, vol. 17, no. 4, pp. 580–587, 2014.

[28] G. Herbet, M. Maheu, E. Costi, G. Lafargue, and H. Duffau, "Mapping neuroplastic potential in brain-damaged patients," *Brain*, vol. 139, no. 3, pp. 829–844, 2016.

[29] V. T. Trinh, D. K. Fahim, K. Shah et al., "Subcortical injury is an independent predictor of worsening neurological deficits following awake craniotomy procedures," *Neurosurgery*, vol. 72, no. 2, pp. 160–169, 2013.

[30] J. S. Wefel, K. R. Noll, G. Rao, and D. P. Cahill, "Neurocognitive function varies by IDH1 genetic mutation status in patients with malignant glioma prior to surgical resection," *Neuro Oncology*, 2016.

[31] N. Sanai and M. S. Berger, "Glioma extent of resection and its impact on patient outcome," *Neurosurgery*, vol. 62, no. 4, pp. 753–764, 2008.

[32] K. J. Meador, "Cognitive outcomes and predictive factors in epilepsy," *Neurology*, vol. 58, no. 8, pp. S21–S26, 2002.

[33] M. Klein, N. H. J. Engelberts, H. M. Van der Ploeg et al., "Epilepsy in low-grade gliomas: The impact on cognitive function and quality of life," *Annals of Neurology*, vol. 54, no. 4, pp. 514–520, 2003.

[34] M. J. B. Taphoorn and M. Klein, "Cognitive deficits in adult patients with brain tumours," *The Lancet Neurology*, vol. 3, no. 3, pp. 159–168, 2004.

[35] L. Douw, "Cognitive and radiological effects of radiotherapy in patients with low-grade glioma: long-term follow-up," *Lancet Neurol*, vol. 8, no. 9, pp. 810–818, 2009.

[36] J. P. Szaflarski, J. R. Binder, E. T. Possing, K. A. McKiernan, B. D. Ward, and T. A. Hammeke, "Language lateralization in left-handed and ambidextrous people: fMRI data," *Neurology*, vol. 59, no. 2, pp. 238–244, 2002.

[37] C. Méndez Orellana, E. Visch-Brink, M. Vernooij et al., "Crossed Cerebrocerebellar Language Lateralization: An Additional Diagnostic Feature for Assessing Atypical Language Representation in Presurgical Functional MR Imaging," *American Journal of Neuroradiology*, vol. 36, no. 3, pp. 518–524, 2015.

[38] E. De Witte, *Speaking the language of the brain. A neurolinguistic approach to the assessment of braintumour patients undergoing awake surgery. Doctoral Dissertation [Doctoral, thesis]*, Brussels University Press: VUBPRESS, 2015.

Adult Primary Spinal Epidural Extraosseous Ewing's Sarcoma: A Case Report and Review of the Literature

Mark Bustoros,[1] Cheddhi Thomas,[2] Joshua Frenster,[1] Aram S. Modrek,[1] N. Sumru Bayin,[1] Matija Snuderl,[2,3,4] Gerald Rosen,[3,5] Peter B. Schiff,[3,6] and Dimitris G. Placantonakis[1,3,4,7]

[1] *Department of Neurosurgery, NYU School of Medicine, New York, NY 10016, USA*
[2] *Department of Pathology, NYU School of Medicine, New York, NY 10016, USA*
[3] *Perlmutter Cancer Center, NYU Langone Medical Center, New York, NY 10016, USA*
[4] *Brain Tumor Center, NYU Langone Medical Center, New York, NY 10016, USA*
[5] *Department of Medicine, NYU School of Medicine, New York, NY 10016, USA*
[6] *Department of Radiation Oncology, NYU School of Medicine, New York, NY 10016, USA*
[7] *Kimmel Center for Stem Cell Biology, NYU School of Medicine, New York, NY 10016, USA*

Correspondence should be addressed to Dimitris G. Placantonakis; dimitris.placantonakis@nyumc.org

Academic Editor: Abbass Amirjamshidi

Background. Extraosseous Ewing's sarcoma in the spinal epidural space is a rare malignancy, especially in adults. *Case Presentation.* A 40-year-old male presented with back pain and urinary hesitancy. MRI revealed a thoracic extradural mass with no osseous involvement. He underwent surgery for gross total resection of the mass, which was diagnosed as Ewing's sarcoma. He was subsequently treated with chemoradiotherapy. He remains disease-free 1 year after surgery. Review of the literature indicated only 45 previously reported cases of spinal epidural extraosseous Ewing's sarcoma in adults. *Conclusions.* Extraosseous Ewing's sarcoma in the spinal epidural space is a rare clinical entity that should be included in the differential for spinal epidural masses. Its treatment is multidisciplinary but frequently requires surgical intervention due to compressive neurologic symptoms. Gross total resection appears to correlate with improved outcomes.

1. Introduction

Ewing's sarcoma (ES) is a malignant bone tumor of childhood and adolescence that occurs primarily in the diaphysis of long bones, such as femur, tibia, fibula, and humerus, but may also occur in other bony structures and cartilage tissue. This tumor was named after James Ewing, who in the 1920s described this small round blue cell tumor as being a separate entity from other histologically similar malignancies, such as lymphoma or neuroblastoma. It is the second most common malignant bone tumor after osteosarcoma, with the highest incidence in the second decade of life [1, 2]. The American Cancer Society estimates that 225 new cases are diagnosed annually in North America [1].

ES is the main member of a group of tumors known as Ewing's Sarcoma Family Tumors (ESFTs), which also contains peripheral primitive neuroectodermal tumors (pPNET). ES and pPNET are small round blue cell tumors; they were originally described as different entities; however, they are now recognized to represent ends of the morphologic spectrum of the ESFTs due to their close molecular relationship [3–7]. Some authors even assume pPNET and ES to be the same tumor with variable neural differentiation, a view that has been recently supported by immunohistochemical and cytogenetic findings [3]. The ESFT now includes osseous Ewing's sarcoma, EES, pPNET and Askin's tumor [7–9].

Ewing's sarcoma has two forms: the more common osseous Ewing's sarcoma (OES) and the relatively rare extraosseous Ewing's sarcoma (EES). EES has been reported in various tissues, including the chest wall, larynx, kidney, and esophagus. EES was first described by Tefft et al. in 1969, when they reported four patients with paravertebral soft tissue tumors

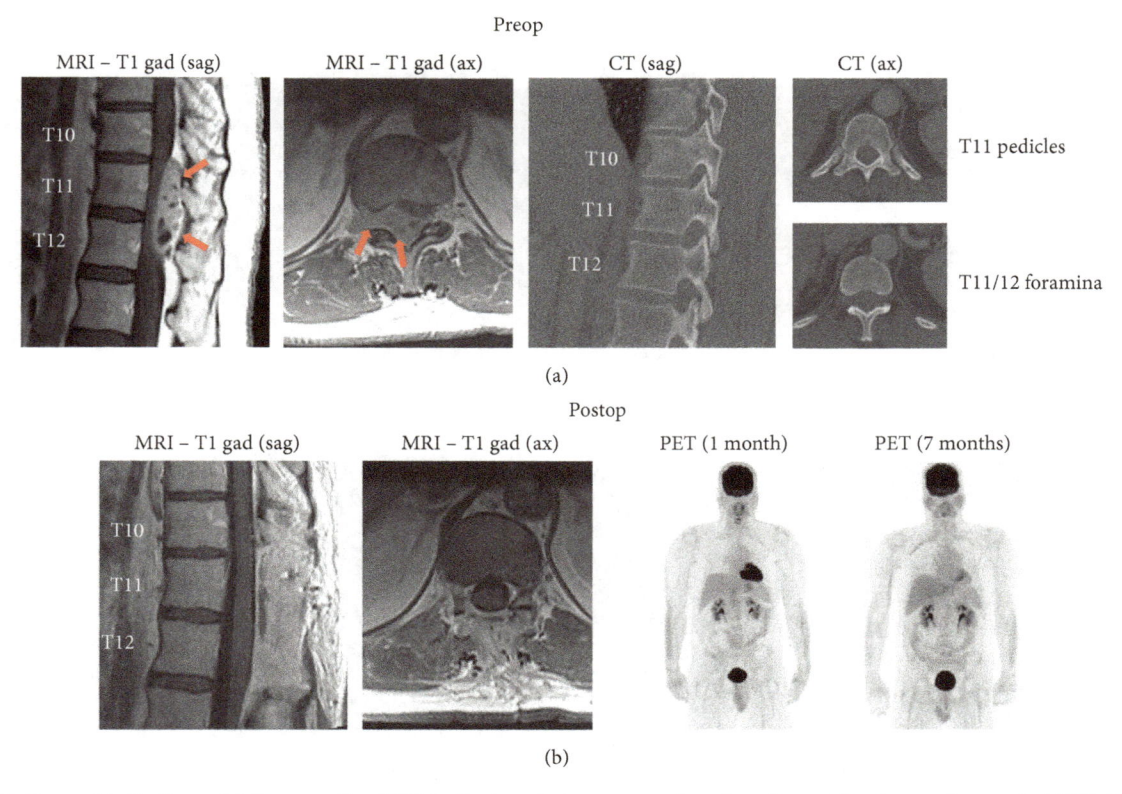

FIGURE 1: Radiographic findings. (a) Preoperative MRI indicates a heterogeneously enhancing epidural mass (arrows) at T10–12 extending from the spinal canal into the right T11-12 foramen. CT shows that the osseous elements are intact. (b) Postoperative imaging shows T10–12 laminectomies and gross total resection of the lesion. PET imaging 1 and 7 months after resection shows no abnormal FDG uptake. Sag: sagittal, ax: axial, and gad: gadolinium.

histologically resembling ES [10]. Angervall and Enzinger in 1975 were the first to name this entity EES when they reviewed 39 patients with malignant soft tissue paravertebral tumors not arising from bone but having similar histologic characteristics to OES [11].

Spinal epidural EES in adults is a rare presentation among those locations where EES may occur. Here, we present an adult patient we recently treated, who represents only the 46th case of adult spinal epidural EES in the literature. Neurosurgeons should be aware of this rare clinical entity, which often presents with myelopathic and radicular symptoms associated with an epidural mass on imaging studies. Our review sheds light on the diagnosis, management, and prognosis of these cases.

2. Case Presentation

The patient is a 40-year-old male, previously healthy, who presented to the emergency department with several weeks of back pain and some urinary hesitancy lasting a few days. MRI of the thoracic spine indicated a heterogeneously enhancing extradural mass within the spinal canal at T10–T12, causing severe cord compression (Figure 1(a)). The mass was extended through the right neural foramina at T11-12 and T12-L1. CT did not suggest osseous involvement (Figure 1(a)). There were no other spinal lesions on MRI. CT of the chest, abdomen, and pelvis did not reveal any extraspinal sites suspicious for tumor growth. There were a number of somewhat enlarged periceliac lymph nodes of uncertain significance.

The patient underwent a T10–12 laminectomy for gross total resection of the tumor (Figure 1(b)), with preservation of motor and sensory function, resolution of urinary hesitancy, and significant improvement in the back pain. Resection of the foraminal component of the tumor required ligation and amputation of the right T11 nerve root.

Pathologic examination indicated a small round blue cell neoplasm (Figure 2(a)) composed of primitive densely packed cells with a very high mitotic index (60–70% of cells positive for Ki67) (Figure 2(b)). Molecular studies showed the EWSR1 rearrangement, confirming the diagnosis of Ewing's sarcoma. The tumor itself was negative for S100/chromogranin/synaptophysin and CD45/CD20, thus ruling out the small round blue cell tumors: pPNET and lymphoma, respectively. Microscopic analysis of the resected right T11 nerve root showed tumor invasion through the perineurium (Figures 2(c) and 2(d)).

Postoperative MRI and PET scan did not reveal residual or metastatic tumor (Figure 1(b)). The previously noted periceliac lymph nodes did not show increased FDG uptake on PET scan. Six weeks after surgery he started adjuvant chemotherapy consisting of ifosfamide (supplemented with mesna), cyclophosphamide, doxorubicin, and irinotecan.

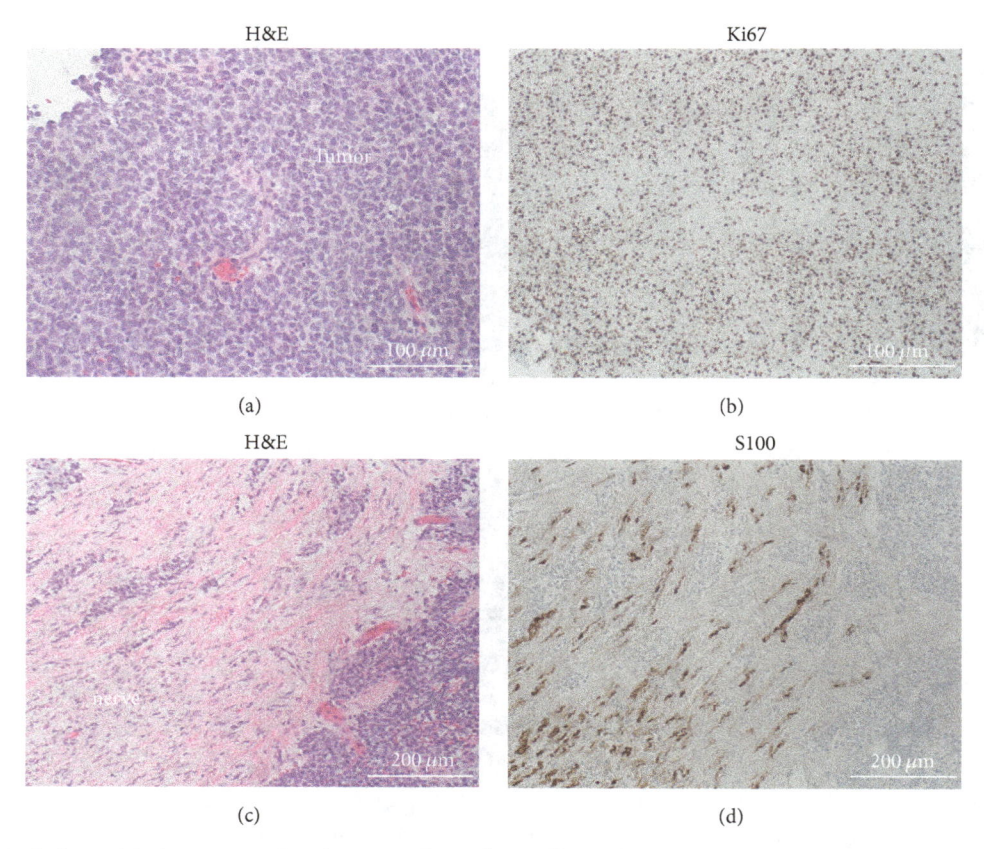

FIGURE 2: Histologic findings. (a) H&E stain within the tumor shows the small round blue cell appearance. (b) Ki67 immunostaining indicates a very high mitotic index (60–70%). (c) H&E stain demonstrates tumor invasion through the perineurium and into the right T11 nerve root. (d) Tumor invasion in the T11 nerve root is demonstrated by tumor cells interspersed within S100-positive Schwann cells. The tumor itself was S100-negative. H&E: hematoxylin & eosin.

Eleven weeks after surgery he began adjuvant radiotherapy (45 Gy in 25 doses). He has tolerated all treatments well. He has no evidence of disease on repeat PET scan and MRI of the thoracic spine one year after surgery.

3. Discussion

3.1. Epidemiology. Spinal epidural EES in adults represents a very small fraction of spinal epidural masses and a rare presentation among those locations where EES may occur. We performed literature searches on PubMed to identify reports of spinal EES. We identified 119 cases of spinal EES in the literature from 1969 to 2015. In 43 of these cases the tumor was intradural, while it was localized to the epidural space in 76 cases. Of the epidural EES cases, 31 cases were pediatric patients and 45 were adults (Table 1). Treatment of these patients commonly required a combination of surgery, chemotherapy, and radiotherapy. The case we present here is the 77th reported case of spinal epidural EES and only the 46th case of adult epidural EES in the literature.

The review of the literature on combined pediatric and adult spinal EES/pPNET showed that the lumbar region is the most common site, followed by the thoracic and cervical spine, with the sacral region being the least common (5% of cases) [7, 12]. However, in our analysis of the 46 adult epidural EES/pPNET cases (including our case), we found that the most common site was the thoracic spine (17 cases), followed by lumbar (13 cases), cervical (13 cases), and sacral segments (3 cases).

Spinal EES in adults shows a predilection for males (61% of the cases), with a male : female ratio of 1.6 : 1, similar to that of OES [13, 14]. The average age at diagnosis was 29 years in contrast to 12 years for OES, and the oldest age reported was 65 years [12]. Interestingly, although it is stated that ES is rare in the Asian population [13, 14], we have found that half of the spinal EES patients in our study are Asians. However, no comprehensive epidemiological conclusions can be extracted due to the paucity of cases reported in the literature.

The mean diagnostic delay calculated from the previous cases is 4.5 months [7], which is explained by nonspecific symptoms at disease onset. The symptoms commonly include back and/or radicular pain in all patients, paresis in about 70%, sensory disturbances in 35%, and to lesser extent bladder and bowel dysfunction in about 12% of patients [7, 15]. One case presented with infection superimposed upon spinal epidural EES [16]. Distant metastases occurred in nearly 40% of the cases, either during or after diagnosis. Lung, spine, and brain were the most frequent sites of metastasis [7].

TABLE 1: Cases of adult primary spinal epidural EES/PNET tumors in the literature.

Author	Year	Age (years)/sex (M or F)	Location/diagnosis	Treatment	Follow-up (months)	Outcome	CD99	t(11:22)	Country*
Angervall and Enzinger [11]	1975	20/M	T2–T5/EES	STR/RT/CT	12	DOD	NA	NA	Sweden
Angervall and Enzinger [11]	1975	18/F	L5/EES	GTR/RT/CT	6	DOD	NA	NA	Sweden
Scheithauer and Egbert [29]	1978	18/M	L1/EES	GTR/RT/CT	16	NED	NA	NA	USA
Scheithauer and Egbert [29]	1978	27/F	T4–T6/EES	STR/RT/CT	132	NED	NA	NA	USA
Mahoney et al. [30]	1978	23/M	S1/EES	Biopsy/RT/CT	12	DOD	NA	NA	USA
Fink and Meriwether [31]	1979	19/M	L2-L3/EES	STR/RT/CT	12	NED	NA	NA	USA
N'Golet et al. [32]	1982	29/M	T1–T3/EES	GTR/RT/CT	6	NED	NA	NA	France
N'Golet et al. [32]	1982	47/F	L4/EES	GTR/RT/CT	4	DOD	NA	NA	France
Sharma et al. [33]	1986	18/M	T10/EES	STR/RT/CT	42	DOD	NA	NA	India
Liu et al. [34]	1987	26/F	L5-S1/PNET	STR/RT	6	NED	NA	NA	Taiwan
Christie et al. [35]	1997	36/F	L2-L3/EES	STR/RT	96	DOD	NA	NA	Australia
Dorfmüller et al. [3]	1999	18/M	L3-L4/PNET	GTR/RT/CT	23	NED	+	+	Austria
Kennedy et al. [36]	2000	24/M	C1–C5/EES	STR/RT/CT	13	NED	NA	NA	Ireland
Shin et al. [37]	2001	38/M	C5-C6/EES	STR/CT	17	NED	+	NA	South Korea
Shin et al. [37]	2001	22/F	C7-T1/EES	STR/CT	48	NED	+	NA	South Korea
Morandi et al. [38]	2001	22/F	T4-T5/EES	GTR/RT/CT	66	NED	+	NA	France
Morandi et al. [38]	2001	25/F	L1-S2/EES	STR/CT	7	DOD	+	NA	France
Mukhopadhyay et al. [15]	2001	29/F	C3–C5/EES	STR/RT/CT	30	NED	+	NA	India
Mukhopadhyay et al. [15]	2001	18/M	T8-T9/EES	STR/RT/CT	18	NED	+	NA	India
Mukhopadhyay et al. [15]	2001	22/M	L5-S1/EES	Biopsy/RT/CT	15	NED	+	NA	India
Mukhopadhyay et al. [15]	2001	31/M	L3-L4/EES	STR/RT/CT	32	NED	+	NA	India
Gandhi et al. [39]	2003	33/M	T5–T10/EES	GTR/RT/CT	3	NED	+	NA	Canada
Weber et al. [40]	2004	26/M	L1-L2/PNET	GTR/RT/CT	16	NED	+	NA	Switzerland
Koudelova et al. [41]	2006	28/F	L1-L2/PNET	STR/RT/CT	24	NED	NA	NA	Czech Republic
Isefuku et al. [5]	2006	20/M	L5-S1/EES	STR/CT	15	DOD	+	+	Japan
Ozturk et al. [8]	2007	18/M	C6-T1/EES	GTR/CT	13	NED	+	NA	Turkey
Lakhdar et al. [16]	2008	24/F	C6-C7/EES	GTR/CT/RT	NA	NA	NA	NA	Morocco
Bozkurt et al. [42]	2007	28/M	C3–C5/EES	GTR/RT/CT	18	NED	+	NA	Turkey
Feng et al. [43]	2008	24/M	T8–T10/PNET	GTR/RT	14	NED	NA	NA	China

TABLE 1: Continued.

Author	Year	Age (years)/sex (M or F)	Location/diagnosis	Treatment	Follow-up (months)	Outcome	CD99	t(11;22)	Country*
Musahl et al. [44]	2008	27/M	S1-S2/PNET	GTR/RT/CT	24	NED	NA	NA	USA
Theeler et al. [9]	2009	28/F	T6/NS	GTR/CT	2	NED	+	+	USA
Kiatsoontorn et al. [45]	2009	25/M	T7/PNET	GTR/RT/CT	6	NED	+	NA	Japan
Jingyu et al. [19]	2009	58y/M	T4/PNET	GTR Only	25	NED	+	NA	China
Duan et al. [4]	2011	26/F	T4–T7/PNET	STR/RT/CT	3	NED	+	NA	China
Duan et al. [4]	2011	34/M	T12/PNET	STR Only	1	NED	+	NA	China
Yasuda et al. [20]	2011	37/F	T8-T9/EES	STR/RT/CT	22	DOD	+	+	Japan
Bostelmann et al. [46]	2011	29/M	C7/EES	STR/RT/CT	6	DOD	+	NA	Germany
Saeedinia et al. [7]	2012	44/F	S1–S3/NS	GTR/RT	9	NED	+	NA	Iran
Zhu et al. [21]	2012	46/M	C3–C6/EES	STR/RT/CT	12	DOD	+	NA	China
Zhu et al. [21]	2012	27/M	C1–C4/EES	GTR/RT/CT	10	NED	+	NA	China
Zhu et al. [21]	2012	27/M	C7/EES	GTR/RT/CT	24	NED	+	NA	China
Zhu et al. [21]	2012	24y/M	C5/EES	STR/RT/CT	7	DOD	+	NA	China
Kazanci et al. [12]	2015	34/F	T4–T6/EES	GTR/RT/CT	18	NED	+	NA	Turkey
Kazanci et al. [12]	2015	65/F	T7-T8/EES	GTR/RT/CT	14	NED	+	NA	Turkey
García-Moreno et al. [47]	2015	45/F	C6-T3/EES	STR/RT/CT	8	NED	+	+	Spain
Present case	2015	40/M	T10–T12/EES	GTR/RT/CT	12	NED	NA	+	USA

M: male. F: female. EES: extraskeletal Ewing's sarcoma. PNET: peripheral neuroectodermal tumor. GTR: gross total resection. STR: subtotal (partial) resection. RT: radiotherapy. CT: chemotherapy. NED: no evidence of disease. DOD: dead of disease. NS: not specified.
*Country: the country where the cases were reported and studied.

3.2. Histopathology. Ewing's sarcoma shows vague lobular proliferation of uniform small round blue cells with clear to lightly eosinophilic cytoplasm, evenly dispersed chromatin, and indistinct nucleoli. Peripheral PNET may specifically contain neuroblastic pseudorosettes termed Homer-Wright rosettes [3, 15, 17].

Immunohistochemical studies show that EES/PNETs strongly express cell surface glycoprotein CD99 (MIC2). This biomarker is considered one of the most accurate diagnostic tools and is positive in more than 90% of EES/pPNET cases. However, it is not exclusively specific for these tumors [18].

Approximately 25% of EES/pPNETs demonstrate aberrant expression of keratins, typically considered an epithelial marker. Expression of at least two different neuroglial antigens, such as neuron-specific enolase (NSE), protein S100, chromogranin, or synaptophysin, is required to distinguish pPNET from ES, with the former typically showing more neuronal differentiation [3, 4, 6, 15, 17, 19]. The tumor of the patient presented here was negative for S100, chromogranin, and synaptophysin, suggesting that the EES diagnosis was favored over pPNET.

At the genetic level, more than 90% of ES/pPNETs contain the same t(11;22)(q24;q12) translocation. Other translocations occur in 5–10% of cases [13]. The t(11;22)(q24;q12) translocation results in the formation of a chimeric gene (EWSR1-FLI1), which has been found to act as an oncogenic transcription factor in ES and pPNET [5, 6, 20]. This translocation can be detected by fluorescent in situ hybridization (FISH) in the nuclei of neoplastic cells. In its latest guidelines, ESMO (European Society for Medical Oncology) recommends that molecular studies be done to confirm the diagnosis of ESFTs through detection of this stereotypical translocation by FISH or RT-PCR [13].

3.3. Imaging Studies. Imaging studies are quintessential in such cases. MRI plays a prominent role in diagnosis, determination of the anatomic relationships with surrounding structures, and preoperative surgical planning. Commonly, EES/pPNET tumors have hypo- or isointense signal on T1-weighted imaging and a hyperintense signal on T2-weighted imaging and enhance heterogeneously. However, these MRI findings are nonspecific. In 15 case reports documenting MRI features of spinal epidural EES, the tumors were dumbbell-shaped and extended from the central canal toward widened foramina. In 3 cases, scalloping of bone was seen [20, 21].

Some reports suggest that the combination of FDG-PET with conventional imaging is a superior and valuable tool for disease staging and detecting metastases [22, 23].

In a recent study, O'Neill et al. proposed the concept of targeted imaging, using ^{64}Cu-radiolabeled anti-CD99 antibody to detect these tumors and potential metastases. They found higher sensitivity with this approach as compared to FDG-PET in preclinical models [24].

3.4. Treatment and Prognosis. Surgical intervention is considered the primary and main approach in the management of these cases, particularly to relieve cord compression symptoms, as well as for cytoreductive purposes. Our analysis of previous cases showed that gross total resection (GTR) correlates with a much better outcome and decrease in recurrence rate than subtotal (partial) resection. Of the reported 46 cases in this paper, 45% had a subtotal resection (STR), while 55% of the cases had a GTR. Although partial resection has an increased risk of recurrence, complete resection is often precluded by tumor infiltration to the surrounding neural and paraspinal tissues.

Evidence from the literature strongly supports the use of local RT and systemic chemotherapy for treatment of EES/pPNET. Chemotherapy regimens for OES are often followed in adults with EES/pPNET. In the past, a traditional regimen was VACA (vincristine, actinomycin, cyclophosphamide, and/or doxorubicin). The addition of ifosfamide and/or etoposide to that regimen was the subject of many studies. In 1998, Ferrari et al. reported that ifosfamide/etoposide added to the induction, and maintenance phase of chemotherapy along with VACA resulted in a significantly better outcome in terms of histologic response and overall survival (OS) [25]. Other studies showed that adding ifosfamide and/or etoposide resulted in significant higher 5-year progression-free survival (PFS) and OS in nonmetastatic ESFTs. However, it did not improve outcomes in metastatic cases [15, 26].

Currently, the guidelines for treatment of ESFTs consider VAC/IE as the preferred first-line regimen for localized disease, concurrently with radiotherapy (45 Gy in 25 fractions). Regimens such as VAdriaC (vincristine, adriamycin, and cyclophosphamide) are used to treat metastatic disease [27]. Most of the recent adult spinal epidural EES/pPNET cases we reviewed followed such protocols postoperatively. We found that neoadjuvant chemotherapy was not used in any of these cases, despite its frequent use in the treatment of OES and other forms of EES. We postulate that neoadjuvant therapy may be of limited use in spinal epidural EES, due to the superior need for surgical decompression of the spinal cord.

Patients who underwent combined chemoradiotherapy after GTR or STR had better 1-year survival rates than patients treated with surgery, chemotherapy, or radiotherapy alone (88% versus 70%, resp.) [7]. In our study, 34 (74%) patients received combined chemoradiotherapy after GTR or STR; 2 (4%) cases underwent surgery only while chemotherapy and radiotherapy were given alone after surgery to 6 (13%) and 4 (9%) cases, respectively.

The prognosis of adult spinal epidural EES/pPNET is poor compared to OES. A study at Dana-Farber Cancer Center concluded that age plays an important prognostic factor, as survival rates are reduced in older adults. Also, primary extraosseous tumor and metastatic disease at diagnosis were adverse prognostic factors, even though both chemotherapy and radiotherapy were administered to patients with those three risk factors [28]. Another study reported that the 2-year survival rate in all spinal EES/pPNET cases was only 50% [7]. Furthermore, the 5-year survival rate in spinal epidural EES/pPNET is considered poor compared to other malignancies within the ESFT family. The 5-year survival rate of EES has been between 38% and 67%; however, the 5-year survival rate in spinal EES/pPNET ranged between 0 and 37.5% [20] (see also the follow-up and outcome data in Table 1).

4. Conclusions

Although primary spinal epidural EES/pPNET in adults is extremely rare, it should be considered in the differential diagnosis of patients with a history of nonspecific back pain and/or radicular pain, especially if accompanied by abnormal neurological examination and an epidural mass on MRI. The disease has an aggressive course, as evidenced by a high incidence of metastases and low survival rates reported in the literature. Early recognition of the disease entity and definitive management is essential. A multidisciplinary approach is the best strategy to manage epidural EES/pPNET, with surgical excision often being the initial intervention, due to neurological symptoms arising from spinal cord compression. Surgical resection should be followed by a combination of adjuvant chemotherapy and radiotherapy to improve overall outcome.

Competing Interests

The authors declare that they have no competing interests.

References

[1] N. Esiashvili, M. Goodman, and R. B. Marcus Jr., "Changes in incidence and survival of Ewing sarcoma patients over the past 3 decades: surveillance epidemiology and end results data," *Journal of Pediatric Hematology/Oncology*, vol. 30, no. 6, pp. 425–430, 2008.

[2] R. D. Riley, S. A. Burchill, K. R. Abrams et al., "A systematic review of molecular and biological markers in tumours of the Ewing's sarcoma family," *European Journal of Cancer*, vol. 39, no. 1, pp. 19–30, 2003.

[3] G. Dorfmüller, F. G. Würtz, H. W. Umschaden, R. Kleinert, and P. F. Ambros, "Intraspinal primitive neuroectodermal tumour: report of two cases and review of the literature," *Acta Neurochirurgica*, vol. 141, no. 11, pp. 1169–1175, 1999.

[4] X. H. Duan, X. H. Ban, B. Liu et al., "Intraspinal primitive neuroectodermal tumor: imaging findings in six cases," *European Journal of Radiology*, vol. 80, no. 2, pp. 426–431, 2011.

[5] S. Isefuku, M. Seki, T. Tajino et al., "Ewing's sarcoma in the spinal nerve root: a case report and review of the literature," *Tohoku Journal of Experimental Medicine*, vol. 209, no. 4, pp. 369–377, 2006.

[6] I. Machado, J. A. López-Guerrero, and A. Llombart-Bosch, "Biomarkers in the Ewing sarcoma family of tumors," *Current Biomarker Findings*, vol. 4, pp. 81–92, 2014.

[7] S. Saeedinia, M. Nouri, M. Alimohammadi, H. Moradi, and A. Amirjamshidi, "Primary spinal extradural Ewing's sarcoma (primitive neuroectodermal tumor): report of a case and meta-analysis of the reported cases in the literature," *Surgical Neurology International*, vol. 3, article 55, 2012.

[8] E. Ozturk, H. Mutlu, G. Sonmez, F. Vardar Aker, C. Cinar Basekim, and E. Kizilkaya, "Spinal epidural extraskeletal Ewing sarcoma," *Journal of Neuroradiology*, vol. 34, no. 1, pp. 63–67, 2007.

[9] B. J. Theeler, J. Keylock, S. Yoest, and M. Forouhar, "Ewing's sarcoma family tumors mimicking primary central nervous system neoplasms," *Journal of the Neurological Sciences*, vol. 284, no. 1-2, pp. 186–189, 2009.

[10] M. Tefft, G. F. Vawter, and A. Mitus, "Paravertebral 'round cell' tumors in children," *Radiology*, vol. 92, no. 7, pp. 1501–1509, 1969.

[11] L. Angervall and F. M. Enzinger, "Extraskeletal neoplasm resembling Ewing's sarcoma," *Cancer*, vol. 36, no. 1, pp. 240–251, 1975.

[12] A. Kazanci, O. Gurcan, A. G. Gurcay, S. Senturk, A. E. Yildirim, A. Kilicaslan et al., "Primary ewing sarcoma in spinal epidural space: report of three cases and review of the literature," *Primer Spinal Epidural Ewing Sarkoma*, vol. 32, no. 1, pp. 250–261, 2015.

[13] Group ESESNW, "Bone sarcomas: ESMO clinical practice guidelines for diagnosis, treatment and follow-up," *Annals of Oncology*, vol. 25, supplement 3, pp. iii113–iii123, 2014.

[14] A. V. Maheshwari and E. Y. Cheng, "Ewing sarcoma family of tumors," *Journal of the American Academy of Orthopaedic Surgeons*, vol. 18, no. 2, pp. 97–107, 2010.

[15] P. Mukhopadhyay, M. Gairola, M. C. Sharma, S. Thulkar, P. K. Julka, and G. K. Rath, "Primary spinal epidural extraosseous Ewing's sarcoma: report of five cases and literature review," *Australasian Radiology*, vol. 45, no. 3, pp. 372–379, 2001.

[16] F. Lakhdar, R. Gana, M. Laghmari, F. Moufid, R. Maaqili, and F. Bellakhdar, "Infected cervical epidural Ewing's sarcoma (case report)," *Journal of Neuroradiology*, vol. 35, no. 1, pp. 51–55, 2008.

[17] D. Schmidt, C. Herrmann, H. Jurgens, and D. Harms, "Malignant peripheral neuroectodermal tumor and its necessary distinction from Ewing's sarcoma: a report from the Kiel Pediatric Tumor Registry," *Cancer*, vol. 68, no. 10, pp. 2251–2259, 1991.

[18] S. H. Olsen, D. G. Thomas, and D. R. Lucas, "Cluster analysis of immunohistochemical profiles in synovial sarcoma, malignant peripheral nerve sheath tumor, and Ewing sarcoma," *Modern Pathology*, vol. 19, no. 5, pp. 659–668, 2006.

[19] C. Jingyu, S. Jinning, M. Hui, and F. Hua, "Intraspinal primitive neuroectodermal tumors: report of four cases and review of the literature," *Neurology India*, vol. 57, no. 5, pp. 661–668, 2009.

[20] T. Yasuda, K. Suzuki, M. Kanamori et al., "Extraskeletal Ewing's sarcoma of the thoracic epidural space: case report and review of the literature," *Oncology Reports*, vol. 26, no. 3, pp. 711–715, 2011.

[21] Q. Zhu, J. Zhang, and J. Xiao, "Primary dumbbell-shaped Ewing's sarcoma of the cervical vertebra in adults: four case reports and literature review," *Oncology Letters*, vol. 3, no. 3, pp. 721–725, 2012.

[22] D. S. Hawkins, S. M. Schuetze, J. E. Butrynski et al., "[18F]fluorodeoxyglucose positron emission tomography predicts outcome for ewing sarcoma family of tumors," *Journal of Clinical Oncology*, vol. 23, no. 34, pp. 8828–8834, 2005.

[23] G. Treglia, M. Salsano, A. Stefanelli, M. V. Mattoli, A. Giordano, and L. Bonomo, "Diagnostic accuracy of 18F-FDG-PET and PET/CT in patients with Ewing sarcoma family tumours: a systematic review and a meta-analysis," *Skeletal Radiology*, vol. 41, no. 3, pp. 249–256, 2012.

[24] A. F. O'Neill, J. L. Dearling, Y. Wang et al., "Targeted imaging of ewing sarcoma in preclinical models using a 64Cu-labeled anti-CD99 antibody," *Clinical Cancer Research*, vol. 20, no. 3, pp. 678–687, 2014.

[25] S. Ferrari, M. Mercuri, P. Rosito et al., "Ifosfamide and actinomycin-D, added in the induction phase to vincristine, cyclophosphamide and doxorubicin, improve histologic response and prognosis in patients with non metastatic Ewing's sarcoma of the extremity," *Journal of Chemotherapy*, vol. 10, no. 6, pp. 484–491, 1998.

[26] W. H. Meyer, L. Kun, N. Marina et al., "Ifosfamide plus etoposide in newly diagnosed Ewing's sarcoma of bone," *Journal of Clinical Oncology*, vol. 10, no. 11, pp. 1737–1742, 1992.

[27] J. S. Miser, M. D. Krailo, N. J. Tarbell et al., "Treatment of metastatic Ewing's sarcoma or primitive neuroectodermal tumor of bone: evaluation of combination ifosfamide and etoposide—a children's cancer group and pediatric oncology group study," *Journal of Clinical Oncology*, vol. 22, no. 14, pp. 2873–2876, 2004.

[28] E. H. Baldini, G. D. Demetri, C. D. M. Fletcher, J. Foran, K. C. Marcus, and S. Singer, "Adults with Ewing's sarcoma/primitive neuroectodermal tumor: adverse effect of older age and primary extraosseous disease on outcome," *Annals of Surgery*, vol. 230, no. 1, pp. 79–86, 1999.

[29] B. W. Scheithauer and B. M. Egbert, "Ewing's sarcoma of the spinal epidural space: report of two cases," *Journal of Neurology, Neurosurgery & Psychiatry*, vol. 41, no. 11, pp. 1031–1035, 1978.

[30] J. P. Mahoney, W. E. Ballinger Jr., and R. W. Alexander, "So-called extraskeletal Ewing's sarcoma. Report of a case with ultrastructural analysis," *American Journal of Clinical Pathology*, vol. 70, no. 6, pp. 926–931, 1978.

[31] L. H. Fink and M. W. Meriwether, "Primary epidural Ewing's sarcoma presenting as a lumbar disc protrusion. Case report," *Journal of Neurosurgery*, vol. 51, no. 1, pp. 120–123, 1979.

[32] A. N'Golet, B. Pasquier, D. Pasquier, A. Lachard, and P. Couderc, "Extraskeletal Ewing's sarcoma of the epidural space. A report of two new cases with literature review," *Archives d'Anatomie et de Cytologie Pathologiques*, vol. 30, no. 1, pp. 10–13, 1982.

[33] B. S. Sharma, V. K. Khosla, and A. K. Banerjee, "Primary spinal epidural Ewing's sarcoma," *Clinical Neurology and Neurosurgery*, vol. 88, no. 4, pp. 299–302, 1986.

[34] H.-M. Liu, W. C. Yang, R. L. Garcia, J. M. Noh, V. Malhotra, and N. E. Leeds, "Intraspinal primitive neuroectodermal tumor arising from the sacral spinal nerve root," *The Journal of Computed Tomography*, vol. 11, no. 4, pp. 350–354, 1987.

[35] D. R. H. Christie, A. M. Bilous, and P. J. A. Carr, "Diagnostic difficulties in extraosseous Ewing's sarcoma: a proposal for diagnostic criteria," *Australasian Radiology*, vol. 41, no. 1, pp. 22–28, 1997.

[36] J. G. Kennedy, S. Eustace, R. Caulfield, D. J. Fennelly, B. Hurson, and K. S. O'Rourke, "Extraskeletal Ewing's sarcoma: a case report and review of the literature," *Spine*, vol. 25, no. 15, pp. 1996–1999, 2000.

[37] J. H. Shin, H. K. Lee, S. C. Rhim, K.-J. Cho, C. G. Choi, and D. C. Suh, "Spinal epidural extraskeletal Ewing sarcoma: MR findings in two cases," *American Journal of Neuroradiology*, vol. 22, no. 4, pp. 795–798, 2001.

[38] X. Morandi, L. Riffaud, C. Haegelen, G. Lancien, P. Kerbrat, and Y. Guegan, "Extraosseous Ewing's sarcoma of the spinal epidural space," *Neurochirurgie*, vol. 47, no. 1, pp. 38–44, 2001.

[39] D. Gandhi, M. Goyal, E. Belanger, A. Modha, J. Wolffe, and W. Miller, "Primary epidural Ewing's sarcomas: case report and review of literature," *Canadian Association of Radiologists Journal*, vol. 54, no. 2, pp. 109–113, 2003.

[40] D. C. Weber, H. P. Rutz, A. J. Lomax et al., "First spinal axis segment irradiation with spot-scanning proton beam delivered in the treatment of a lumbar primitive neuroectodermal tumour," *Clinical Oncology*, vol. 16, no. 5, pp. 326–331, 2004.

[41] J. Koudelova, M. Kunesova, K. Koudela Jr., J. Matejka, P. Novak, and J. Prausova, "Peripheral primitive neuroectodermal tumor—PNET," *Acta Chirurgiae Orthopaedicae et Traumatologiae Cechoslovaca*, vol. 73, no. 1, pp. 39–44, 2006.

[42] G. Bozkurt, S. Ayhan, C. C. Turk, A. Akbay, F. Soylemezoglu, and S. Palaoglu, "Primary extraosseous Ewing sarcoma of the cervical epidural space. Case illustration," *Journal of Neurosurgery: Spine*, vol. 6, no. 2, article 192, 2007.

[43] J. F. Feng, Y. M. Liang, Y. H. Bao, Y. H. Pan, and J. Y. Jiang, "Multiple primary primitive neuroectodermal tumours within the spinal epidural space with non-concurrent onset," *Journal of International Medical Research*, vol. 36, no. 2, pp. 366–370, 2008.

[44] V. Musahl, J. A. Rihn, F. E. Fumich, and J. D. Kang, "Sacral intraspinal extradural primitive neuroectodermal tumor," *Spine Journal*, vol. 8, no. 6, pp. 1024–1029, 2008.

[45] K. Kiatsoontorn, T. Takami, T. Ichinose et al., "Primary epidural peripheral primitive neuroectodermal tumor of the thoracic spine—case report," *Neurologia Medico-Chirurgica*, vol. 49, no. 11, pp. 542–545, 2009.

[46] R. L. M. Bostelmann, H. J. Steiger, S. Eicker, and J. F. Cornelius, "Rapid progressive primary extraosseous Ewing sarcoma of the cervical intra- and epidural space," in *Proceedings of the 62nd Annual Meeting of the German Society of Neurosurgery (DGNC), Joint Meeting with the Polish Society of Neurosurgeons (PNCH)*, vol. 7, Hamburg, Germany, May 2011.

[47] R. García-Moreno, L. M. Bernal-García, M. Pineda-Palomo, M. Botana-Fernández, I. J. Gilete-Tejero, and J. M. Cabezudo-Artero, "Epidural extraskeletal Ewing sarcoma. Case report and literature review," *Neurocirugia*, vol. 26, no. 3, pp. 151–156, 2015.

Retained Glass Fragment in the Cervical Spinal Canal in a Patient with Acute Transverse Myelitis: A Case Report and Literature Review

Simonas Jesmanas,[1] Kristina Norvainytė,[1] Rymantė Gleiznienė,[2] and Algirdas Mačionis[3]

[1] Faculty of Medicine, Medical Academy, Lithuanian University of Health Sciences, Kaunas, Lithuania
[2] Department of Radiology, Medical Academy, Lithuanian University of Health Sciences, Kaunas, Lithuania
[3] Department of Neurology, Medical Academy, Lithuanian University of Health Sciences, Kaunas, Lithuania

Correspondence should be addressed to Simonas Jesmanas; s.jesmanas@gmail.com

Academic Editor: Abbass Amirjamshidi

A 50-year-old male presented with a one-day history of right leg weakness, numbness, and urinary retention. Weakness was present for two weeks but worsened significantly during the last 24 hours. On the right there was sensory loss in the leg and below the Th8 dermatome. On the left there was sensory loss below the Th10 dermatome and distal loss of temperature sensation. Past medical history revealed a cervical trauma 30 years ago when a glass chip lodged into the left side of the neck. The patient did not seek medical attention after removing it himself. No neurological symptoms followed the incident. No cervical manipulation or other physical trauma occurred before current symptom onset. Magnetic resonance (MR) imaging showed features consistent with myelitis at the level of C4–Th3. At the level of C6–C7, a T1 and T2 hypointense lesion was noted. On computed tomography, this lesion was hyperdense and occupied the spinal canal and the left intervertebral foramen. It was deemed to be a glass fragment. Surgical removal was withheld because the fragment was clinically silent for 30 years, the risk of surgical removal would outweigh the benefits and the patient did not prefer surgical treatment. Acute demyelinating transverse myelitis was diagnosed and treated with methylprednisolone. 10 months later MR features of myelitis resolved and the patient's neurological condition improved. Our case shows that foreign bodies in the cervical spinal canal can remain asymptomatic for up to 30 years. In the case of a long asymptomatic retention period the need for surgical removal of a foreign body must be carefully evaluated, taking into account the probability that a foreign body is the cause of current symptoms, risk of a foreign body causing damage in the future, risk of damage to the spinal cord during removal, and probability of therapeutic success.

1. Introduction

The vertebral column does not provide perfect protection to the spinal cord. Multiple openings, most notably the intervertebral foramina, exist for passage of structures to and from the spinal canal. Those same openings can serve as pathways by which foreign bodies can enter and damage the contents of the spinal canal. Various rarely encountered accidental injuries by metallic, wooden, and other objects or medical intervention can cause traumatic penetrating nonmissile spinal cord injury [1–3]. Spinal cord trauma most often presents with either complete or incomplete tetraplegia or paraplegia with or without accompanying sensory, autonomic (bowel and bladder function) disturbance [1]. Acute demyelinating transverse myelitis can also present with a similar clinical picture, particularly with a sensory level, although there usually will not be a history of trauma and the course is likely to be acute-to-subacute, reaching its peak over several weeks [4]. We present a rare case of a clinically silent glass fragment impaction into the cervical spinal canal which went undiscovered for several decades until an episode of acute demyelinating transverse myelitis and provide a literature review.

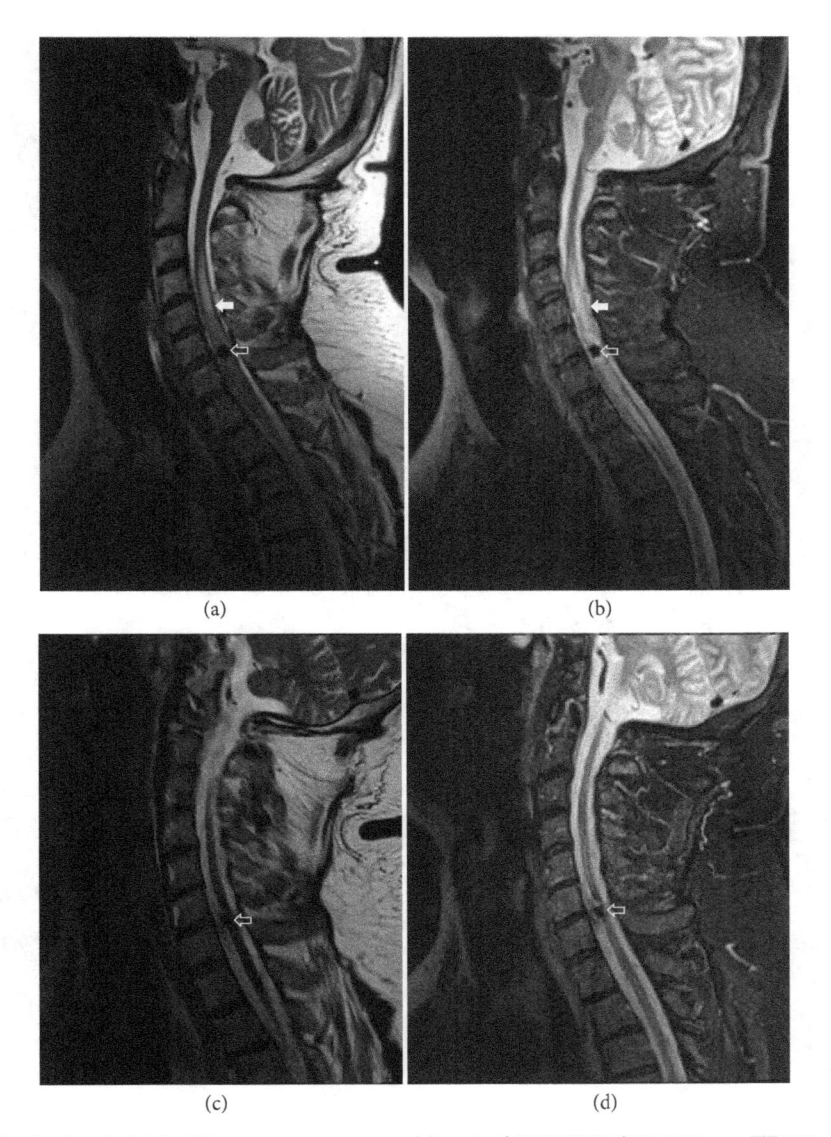

FIGURE 1: **MRI of the cervical spine: initial MRI at symptom onset**: (a) sagittal T2W/TSE (TR 3800 ms, TE 108 ms); (b) sagittal T2W/STIR (TR 4000 ms, TE 39 ms). Images show a hypointense oblong lesion in the spinal cord at the level of C6-C7 (empty arrows). Above and below the lesion the spinal cord shows hyperintense signal consistent with myelitis (filled arrows). **Follow-up MRI 10 months later**: (c) sagittal T2W/TSE (TR 3800 ms, TE 108 ms) and (d) sagittal T2W/STIR (TR 4000 ms, TE 39 ms). Follow-up images show normal spinal cord appearance following the resolution of myelitis and the same hypointense glass lesion (empty arrows).

2. Clinical Case

A 50-year-old male patient presented with a one-day history of right leg weakness, numbness, and urinary retention. There was mild back pain and right leg weakness for two weeks which worsened significantly during the last 24 hours. On neurological examination the patient's right leg was weaker than the left (2/5 and 4/5 on Lovett test, respectively), the patellar reflex was exaggerated, and Babinski sign was positive bilaterally. Also, on the right side, there was sensory loss in the leg and below the Th8 dermatome. On the left, there was sensory loss below Th10 dermatome and distal loss of temperature sensation.

Past medical history revealed a cervical trauma which occurred 30 years ago when a glass chip lodged into the left side of the patient's neck. The patient removed the visible glass shard from his neck and did not seek medical attention; therefore no clinical and radiological investigations were carried out. No neurological symptoms followed this incident.

Computed tomography (CT) of the lumbosacral and thoracic regions showed a mild convexity of the L5-S1 intervertebral disc with no other clinically significant findings ("Siemens SOMATOM Emotion 6") (images not shown). To further explore the possible causes of the patient's symptoms, magnetic resonance imaging (MRI) of the C1–L2 segments was performed ("Siemens MAGNETOM Avanto 1.5 T"). At the level of C4–Th3 the spinal cord was thickened and hyperintense on T2W images, features consistent with myelitis; however there was no appreciable contrast uptake (Figures 1(a) and 1(b)). At the level of C6–C7 an oblong (1.6 x 0.4 cm),

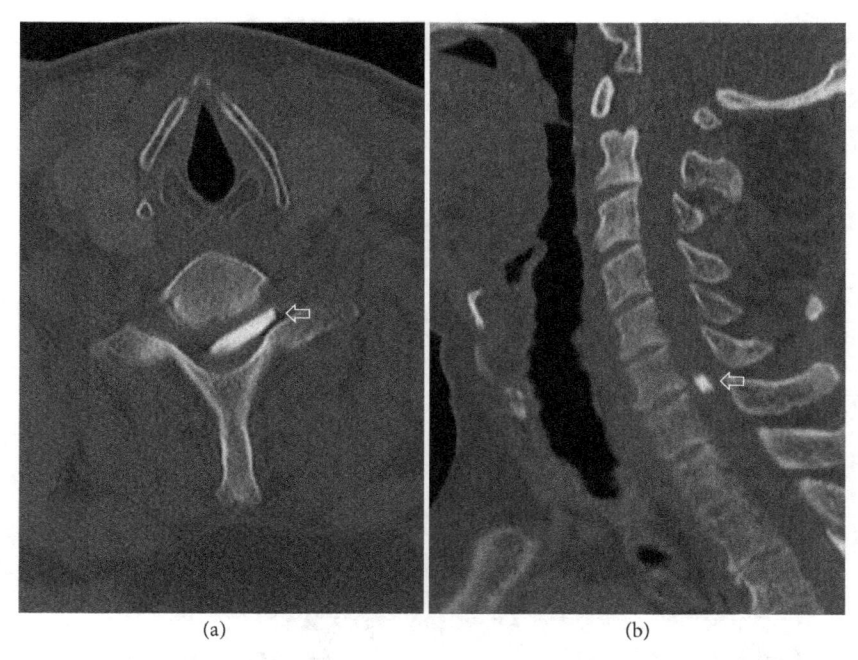

FIGURE 2: **CT of the cervical spine:** bone windows, axial (a) and sagittal reconstruction (b) showing a hyperdense oblong lesion at the level of C6-C7 in the left intervertebral foramen and spinal canal (arrows).

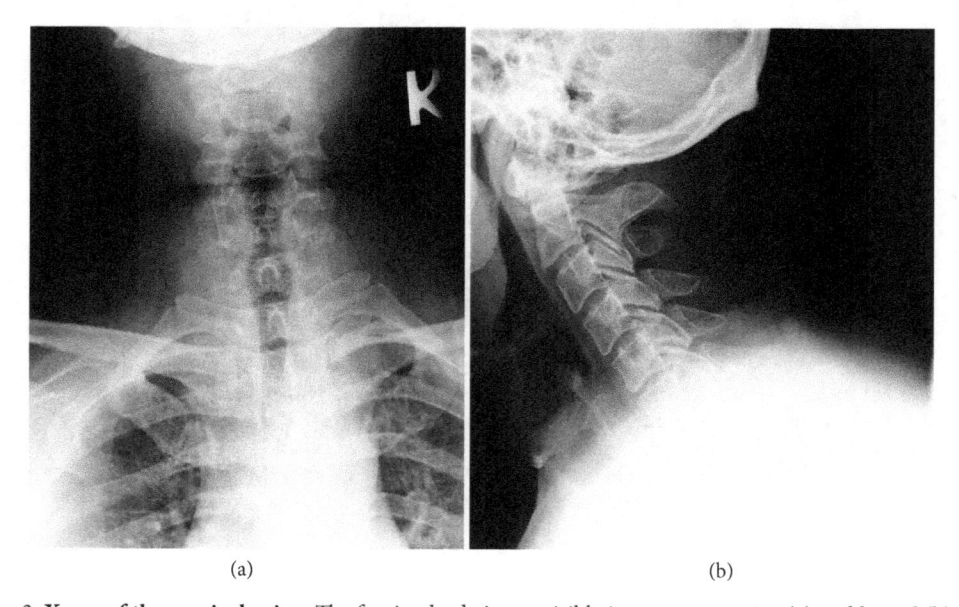

FIGURE 3: **X-ray of the cervical spine.** The foreign body is not visible in posteroanterior (a) and lateral (b) views.

T1 and T2 hypointense lesion was found (Figure 1). Because a foreign body was suspected, CT scan of the C1–Th3 levels was performed and demonstrated a hyperdense lesion occupying the spinal canal and the left intervertebral foramen (Figure 2).

Combining the CT and MRI results with the past medical history of an old injury with a glass fragment, it was determined that the lesion represented a glass foreign body in the spinal canal. The patient also had an X-ray of the cervical spine but the foreign body could not be visualized, most likely due to being located at the level of C6-C7, where it was obscured by the surrounding structures (Figure 3).

Taking into account the clinical picture, an extensive period of time between the trauma and current presentation, and MR imaging findings, an acute demyelinating episode rather than traumatic spinal cord injury was suspected. Further diagnostic work-up would typically have included a lumbar puncture to identify oligoclonal bands, cells, and protein, but it was contraindicated due to the risk of disturbing the foreign body and causing it to migrate upon a sudden decrease in pressure during puncture. Serum Aquaporin-4-specific antibodies could not be performed at the time and were planned for a later time.

The patient fulfilled the inclusion criteria for acute transverse myelitis: bilateral and not necessarily symmetrical sensory, motor, and autonomic spinal cord dysfunction, a clear sensory level, peak of symptoms within 4 hours and 21 days after onset of symptoms, and exclusion of other causes (neoplastic, vascular, and compressive) [5]. Compressive cause was excluded because the spinal cord pathology seen on MRI extends far from the location of the glass shard, which would be unlikely given the size of the foreign object and its possible effect upon the spinal cord if it migrated within the spinal canal. Thus, because the glass fragment lay dormant for the last 30 years, it was deemed not to be the direct cause of the patients' symptoms.

Treatment with methylprednisolone 500 mg intravenously daily for 6 days was initiated.

After consultation with the neurosurgeons it was decided not to remove the foreign body from the spinal canal, because the risks of surgery would outweigh the benefits. At the time of consultation, the patient was already showing improvement on medical management. Given that the situation was not hyperacute, the symptoms were better explained by the inflammatory and demyelinating reaction within the spinal cord rather than direct contact with the foreign body. Also, it could not be guaranteed that removing the glass shard would result in symptomatic improvement. Upon removal of the foreign body some diffuse bleeding would be expected, which combined with the already inflamed spinal cord parenchyma would likely further compromise the spinal cord, potentially causing vascular complications and myelomalacia, all of which would further decrease the chance of clinical improvement. Risk of general surgical complications (postoperative infection, bleeding, and thromboembolism) further argued against surgical treatment. An absolute indication for surgical treatment would be an infectious complication of the foreign body, which was not present. The patient agreed with the treating physicians that surgery would not be the best option and did not want the operation. If current medical treatment would have proven unsuccessful, and the patient's clinical condition worsened, surgery would have been indicated.

During the course of treatment the patient's condition improved. Sensory loss diminished, and the right leg strength improved to 4/5 on Lovett test, but urinary retention remained. Intermittent catheterization was prescribed.

The patient returned for a follow-up visit 10 months later with a stable and improved neurological state. Lower limb strength was 3/5 proximally and 4/5 distally, with positive bilateral Babinski sign. Minimal intermittent urinary retention remained but did not significantly impair the patients' quality of life. The patient resumed his activities of daily living and continues to work as a security guard. Follow-up MRI of the cervical spine shows the same oblong hypointense object and normal spinal cord after the resolution of myelitis (Figures 1(c) and 1(d)).

Further follow-up is scheduled every 6 to 12 months, with an outpatient brain MRI to identify any other demyelinating lesions that may be present in case this episode was part of neuromyelitis optica (NMO), acute demyelinating encephalomyelitis (ADEM), or multiple sclerosis (MS).

3. Discussion and Literature Review

3.1. Glass Foreign Bodies and Delayed Symptom Onset. In total we found 17 cases of glass spinal injuries reported in the literature [6–22].

Of particular interest to our case is the sometimes observed significant time lag between injury and symptom onset or complete absence of neurological symptoms after apparently substantial disruption of the spinal cord by a foreign body. 5 out of 17 cases presented months or years after the injury, ranging from 3.5 months to 21 years [8, 11, 16, 18, 19]. In our described case, the time until discovery of a glass fragment was greater than in any of the studies reported in the literature. Vadasz et al. noted that the delay between the initial injury and symptom onset can be either subacute, due to CSF leak, meningitis, or abscess, or chronic, due to myelomalacia and spinal cyst formation [12].

While our patient had the foreign body for several decades, clinical and imaging findings were most consistent with an acute demyelinating myelitis. Some authors have reasoned that slow migration of the foreign body can cause spinal cord damage to manifest [11, 18, 19], but we think this was unlikely in our case. The small amount of kinetic energy arising from a slow migration of a relatively small object would be unlikely to cause such extensive spinal cord involvement seen on the spinal MRI. Indeed, in such a scenario the MRI appearance should resemble that of localized compressive myelopathy due to intervertebral disc pathology or chronic localized spinal stenosis of other etiologies.

Acute transverse myelitis is usually acute or subacute in onset, and neurological symptoms tend to worsen and reach their peak after a few weeks [4]. The name "transverse" myelitis is rather historical in nature, because demyelination does not always completely encompass the spinal cord transversely. However, the presence of a sensory level and an acute-to-subacute course are crucial, which were present in our patient. It can be further divided into complete or partial, with the latter including hemicord (Brown-Sequard), central cord, dorsal column, or specific tract disruption [4]. Longitudinally extensive transverse myelitis, which involves more than 3 segments, was detected in our case. The symptoms were mostly localized to the right spinal cord producing a mostly hemicord clinical picture, with at least some central and contralateral cord involvement producing a mixed symptomatology. The glass foreign body hypothetically could have been a predisposing factor for an autoimmune demyelinating process of the spinal cord; however, we cannot confidently exclude a simple coincidence. Therefore, in our view, the foreign body has remained asymptomatic despite the patients' current condition.

It is interesting to note that in cases when the cervical spine was injured, the symptoms were logically explained by the location: quadriparesis and anesthesia or hypoesthesia [7, 13, 21], hemiparesis on the left and hypoesthesia with spared deep sensations on the right [8, 10], and dysesthesia in the arms [16, 18]. However, in our case, the absence of any upper extremity symptoms is surprising, because the glass shard is at the level of the segments supplying the brachial plexus and lodged into the C6/C7 intervertebral foramen, where it most likely should have damaged the corresponding nerve root. One possible explanation of the absence of nerve root symptoms would be that this patient had anomalous nerve root origin, whereby no root was present in the C6/C7 intervertebral foramen; however such anomalies are more common in the lumbosacral region [23].

3.2. Removal of Retained Glass Foreign Bodies from the Spinal Canal. The management of glass fragments in the described cases was always surgical (laminectomy, removal of the fragments, and dural closure) if the patient presented to the hospital immediately after injury and exhibited signs of neurological damage and the glass fragment was successfully visualized with imaging [7–10, 13, 15, 20–22]. One patient died due to cardiopulmonary insufficiency [7], while others survived, but some exhibited varying degrees of neurological dysfunction [10, 13, 20, 21].

Some authors reasoned that delayed presentation in the presence of a foreign body is usually precipitated by a small injury, which disturbs the foreign body, causes it to move to a greater or lesser extent and triggers the onset of symptoms by affecting spinal cord function [11, 18, 19]. The decision reached by Oertel et al. to withhold surgical removal of the glass fragment after it was lodged for 12 years seems to support this conclusion, as the authors noted that fibrous tissue had already formed and seemed to be protecting surrounding the spinal cord and nerve roots [16]. Symptoms probably appeared because of progressively narrowing vertebral canal due to degeneration [16]. Removal of the fragment would disrupt the protective tissue and may in itself cause neurological damage; however the possibility of the fragment being displaced and causing symptoms on its own cannot be absolutely excluded [16]. In other cases with a delayed presentation, the surgeons chose to operate and remove the fragments due to severe neurological impairment and achieved therapeutic success [8, 19]. In our case surgical treatment was withheld for the reasons outlined in the case description.

Akcakaya et al. emphasized that usually foreign body removal is indicated if there is a possibility of toxicity, for example, if it is composed of lead or copper [18]. When foreign bodies remain in the vertebral canal for a long period of time, they can slowly degrade or corrode and cause sustained tissue irritation, which can lead to chronic inflammation and progressive damage to nerve roots or spinal cord itself, causing pain or a delayed neurological deficit [24]. While we do not have any evidence to support our hypothesis, we think it is plausible that the glass fragment could have played some part in predisposing the patient to develop acute demyelinating transverse myelitis, by causing either localized chronic irritation or immunological disturbance.

3.3. Imaging. Glass of at least 2 mm in size should always be visible on X-rays due to its higher density and effective atomic number when compared with soft tissues [3, 25]. However, as our case illustrates, if there is sufficient obstruction of the view by surrounding radiopaque structures, it may be obscured. On CT it is always hyperdense. MR signal is derived from hydrogen protons, but glass has no hydrogen atoms; therefore it produces no signal and is dark on both T1 and T2. Even if MR does not provide good visualization of the foreign body itself, it can be useful to show the reactive changes of the surrounding tissues, lacerations, signs of infection, inflammation, and demyelination [26].

MR features of acute spinal cord injury (SCI) include smooth enlargement of the cord contour, hyperintensity on T2W and hypointensity on T1W, and hemorrhage [27]. In cases of subacute SCI a progressive decrease in overall spinal cord area above the lesion level can be seen on MRI [28]. Eventually, this decrease may lead to the spinal cord atrophy, the most common finding in patients imaged more than 20 years after the initial trauma [27]. In a patient with history of previous spinal injury and new onset of neurological deficits, there is a possibility of posttraumatic syringomyelia [29]. Neither atrophy nor syringomyelia was present in our patient. Myelomalacia demonstrates similar findings to myelitis [27] and would be more likely without the acute-to-subacute clinical picture. Longitudinally extensive transverse myelitis encompasses more than 3 segments and exhibits T2W hyperintensity and sometimes T1W hypointensity, swelling, and none or variable enhancement [30], and it was the best fit in our case.

Idiopathic demyelinating transverse myelitis should be distinguished from transverse myelitis occurring with other demyelinating conditions, specifically neuromyelitis optica (NMO), multiple sclerosis (MS), and acute demyelinating encephalomyelitis (ADEM). MS lesions are usually multiple, located in the peripheral spinal cord, and less extensive, exhibiting a distribution in space and time [31]. Follow-up imaging of the spinal cord and MR of the brain are important to look for widely distributed or new demyelinating lesions which would support the diagnosis of MS. Immunologic testing for aquaporin-4 antibodies and visually evoked potentials are also important in ruling out NMO [31]. Our patient will continue to be followed and evaluated for signs and symptoms of ADEM, NMO, and MS.

4. Conclusion

In conclusion, we report a very rare case of a 50-year-old male with a glass shard in the cervical spinal canal which has remained clinically silent for 30 years until an episode of acute demyelinating transverse myelitis. Physicians must keep in mind that foreign bodies in the spinal canal can produce no neurological symptoms for up to 30 years. In the case of a long asymptomatic retention period the need for surgical removal of a foreign body must be carefully evaluated, taking into account the estimated probability that a foreign body is the cause of current symptoms or just an incidental finding, risk of a foreign body causing damage in the future, risk of further damage to the spinal cord during removal, and probability of therapeutic success.

References

[1] L. Snyder, L. Tan, C. Gerard, and R. Fessler, "Spinal cord trauma," in *Bradley's Neurology in Clinical Practice*, R. Daroff, J.

Jankovic, J. Mazziotta, and S. Pomeroy, Eds., pp. 881–902, Elsevier Inc., London, UK, 7th edition, 2017.

[2] A. Kumar, P. N. Pandey, A. Ghani, and G. Jaiswal, "Penetrating spinal injuries and their management," *Journal of Craniovertebral Junction & Spine*, vol. 2, no. 2, pp. 57–61, 2011.

[3] T. B. Hunter and M. S. Taljanovic, "Foreign bodies," *RadioGraphics*, vol. 23, no. 3, pp. 731–757, 2003.

[4] S. C. Beh, B. M. Greenberg, T. Frohman, and E. M. Frohman, "Transverse myelitis," *Neurologic Clinics*, vol. 31, no. 1, pp. 79–138, 2013.

[5] "Proposed diagnostic criteria and nosology of acute transverse myelitis," *Neurology*, vol. 59, no. 4, pp. 499–505, 2002.

[6] E. Topliff and J. Daly, "Accidental puncture of the cerebrospinal canal," *Canadian Medical Association Journal*, vol. 24, no. 6, pp. 836–838, 1931.

[7] A. Z. Buczynski and J. Makowski, "A case of traumatic transection of cervical spinal cord by glass," *Paraplegia*, vol. 12, no. 3, pp. 167–169, 1974.

[8] Y. Miyazaki and K. Inaba, "Transfixion of cervical cord by a glass fragment. Report of a case (Japanese)," *Journal of Neurological Surgery*, vol. 4, no. 8, pp. 799–803, 1976.

[9] P. Baghai and P. E. Sheptak, "Penetrating spinal injury by a glass fragment: case report and review," *Neurosurgery*, vol. 11, no. 3, pp. 419–422, 1982.

[10] T. Isu, Y. Iwasaki, H. Sasaki, and H. Abe, "Spinal cord and root injuries due to glass fragments and acupuncture needles," *World Neurosurgery*, vol. 23, no. 3, pp. 255–260, 1985.

[11] I. Reid, G. O. Neill, and C. N. Pidgeon, "Retained glass fragment in the spinal canal," *Irish Journal of Medical Science*, vol. 158, no. 11, p. 280, 1989.

[12] A. G. Vadasz, C. F. Torres, and J. K. Chang, "Accidental penetrating cervical cord injury in a young child," *Pediatric Emergency Care*, vol. 12, no. 6, pp. 428–431, 1996.

[13] C. R. Tomaras, R. W. Grundmeyer, T. S. Chow, and T. W. Trask, "Unusual foreign body causing quadriparesis: case report," *Neurosurgery*, vol. 40, no. 6, pp. 1291–1294, 1997.

[14] S. L. Almond, E. C. Jesudason, P. D. Losty, and C. L. Malluci, "Occult intraspinal glass injury," *Archives of Disease in Childhood*, vol. 88, no. 9, p. 801, 2003.

[15] D. J. Opel, D. A. Lundin, K. L. Stevenson, and E. J. Klein, "Glass foreign body in the spinal canal of a child: case report and review of the literature," *Pediatric Emergency Care*, vol. 20, no. 7, pp. 468–472, 2004.

[16] M. F. Oertel, I. Kreitschmann-Andermahr, Y.-M. Ryang, J. M. Gilsbach, and M. C. Korinth, "The awakened intraspinal glass shard," *Acta Neurochirurgica*, vol. 151, no. 1, pp. 99–101, 2009.

[17] E. R. Anderson, H. I. Grant III, and M. Weissman, "Penetrating glass injury to the sacral spine," *Clinical Medicine & Research*, vol. 8, no. 2, pp. 114–115, 2010.

[18] M. O. Akcakaya, Y. Aras, A. G. Yorukoglu, C. Ovalioglu, and A. Sencer, "Cervical intradural glass fragment: a rare cause of neuropathic pain," *Turkish Neurosurgery*, vol. 22, no. 5, pp. 667–670, 2012.

[19] K. Yoshioka, N. Kawahara, H. Murakami et al., "A glass foreign body migrating into the lumbar spinal canal: a case report," *Journal of Orthopaedic Surgery*, vol. 20, no. 2, pp. 257–259, 2012.

[20] M. Komarowska, W. Debek, J. A. Wojnar, A. Hermanowicz, and M. Rogalski, "Brown-Séquard syndrome in a 11-year-old girl due to penetrating glass injury to the thoracic spine," *European Journal of Orthopaedic Surgery and Traumatology*, vol. 23, no. 2, pp. S141–S143, 2013.

[21] R. Selvan, R. Ramkumar, S. Subikshavarthni, and J. Parthiban, "Unique case of glass piece injury to cervical spinal cord: a very rare presentation," *The Journal of Spinal Surgery*, vol. 3, pp. 63–65, 2016.

[22] İ. Toker, Ö. D. Atilla, T. Y. Kılıç, O. Taş, and S. Hacar, "A rare lumbar spinal column injury: glass injury," *The Journal of Tepecik Education and Research Hospital*, vol. 26, no. 3, pp. 250–252, 2016.

[23] S. M. Burke, M. G. Safain, J. Kryzanski, and R. I. Riesenburger, "Nerve root anomalies: implications for transforaminal lumbar interbody fusion surgery and a review of the Neidre and Macnab classification system," *Neurosurgical Focus*, vol. 35, no. 2, Article ID E9, 2013.

[24] G. Guarnieri, L. Genovese, and M. Muto, "Retained intraspinal foreign bodies," in *Imaging of Foreign Bodies*, A. Pinto and L. Romano, Eds., pp. 94–98, Springer-Verlag Italia Inc., Milan, Italt, 1st edition, 2014.

[25] A. H. Felman and M. S. Fisher, "The radiographic detection of glass in soft tissue," *Radiology*, vol. 92, no. 7, pp. 1529–1531, 1969.

[26] M. Jarraya, D. Hayashi, R. V. De Villiers et al., "Multimodality imaging of foreign bodies of the musculoskeletal system," *American Journal of Roentgenology*, vol. 203, no. 1, pp. W92–W102, 2014.

[27] A. L. Goldberg and S. M. Kershah, "Advances in imaging of vertebral and spinal cord injury," *The Journal of Spinal Cord Medicine*, vol. 33, no. 2, pp. 105–116, 2010.

[28] P. Grabher, M. F. Callaghan, J. Ashburner et al., "Tracking sensory system atrophy and outcome prediction in spinal cord injury," *Annals of Neurology*, vol. 78, no. 5, pp. 751–761, 2015.

[29] A. Agrawal, M. Shetty, L. Pandit, L. Shetty, and U. Srikrishna, "Post-traumatic syringomyelia," *Indian Journal of Orthopaedics*, vol. 41, no. 4, pp. 398–400, 2007.

[30] C. Goh, P. M. Desmond, and P. M. Phal, "MRI in transverse myelitis," *Journal of Magnetic Resonance Imaging*, vol. 40, no. 6, pp. 1267–1279, 2014.

[31] S.-J. Moon, J.-K. Lee, T.-W. Kim, and S.-H. Kim, "Idiopathic transverse myelitis presenting as the Brown-Sequard syndrome," *Spinal Cord*, vol. 47, no. 2, pp. 176–178, 2009.

Simultaneous Combined Myositis, Inflammatory Polyneuropathy, and Overlap Myasthenic Syndrome

Stéphane Mathis,[1] Laurent Magy,[2] Philippe Corcia,[3] Karima Ghorab,[2] Laurence Richard,[2] Jonathan Ciron,[4] Mathilde Duchesne,[2] and Jean-Michel Vallat[2]

[1]Department of Neurology, Nerve-Muscle Unit, CHU Bordeaux (Groupe Hospitalier Pellegrin), place Amélie-Raba-Léon, 33000 Bordeaux, France
[2]Department of Neurology, Centre de Référence "Neuropathies Périphériques Rares", CHU Limoges, 2 avenue Martin Luther King, 87042 Limoges, France
[3]Department of Neurology, CHU Bretonneau, 2 boulevard Tonnellé, 37044 Tours, France
[4]Department of Neurology, CHU Poitiers, 2 rue de la Milétrie, 86021 Poitiers, France

Correspondence should be addressed to Stéphane Mathis; stephane.mathis@chu-bordeaux.fr

Academic Editor: Tapas Kumar Banerjee

Immune-mediated neuromuscular disorders include pathologies of the peripheral nervous system, neuromuscular junction, and muscles. If overlap syndromes (or the association of almost two autoimmune disorders) are recognized, the simultaneous occurrence of several autoimmune neuromuscular disorders is rare. We describe two patients presenting the simultaneous occurrence of inflammatory neuropathy, myositis, and myasthenia gravis (with positive acetylcholine receptor antibodies). For each patient, we carried out a pathological analysis (nerve and muscle) and an electrophysiological study (and follow-up). To our knowledge, this is the first description of such a triple immune-mediated neuromuscular syndrome. We compared our observations with a few other cases of simultaneous diagnosis of two inflammatory neuromuscular disorders.

1. Introduction

Neuromuscular disorders are a heterogeneous group of diseases affecting the peripheral nervous system (including anterior horn cells, nerve roots, plexus, and peripheral nerves), the neuromuscular junction, and muscles. These different entities are well described, and the clinical manifestations and some hallmark signs usually help to make the diagnosis [1]. However, such a diagnosis may sometimes be difficult in an atypical presentation or overlap syndrome: for example, some entities can combine myopathy and neuropathy, such as "critical illness neuromuscular dysfunction." We report here two patients with a subacute presentation of simultaneous myasthenia gravis, inflammatory polyneuropathy, and myositis, and we discuss this rare occurrence of immune-mediated neuromuscular disorders.

2. Case Reports

2.1. Patient 1. This 67-year-old woman complained of severe asthenia, loss of weight, and overall muscular weakness for five months. Her medical history only showed osteoporosis (without any fracture). On clinical examination we found drop head, bilateral facial weakness, and also swallowing, breathing, and speech troubles (these symptoms were present for two months). We observed a generalized decrease of the muscular strength: the motor weakness was proximal and distal in the four limbs but predominantly in the upper limbs (Medical Research Council (MRC): grade 3 in the upper limbs and grade 4 in the lower limbs). Amyotrophy was moderate and restricted to the hands. She also complained of paresthesia in her hands (for five months), but we found neither sensory deficit nor ataxia. Deep tendon reflexes were weak in the upper limbs but normal in the lower limbs. We observed no cramp or fasciculation. No pyramidal or cerebellar signs were found. She presented a Raynaud phenomenon for one month, but no cutaneous abnormality was observed. She also had a deformity of the hand joints (distal and proximal interphalangeal joints) but without any inflammatory sign and a kyphoscoliosis. We found neither adenopathy nor organomegaly. The cardiovascular and pulmonary examinations were normal.

Ancillary tests showed a high level of creatine kinase (ranging between 400 and 1200 IU/L) and C-reactive protein (91 mg/L) and mild hepatic cytolysis (alanine aminotransferase: 87 U/L; aspartate aminotransferase: 66 U/L). No monoclonal gammopathy was present. The immunological tests showed a positivity of antinuclear factors (titer > 1/640), but anti-double stranded DNA, anti-SM, anti-nucleosome, and anti-cardiolipin antibodies were negative; no cryoglobulinemia was detected. Anti-glycolipid, anti-MAG, and anti-neuronal antibodies were negative, but anti-acetylcholine receptor (anti-AchR) antibodies were positive (14.4 nmol/L; reference range < 0.2 nmol/L). Thyroid stimulating hormone (TSH) level was normal. The various serologies (HIV, hepatitis B and hepatitis C, Borrelia burgdorferi, Herpes, VZV, and HTLV) were negative. On lumbar puncture, no cell, no infection, and a normal protein (41 g/dL) and glucose (64 g/dL) levels were found in cerebrospinal fluid (CSF). A whole-body CT-scan did not detect any thymoma or underlying cancer or infection. The electrophysiological study showed decreased CMAP (compound muscle action potentials) amplitude in the upper limbs, with normal motor nerve conduction velocities, distal latencies, and F-wave latencies in the four limbs (Table 1). We also observed moderate decreased SNAP (sensory nerve action potentials) amplitude in the upper limbs and severe reduction in the lower limbs (Table 1). In the upper limbs, needle electromyography showed early recruitment with small and spiky motor units on the deltoid muscles (myogenic pattern) but also a reduced recruitment of the motor units in first dorsal interosseous muscles (neurogenic pattern); there was no spontaneous activity. Repetitive nerve stimulation testing was performed and showed a marked decremental response at 3 Hz stimulation in genioglossus (−48.1%) and also right (−23.7%) and left (−24.3%) abductor digiti minimi. Sural nerve and deltoid muscle biopsies were performed.

This patient has been treated with a cure of intravenous immunoglobulins (IVIg: 0.4 g per day during 5 days) before starting oral steroids (1 mg/kg/day) and then tapering over three months; acetylcholinesterase inhibitors were also added. After 6 months, we observed a dramatic improvement with MRC score graded 5 (proximal and distal) in the four limbs (except on quadriceps: 4/5), with no drop head (but a mild difficulty of the flexion of the head against resistance) and no facial weakness, but still some paresthesia in the feet. Two years after the onset of the symptoms, we observed electrophysiological improvement (amplitude of potentials) on both motor and sensory nerves (Table 1); however, there was still some slowing of motor nerve conduction velocities, demonstrating a mild demyelinating process.

2.2. Patient 2. This 79-year-old man complained of generalized weakness for three months. His medical history included shoulder pain and acromioclavicular joint dislocation (seven years earlier); eight years earlier, he presented myocardial infarction (he has been treated by aspirin, statins, and antihypertensive drugs). The first symptoms were lumbar pain and muscular weakness, with progressive worsening for three months although the patient was still autonomous and able to walk. The motor testing found proximal weakness in the four limbs (MRC: grade 3) but no distal weakness; we also observed moderate atrophy of quadriceps and pectoral muscles (without severe muscular pain). Deep tendon reflexes were absent in the lower limbs and weak in the upper limbs. Some difficulties in swallowing were reported (for three months), but he presented no other cranial nerve symptom. He did not complain of any paresthesia, and we did not observe any sensory impairment (in all modalities). There was no pyramidal sign.

The ancillary tests showed a moderate increase of creatine kinase (249 U/L) with normal c-reactive protein (2 mg/L) and also a high level of cholesterol (total cholesterol was 2.36 g/L, and LDL-cholesterol was 1.58 g/L). Antinuclear factors were positive (titer: 1/320), as were anti-DNA antibodies (55 U/L), and anti-SM, anti-nucleosome, and anti-cardiolipin antibodies were negative; no cryoglobulinemia was detected. Antiglycolipid, anti-MAG, and anti-neuronal antibodies were negative; anti-AchR antibodies were positive (16 nmol/L; reference range < 0.2 nmol/L). There was no monoclonal gammopathy. The spinal MRI was normal (except for moderate lumbar and cervical arthrosis), and we found no thymoma on thoracic CT-scan. The electrophysiological study showed reduced CMAP amplitude in the lower limbs (with increased F-wave latencies but normal nerve conduction velocities) and only a bilateral carpal tunnel syndrome in the upper limbs (Table 1). We also observed reduced SNAP amplitude in the lower limbs (Table 1). In the lower limbs, needle electromyography showed early recruitment with spiky motor units on the quadriceps muscles (myogenic pattern) but also a reduced recruitment of the motor units in tibialis anterior (neurogenic pattern); there was no spontaneous activity. Repetitive nerve stimulation showed a marked decremental response at 3 Hz stimulation in the trapezius muscles (−20%). Sural nerve and deltoid muscle biopsies were performed.

This patient was treated with three monthly doses of IVIg (0.4/g/day for 5 days) and oral steroids (1 mg/kg/day; tapering after 3 months); acetylcholinesterase inhibitors were also added. After 6 months, we observed a moderate improvement in the four limbs with MRC score graded 4 in proximal and still 5 in distal. Four years after the onset of the first symptoms, we observed a mild decrease of amplitude of both CMAP and SNAP (Table 1).

2.3. Pathological Findings. After informed consent, nerve and muscle biopsies were performed in the two patients and processed as described elsewhere [35].

On sural nerve of both patients, we observed a pathological pattern of primary demyelinating polyneuropathy, with a moderate loss of myelinated fibers, too thin myelin sheath, and also "onion bulb" formations (Figures 1 and 2).

TABLE 1: Motor and sensory nerve conduction studies: follow-up of our two patients.

	Nerve	DA	DL	NCV	F	CB
Patient 1						
ENMG1 (year 0)						
Motor nerves						
Right	Median	1.46 mV	4.74 ms	56.3 m/s	30 ms	No
	Ulnar	4 mV	4.34 ms	65.8 m/s	31.4 ms	No
	Peroneal	5.2 mV	4.1 ms	46.9 m/s	51.9 ms	No
	Tibial	15 mV	4.58 ms	ND	52.7 ms	ND
Left	Median	2.6 mV	3.4 ms	55 m/s	31.8 ms	No
	Ulnar	3.9 mV	3.87 ms	60 m/s	31 ms	No
	Peroneal	5.2 mV	4.03 ms	41.3 m/s	50.4 ms	No
	Tibial	9.9 mV	4.58 ms	ND	54.8 ms	ND
Sensory nerves						
Right	Median	8.5 μV	—	45.5 m/s	—	—
	Ulnar	5.8 μV	—	57.1 m/s	—	—
	Peroneal	0 μV	—	—	—	—
	Sural	0 μV	—	—	—	—
Left	Median	6.5 μV	—	42.7 m/s	—	—
	Ulnar	8 μV	—	51.6 m/s	—	—
	Peroneal	0 μV	—	—	—	—
	Sural	4 μV	—	36.8 m/s	—	—
ENMG2 (year 1)						
Motor nerves						
Right	Median	2.9 mV	3.55 ms	46.3 m/s	ND	No
	Ulnar	7.5 mV	2.13 ms	57.5 m/s	30.5 ms	No
	Peroneal	7.4 mV	13.2 ms	43.3 m/s	54.1 ms	No
	Tibial	19.4 mV	3.32 ms	ND	51.4 ms	ND
Left	Median	5.8 mV	2.76 ms	55.1 m/s	27 ms	No
	Ulnar	6.5 mV	2.92 ms	71.8 m/s	27.3 ms	No
	Peroneal	4 mV	10.7 ms	42.5 m/s	50.7 ms	No
	Tibial	8.4 mV	3.32 ms	ND	56.1 ms	ND
Sensory nerves						
Right	Median	9 μV	—	49.8 m/s	—	—
	Ulnar	4.9 μV	—	46 m/s	—	—
	Peroneal	0 μV	—	—	—	—
	Sural	2.8 μV	—	44.2 m/s	—	—
Left	Median	9.2 μV	—	33.7 m/s	—	—
	Ulnar	10.6 μV	—	47.9 m/s	—	—
	Peroneal	0 μV	—	—	—	—
	Sural	0 μV	—	—	—	—
ENMG3 (year 2)						
Motor nerves						
Right	Median	4.1 mV	3.24 ms	41.4 m/s	27.2 ms	No
	Ulnar	ND	ND	ND	ND	No
	Peroneal	6.3 mV	3.16 ms	42.6 m/s	48.3 ms	No
	Tibial	15 mV	3.57 ms	35.6 m/s	51.4 ms	ND

TABLE 1: Continued.

	Nerve	DA	DL	NCV	F	CB
Left	Median	8.2 mV	2.92 ms	53.5 m/s	29.4 ms	No
	Ulnar	ND	ND	ND	ND	No
	Peroneal	2.6 mV	3.79 ms	42.8 m/s	40.6 ms	No
	Tibial	10.8 mV	3.9 ms	33.6 m/s	56.3 ms	ND
Sensory nerves						
Right	Median	6.3 μV	—	48.8 m/s	—	—
	Ulnar	ND	—	ND	—	—
	Peroneal	0 μV	—	—	—	—
	Sural	4 μV	—	54 m/s	—	—
Left	Median	7.9 μV	—	47.2 m/s	—	—
	Ulnar	ND	—	ND	—	—
	Peroneal	0 μV	—	—	—	—
	Sural	0 μV	—	—	—	—

Patient 2
ENMG1 (year 0)
Motor nerves

	Nerve	DA	DL	NCV	F	CB
Right	Median	7.5 mV	4.2 ms	46.9 m/s	33.2 ms	No
	Ulnar	6.4 mV	2.5 ms	60 m/s	32.4 ms	No
	Peroneal	2.3 mV	5.2 ms	42.3 m/s	60.3 ms	No
	Tibial	2 mV	5 ms	42.4 m/s	63.3 ms	ND
Left	Median	8.2 mV	4.4 ms	45 m/s	32.5 ms	No
	Ulnar	7.8 mV	3.1 ms	62.2 m/s	33.1 ms	No
	Peroneal	2.3 mV	5.2 ms	42.7 m/s	60.8 ms	No
	Tibial	1.3 mV	4.5 ms	44.9 m/s	63 ms	ND

Sensory nerves

	Nerve	DA	DL	NCV	F	CB
Right	Median	6.5 μV	—	46.3 m/s	—	—
	Ulnar	3.5 μV	—	32 m/s	—	—
	Peroneal	ND	—	ND	—	—
	Sural	4.6 μV	—	40 m/s	—	—
Left	Median	3 μV	—	43.1 m/s	—	—
	Ulnar	3.3 μV	—	40 m/s	—	—
	Peroneal	ND	—	ND	—	—
	Sural	ND	—	ND	—	—

ENMG2 (year 4)
Motor nerves

	Nerve	DA	DL	NCV	F	CB
Right	Median	6.3 mV	6.14 ms	45.2 m/s	38.5 ms	No
	Ulnar	7.1 mV	2.65 ms	59.5 m/s	35.5 ms	No
	Peroneal	ND	ND	ND	ND	ND
	Tibial	1.18 mV	5.02 ms	ND	61.6 ms	ND
Left	Median	ND	ND	ND	ND	No
	Ulnar	ND	ND	ND	ND	No
	Peroneal	ND	ND	ND	ND	ND
	Tibial	ND	ND	ND	ND	ND

Sensory nerves

	Nerve	DA	DL	NCV	F	CB
Right	Median	0 μV	—	—	—	—
	Ulnar	4.1 μV	—	42 m/s	—	—
	Peroneal	ND	—	ND	—	—
	Sural	2.1 μV	—	38.9 m/s	—	—

TABLE 1: Continued.

	Nerve	DA	DL	NCV	F	CB
Left	Median	ND	—	ND	—	—
	Ulnar	ND	—	ND	—	—
	Peroneal	ND	—	ND	—	—
	Sural	ND	—	ND	—	—

CB: conduction block; DA: distal amplitude; DL: distal latency; F: F wave; μV: microVolt; ms: millisecond; m/s: meter/second; mV: millivolt; NCV: nerve conduction velocity.

(a)

(b)

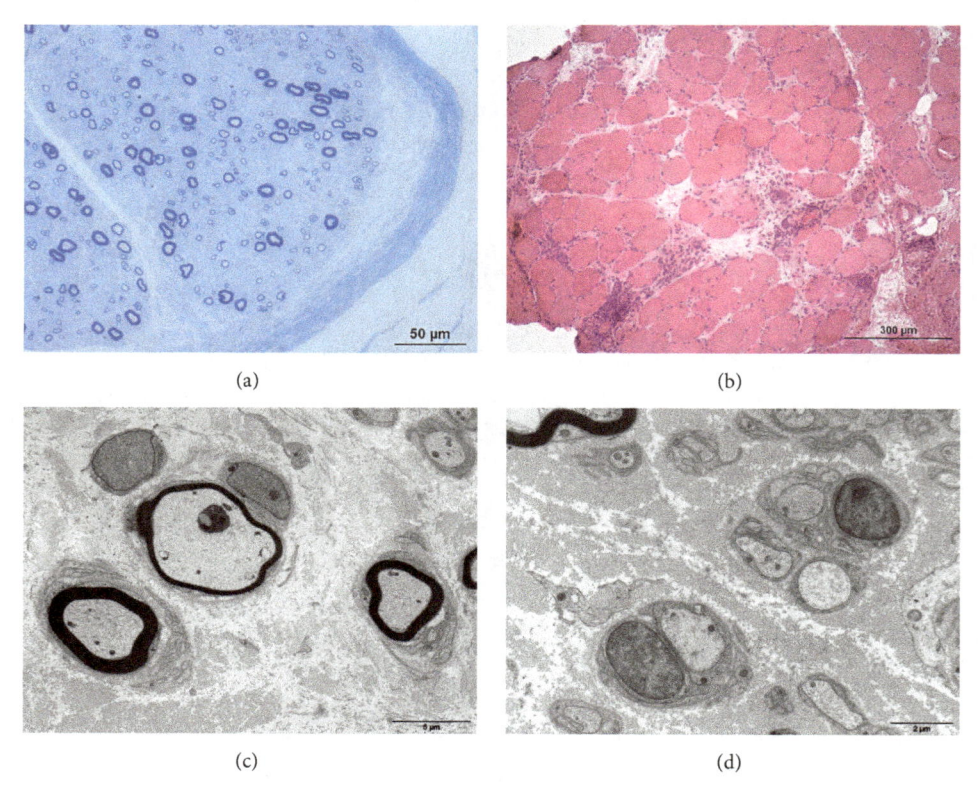

(c)

(d)

FIGURE 1: Pathological findings in patient 1. (a) Transverse semithin section of sural nerve stained with Toluidine Blue: there is a moderate loss of myelinated fibers. Only a few fibers have a too thin myelin sheath compared to their axonal diameter. (b) Frozen section of deltoid muscle stained with hematein-eosin showing important infiltrates of mononuclear cells; the immunostaining confirmed that these cells were mostly T cells and macrophages. (c) Electron micrograph of a sural nerve section showing two fibers surrounded by onion bulb formation and a fiber with a thin myelin sheath. (d) Electron micrograph of a sural nerve section showing an axon that has been completely demyelinated.

No pattern of vasculitis or amyloid deposit was found and no clonal cell was seen on immunostaining.

Deltoid muscle biopsy of both patients evidenced a classical pattern of inflammatory myopathy. The immunostaining confirmed the presence of inflammatory infiltrates (mainly T cells), without clonal cells (Figures 1 and 2). No amyloid deposits or vasculitis was found in muscles.

2.4. Method for the Review of the Literature. We searched MEDLINE, Scopus, and Google Scholar for case reports and case series of patients with at least two simultaneous dysimmune neuromuscular disorders (inflammatory polyneuropathy, myasthenia gravis, or myositis) published since 1975. We include all cases with sufficient clinical, electrophysiological, biological, or pathological data to perform a diagnosis of one of these three dysimmune neuromuscular disorders.

3. Discussion

Idiopathic inflammatory muscle diseases (or myositis) are rare (annual incidence range from 2.1 to 7.7 cases per million) and represent a heterogeneous group of acquired myopathies comprising pure polymyositis, pure dermatomyositis, necrotizing myopathy, inclusion body myositis, overlap myositis, and myositis-specific autoantibodies (and associated diseases), according to the usual classification [36]. They are characterized by mainly proximal motor weakness (acute, subacute, or chronic) of the four limbs on clinical

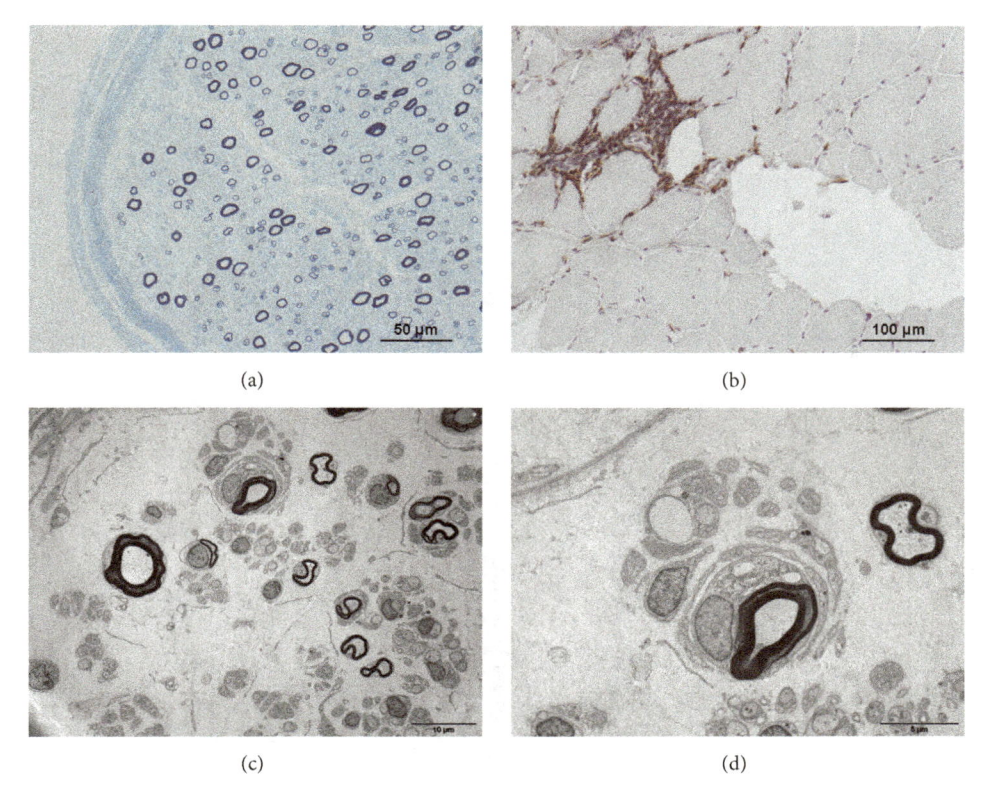

FIGURE 2: Pathological findings in patient 2. (a) Transverse semithin section of a sural nerve stained with Toluidine Blue: there is a moderate loss of myelinated fibers; several fibers have a too thin sheath compared to their axonal diameter. (b) Frozen section of a deltoid muscle stained with anti-CD45 antibody showing the presence of T cell infiltrates. (c) Electron micrograph of a sural nerve section showing a myelinated fiber which is surrounded by an onion bulb formation. (d) Same field as in (c) but at higher magnification.

examination and inflammatory signs on muscle biopsy (with the presence of T cells, macrophages, dendritic cells, B cells, and plasma cells in the muscle tissue) [37]. More than half of the myositis is associated with the presence of autoantibodies [36]. These pathological and biological features suggest that immune mechanisms are involved in their pathogenesis [36]. Myositis patients can also develop additional autoimmune diseases, as seen in the "overlap syndromes" corresponding to the association of at least two different connective tissue diseases (such as the association of systemic sclerosis and myositis, also named "scleromyositis") [38]. Moreover, patients with idiopathic inflammatory myopathies may present various extramuscular signs such as skin manifestation (in dermatomyositis), cardiac disturbances, gastrointestinal disorders, pulmonary symptoms, or general symptoms (such as fever or Raynaud phenomenon) [39]. However, among all these manifestations, concomitant neurological and neuromuscular disorders have been rarely reported.

The association of myositis and neuritis was first described by Senator at the end of the nineteenth century [40]. The term of "neuromyositis" was given to this entity including acute or subacute occurrence of neuropathic signs (distal weakness and sensory disturbances, paresthesia, absent Achilles reflexes, and sometimes ataxia) and muscular signs (muscle hypertrophy then amyotrophy and myalgia), with pathological sign of inflammation in nerves and muscles [41]. Since that time, a decade of cases of "neuromyositis" were reported, usually with inflammatory signs in nerves (perineural infiltrates of lymphocytes or neutrophils) [42–44]; however, some patients may present nonspecific axonal neuropathy with no inflammation in the nerve [10], and recent reports also described nerve vasculitis [7, 18, 25]. These recent observations suggest that "neuromyositis" could be due to a vasculitic process as evidenced by the overexpression of VEGF (vascular endothelial growth factor) in both nerve and muscle of two patients (in comparison to controls) [18]. We did not observe any sign of vasculitis in nerves and muscles of our patients, but we noted pathological signs of demyelinating neuropathy suggesting that the mechanism of "neuromyositis" could be immune-mediated. However, this association may well represent an incidental combination of myositis and neuritis.

The simultaneous occurrence of Guillain-Barré syndrome (GBS) (as well as Miller-Fisher syndrome) and myasthenia gravis (MG) has also been reported in a few cases [3, 6, 9, 11]. The molecular mimicry between the infectious agents and self-antigens may initiate GBS and MG concurrently, as suggested by Krampfl et al. who showed that antibodies from patients with GBS can cross-react against acetylcholine

TABLE 2: Main characteristics of the patients with concurrent acute/subacute autoimmune neuromuscular disorders diagnosed at the same time (ranked in descending chronological order).

References	Type of NMD			Age	Sex	Description of NMD
	N	M	MG			
Our observations [2]						
Patient 1			•	67	F	Simultaneous diagnosis of MG (no thymus abnormality), subacute inflammatory neuropathy, and myositis
Patient 2	•		•	79	M	Simultaneous diagnosis of MG (no thymus abnormality), subacute inflammatory neuropathy, and myositis
Tanaka & Satomi, 2016 [3]	•		•	69	F	Simultaneous diagnosis of MFS (positivity of anti-GQ1b antibodies) and MG
Seton et al., 2013 [4]		•	•	46	F	Simultaneous diagnosis of PM and MG (with thymoma)
Paik et al., 2014 [5]						
Patient 1		•	•	75	F	Simultaneous diagnosis of DM and MG
Patient 2		•	•	44	M	Simultaneous diagnosis of PM and MG (with thymic mass and lymphoid follicular hyperplasia)
Patient 3		•	•	54	M	Simultaneous diagnosis of PM and MG
Patient 4		•	•	38	F	Simultaneous diagnosis of DM and MG (with thymic mass and lymphoid follicular hyperplasia)
Patient 5		•	•	61	M	Simultaneous diagnosis of PM and MG
Patient 6		•	•	24	F	Simultaneous diagnosis of PM and MG
Belin et al., 2013 [6]	•		•	58	M	Simultaneous diagnosis of GBS and MG
Reimann et al., 2011 [7]	•		•	57	M	Simultaneous diagnosis of myositis and neuropathy with pipestem capillaries and vascular activated complement deposition
Hill et al., 2011 [8]		•	•	67	F	Simultaneous diagnosis of DM and MG
Kung et al., 2009 [9]	•		•	36	F	Simultaneous diagnosis of GBS and MG
Nomura et al., 2010 [10]		•	•	52	F	Simultaneous diagnosis of DM and severe axonal neuropathy (nerve biopsy: axonal atrophy, ovoids, no demyelinating feature, no vasculitis)
Kizilay et al., 2008 [11]	•		•	52	M	Simultaneous diagnosis of GBS and MG
Kraus et al., 2007 [12]	•		•	65	M	Development of MG 10 weeks after GBS
Yoshidome et al., 2007 [13]		•	•	62	F	Simultaneous diagnosis of PM and MG
Avni et al., 2006 [14]			•	66	M	MG (with thymoma) diagnosed 2 weeks after treatment for PM (with high level of blood eosinophils)
Shichijo et al., 2005 [15]		•	•	57	M	Simultaneous diagnosis of DM and MG
Farah et al., 2005 [16]	•		•	71	F	Diagnosis of AMSAN two years after a diagnosis of MG
Diaco et al., 2004 [17]		•	•	47	F	Myositis (antisynthetase syndrome) developed in a context of MG

TABLE 2: Continued.

References	N	M	MG	Age	Sex	Description of NMD
Matsui et al., 2003 [18]						
Case 1	•	•		68	F	Simultaneous diagnosis of DM and inflammatory neuropathy
Case 2	•	•		48	F	Simultaneous diagnosis of DM and inflammatory neuropathy
Van de Warrenburg et al., 2002 [19]		•	•	28	F	Simultaneous diagnosis of DM and MG
Otton et al., 2000 [20]	•		•	71	M	Simultaneous diagnosis of MG (with thymoma) sensorimotor neuropathy (no nerve biopsy), and PM
Kornizky et al., 2000 [21]		•	•	69	M	PM in a context of MG
Raschilas et al., 1999 [22]		•	•	66	F	Simultaneous diagnosis of PM and MG (with malignant thymoma)
Kobayashi et al., 1997 [23]		•	•	14	F	PM developed 29 years after MG (in a context of Grave's syndrome)
Ko et al., 1995 [24]		•	•	25	F	Simultaneous diagnosis of PM and MG (with thymoma), with also autoimmune active chronic hepatitis
Vogelgesang et al., 1995 [25]	•	•		9	M	Simultaneous DM and sensorimotor neuropathy (no biopsy)
	•	•		7	F	Simultaneous DM and sensorimotor neuropathy (nerve biopsy: vasculitis)
Hausmanowa-Petrusewicz et al., 1995 [26]		•	•	58	F	DM developed 9 years after MG
Hassel et al., 1992 [27]		•	•	37	M	Simultaneous diagnosis of PM and MG two days after thymectomy (for thymoma)
Carlander et al., 1991 [28]	•		•	45	M	MG with recurrent episodes of GBS
Garcia-Merino et al., 1991 [29]	•		•	68	M	Inflammatory neuropathy (and continuous muscle fiber activity) developed 12 years after a diagnosis of MG (with thymoma)
Behan et al., 1982 [30]		•	•	56	M	Simultaneous diagnosis of PM and MG, with also Hashimoto's thyroiditis, pemphigoid, carcinoma of the bladder, and Norwegian scabies
Boudouresques et al., 1981 [31]	•		•	71	F	MG developed 7 months prior to GBS
Davis & Gallai, 1979 [32]		•	•			MG developed after PM
Vasilescu et al., 1978 [33]						
Case 1		•	•	24	F	Simultaneous diagnosis of DM and MG
Case 2		•	•	46	M	Simultaneous diagnosis of DM and MG
Case 3		•	•	18	F	Simultaneous diagnosis of DM and MG
Case 4		•	•	42	F	Simultaneous diagnosis of DM and MG
De Reuck et al., 1976 [34]		•	•	23	M	Simultaneous diagnosis of PM and MG

AMSAN: acute motor sensory axonal neuropathy; DM: = dermatomyositis; GBS: Guillain-Barré syndrome; M: myositis; MFS: Miller Fisher syndrome; MG: myasthenia gravis; N: acute/subacute neuropathy; NMD: neuromuscular disorder; PM: polymyositis.

receptors from mice [45]. It is also known that various infectious agents (such as viruses) may cause myalgias, rhabdomyolysis, and myositis (muscle biopsy showing degeneration and necrosis with overall little inflammatory infiltrates) [46]. In our cases, despite no evidence of infection or glycolipid antibodies, infectious or postinfectious origin could not be ruled out. Moreover, patient 2 has probably more developed acute onset CIDP (a-CIDP) than GBS.

In a recent study, six patients with concurrent MG and inflammatory myopathy (dermatomyositis or polymyositis) were reported, with also twenty other cases found in the medical literature since 1976: most of these patients had no thymic hyperplasia, and the main myasthenic manifestations were bulbar weakness (83%), limb weakness (83%), ptosis (33%), and diplopia (17%) [5]. The presence of pathological lesions in MG is not recent and was observed early in the beginning of the twentieth century. Carl Weigert first described the relationship between hypertrophy of the thymus and MG but also observed lymphocytic infiltrations ("lymphorrhages") in muscles of patients with MG (that he considered as "metastases of the thymoma") [47]. Lymphorrhages are found more frequently in patients with thymoma [48]. Other features have also been described in muscles of patients with MG, such as neurogenic muscular atrophy and focal myositis: focal myositis seems to occur chiefly in patients with thymoma [49], whereas neurogenic abnormalities are not linked to thymoma [50]. A relation was also established between lymphorrhages and anti-muscle antibodies [48]. Despite this strong relation between lymphorrhages and thymoma, our two patients presented no thymoma. Finally, myositis and myocarditis may be sometimes considered as an uncommon complication of MG. Some authors have described the occurrence of "nucleated giant cells" (probably due to muscle regeneration following inflammatory degeneration and necrosis) in the skeletal muscles and myocardium of patients with myasthenia and thymoma [51–63], but it was not the case in our patients. One explanation could be the presence of "striational antibodies" (recognizing epitopes on skeletal muscle proteins) detected in the serum of some patients with MG (particularly those against titin, ryanodine receptor, and Kv1.4) [64]. However, because such antibodies are not routinely tested, we were unable to test their presence in our patients.

The simultaneous occurrence of three autoimmune neuromuscular disorders is rare, and we found only one similar observation in the literature (a 71-year-old man who presented polymyositis, MG, and neuropathy in a context of T cell lymphoma) [20] (Table 2): electrophysiological features of axonal sensorimotor neuropathy were found, but no nerve biopsy was performed; MG was confirmed by a positivity of AchR antibodies (along with a thymic mass); muscle biopsy was consistent with a chronic inflammatory myopathy (no T cell infiltrates were observed). This observation is similar to ours (but without certainty of inflammation of the nerves), with an immune-mediated mechanism. However, the authors have not given any details about the follow-up of the patient. In our patients, we observed a significant improvement after immunosuppressive (steroids), immunomodulatory (IgIV), and acetylcholinesterase inhibitors. The simultaneous diagnosis of two acute/subacute (<3 months) autoimmune neuromuscular disorders is rare but more frequent than the triple association we have observed. Excluding the association of MG-thymoma-myositis-cardiomyositis (because of nonsimultaneous diagnosis, but successive diagnosis), we have found 41 cases in the medical literature: among these cases, the most frequent association was myositis-myasthenia (27 cases), neuropathy-myasthenia (8 cases), and neuropathy-myositis (6 cases) (Table 2). If it was not the case for our patients, thymoma has been found in some cases. Moreover, even if initial screening is negative, the long-term follow-up for the tumor is needed in such cases.

Finally, our cases illustrate the difficulty in diagnosis of neuromuscular disorders in the presence of overlaps. Although a chance association is possible, we suspect that the coexistence of these three inflammatory disorders relies on common immunological mechanisms: it should be borne in mind that a neuromuscular disorder can hide one or two others. Such associations are evidence for an immune-mediated origin of these diseases, but further studies are needed to confirm this hypothesis. These rare occurrences need to be recognized in order to manage these patients appropriately.

Abbreviations

AchR: Acetylcholine receptor
CMAP: Compound muscle action potential
CSF: Cerebrospinal fluid
CT-scan: Computerized tomography scanner
DNA: Deoxyribonucleic acid
GBS: Guillain-Barré syndrome
IU: International unit
IVIg: Intravenous immunoglobulins
LDL: Light density lipoprotein
MAG: Myelin-associated glycoprotein
MRC: Medical Research Council
MG: Myasthenia gravis
MRI: Magnetic resonance imaging
SNAP: Sensory nerve action potential
VEGF: Vascular endothelial growth factor.

Competing Interests

The authors declare that they have no competing interests.

References

[1] T. Chitnis and S. J. Khoury, "20. Immunologic neuromuscular disorders," *Journal of Allergy and Clinical Immunology*, vol. 111, supplement 2, pp. S659–S668, 2003.

[2] S. Mathis, L. Magy, P. Corcia, K. Ghorab, L. Richard, and J. M. Vallat, "Simultaneous combined myositis, inflammatory polyneuropathy and myasthenic syndrome (2014 Inflammatory Neuropathy Consortium of the Peripheral Nerve Society, Düsseldorf, Germany)," *Journal of the Peripheral Nervous System*, vol. 19, no. 3, p. 274, 2014.

[3] Y. Tanaka and K. Satomi, "Overlap of myasthenia gravis and Miller Fisher syndrome," *Internal Medicine*, vol. 55, no. 14, pp. 1917–1918, 2016.

[4] M. Seton, C. C. Wu, and A. Louissaint Jr., "Case records of the Massachusetts General Hospital. Case 26-2013—a 46-year-old woman with muscle pain and swelling," *The New England Journal of Medicine*, vol. 369, no. 8, pp. 764–773, 2013.

[5] J. J. Paik, A. M. Corse, and A. L. Mammen, "The co-existence of myasthenia gravis in patients with myositis: a case series," *Seminars in Arthritis and Rheumatism*, vol. 43, no. 6, pp. 792–796, 2014.

[6] J. Belin, B. De Toffol, M. Gaudron, A. Beaume, N. Gavrylova, and J. Praline, "Polyradiculonévrite aiguë et myasthénie auto-immune: quand un train peut en cacher un autre," *Revue Neurologique*, vol. 169, no. 6-7, p. 527, 2013.

[7] J. Reimann, C. Kornblum, K. Tolksdorf, W. Brück, and F. K. H. Van Landeghem, "Myopathy and neuropathy with pipestem capillaries and vascular activated complement deposition," *Neurology*, vol. 77, no. 4, pp. 401–403, 2011.

[8] E. K. Hill, P. H. King, and L. C. Hughey, "Dermatomyositis and concomitant overlap myasthenic syndrome: a rare presentation," *Journal of the American Academy of Dermatology*, vol. 65, no. 5, pp. e150–e152, 2011.

[9] S.-L. Kung, J.-M. Su, S.-J. Tsai, T.-M. Lu, and C.-M. Chen, "Concurrent Guillain-Barré syndrome and myasthenia gravis: the first case in Taiwan," *Acta Neurologica Taiwanica*, vol. 18, no. 3, pp. 193–197, 2009.

[10] M. Nomura, T. Watanabe, H. Mikami et al., "Adult dermatomyositis with severe polyneuropathy: does neuromyositis exist?" *Neurological Sciences*, vol. 31, no. 3, pp. 373–376, 2010.

[11] F. Kizilay, H. F. Ryan Jr., and S. J. Oh, "Myasthenia Gravis and Guillain-Barré syndrome occurring simultaneously in the same patient," *Muscle and Nerve*, vol. 37, no. 4, pp. 544–546, 2008.

[12] J. Kraus, I. Teismann, C. Kellinghaus et al., "Temporal coincidence between AMAN type of GBS and myasthenia gravis," *Journal of Neurology*, vol. 254, no. 2, pp. 264–265, 2007.

[13] Y. Yoshidome, S. Morimoto, N. Tamura et al., "A case of polymyositis complicated with myasthenic crisis," *Clinical Rheumatology*, vol. 26, no. 9, pp. 1569–1570, 2007.

[14] I. Avni, Y. Sharabi, M. Sadeh, and A. S. Buchman, "Eosinophilia, myositis, and myasthenia gravis associated with a thymoma," *Muscle and Nerve*, vol. 34, no. 2, pp. 242–245, 2006.

[15] K. Shichijo, T. Mitsui, M. Kunishige, Y. Kuroda, K. Masuda, and T. Matsumoto, "Involvement of mitochondria in myasthenia gravis complicated with dermatomyositis and rheumatoid arthritis: a case report," *Acta Neuropathologica*, vol. 109, no. 5, pp. 539–542, 2005.

[16] R. Farah, R. Farah, and W. Simri, "Acute motor sensory axonal Guillain-Barré syndrome and myasthenia gravis," *European Journal of Internal Medicine*, vol. 16, no. 2, pp. 134–135, 2005.

[17] M. Diaco, F. Ancarani, M. Montalto et al., "Association of myasthenia gravis and antisynthetase syndrome: a case report," *International Journal of Immunopathology and Pharmacology*, vol. 17, no. 3, pp. 395–399, 2004.

[18] N. Matsui, T. Mitsui, I. Endo, Y. Oshima, M. Kunishige, and T. Matsumoto, "Dermatomyositis with peripheral nervous system involvement: activation of vascular endothelial growth factor (VEGF) and VEGF receptor (VEGFR) in vasculitic lesions," *Internal Medicine*, vol. 42, no. 12, pp. 1233–1239, 2003.

[19] B. P. C. Van De Warrenburg, G. J. D. Hengstman, P. E. Vos, R. H. Boerman, H. J. Ter Laak, and B. G. M. Van Engelen, "Concomitant dermatomyositis and myasthenia gravis presenting with respiratory insufficiency," *Muscle and Nerve*, vol. 25, no. 2, pp. 293–296, 2002.

[20] S. H. Otton, G. R. Standen, and I. E. C. Ormerod, "T cell lymphocytosis associated with polymyositis, myasthenia gravis and thymoma," *Clinical and Laboratory Haematology*, vol. 22, no. 5, pp. 307–308, 2000.

[21] Y. Kornizky, I. Heller, A. Isakov, I. Shapira, and M. Topilsky, "Dysphagia with multiple autoimmune disease," *Clinical Rheumatology*, vol. 19, no. 4, pp. 321–323, 2000.

[22] F. Raschilas, L. Mouthon, M.-H. André, J. Azorin, A. Couvelard, and L. Guillevin, "Concomitant polymyositis and myasthenia gravis reveal malignant thymoma. A case report and review of the literature," *Annales de Medecine Interne*, vol. 150, no. 5, pp. 370–373, 1999.

[23] T. Kobayashi, H. Asakawa, Y. Komoike, Y. Nakano, Y. Tamaki, and M. Monden, "A patient with graves' disease, myasthenia gravis, and polymyositis," *Thyroid*, vol. 7, no. 4, pp. 631–632, 1997.

[24] K. F. Ko, T. Ho, and K. W. Chan, "Autoimmune chronic active hepatitis and polymyositis in a patient with myasthenia gravis and thymoma," *Journal of Neurology, Neurosurgery and Psychiatry*, vol. 59, no. 5, pp. 558–559, 1995.

[25] S. A. Vogelgesang, J. Gutierrez, G. L. Klipple, and I. M. Katona, "Polyneuropathy in juvenile dermatomyositis," *Journal of Rheumatology*, vol. 22, no. 7, pp. 1369–1372, 1995.

[26] I. Hausmanowa-Petrusewicz, M. Blaszczyk, and S. Jablońska, "Coexistence of scleromyositis associated with PM-SCL antibody and myasthenia," *Neuromuscular Disorders*, vol. 5, no. 2, pp. 145–147, 1995.

[27] B. Hassel, N. E. Gilhus, J. A. Aarli, and O. R. Skogen, "Fulminant myasthenia gravis and polymyositis after thymectomy for thymoma," *Acta Neurologica Scandinavica*, vol. 85, no. 1, pp. 63–65, 1992.

[28] B. Carlander, J. Touchon, M. Georgesco, and J. Cadilhac, "Myasthenia gravis and recurrent Guillain-Barré syndrome," *Neurology*, vol. 41, no. 11, p. 1848, 1991.

[29] A. García-Merino, A. Cabello, J. S. Mora, and H. Liaño, "Continuous muscle fiber activity, peripheral neuropathy, and thymoma," *Annals of Neurology*, vol. 29, no. 2, pp. 215–218, 1991.

[30] W. M. H. Behan, P. O. Behan, and D. Doyle, "Association of myasthenia gravis and polymyositis with neoplasia, infection and autoimmune disorders," *Acta Neuropathologica*, vol. 57, no. 2-3, pp. 221–229, 1982.

[31] G. Boudouresques, F. Delpuech, R. Giudicelli et al., "Polyradiculonévrite au cours d'une myasthénie avec thymome bénin," *La Nouvelle Presse Médicale*, vol. 10, no. 4, pp. 253–254, 1981.

[32] C. J. F. Davis and V. Gallai, "Myasthenia progressing to polymyositis with respiratory failure," *Acta Neurologica*, vol. 1, no. 5, pp. 365–370, 1979.

[33] C. Vasilescu, G. Bucur, A. Petrovici, and A. Florescu, "Myasthenia in patients with dermatomyositis. Clinical, electrophysiological and ultrastructural studies," *Journal of the Neurological Sciences*, vol. 38, no. 2, pp. 129–144, 1978.

[34] J. De Reuck, E. Thiery, W. De Coster, and H. Van Der Eecken, "Myasthenic syndrome in polymyositis," *European Neurology*, vol. 14, no. 4, pp. 275–284, 1976.

[35] J.-M. Vallat, A. Vital, L. Magy, M.-L. Martin-Negrier, and C. Vital, "An update on nerve biopsy," *Journal of Neuropathology and Experimental Neurology*, vol. 68, no. 8, pp. 833–844, 2009.

[36] P.-O. Carstens and J. Schmidt, "Diagnosis, pathogenesis and treatment of myositis: recent advances," *Clinical and Experimental Immunology*, vol. 175, no. 3, pp. 349–358, 2014.

[37] G. J. D. Hengstman, R. Brouwer, W. T. M. Vree Egberts et al., "Clinical and serological characteristics of 125 Dutch myositis

patients: myositis specific autoantibodies aid in the differential diagnosis of the idiopathic inflammatory myopathies," *Journal of Neurology*, vol. 249, no. 1, pp. 69–75, 2002.

[38] L. Iaccarino, M. Gatto, S. Bettio et al., "Overlap connective tissue disease syndromes," *Autoimmunity Reviews*, vol. 12, no. 3, pp. 363–373, 2013.

[39] J. C. Milisenda, A. Selva-O'Callaghan, and J. M. Grau, "The diagnosis and classification of polymyositis," *Journal of Autoimmunity*, vol. 48-49, pp. 118–121, 2014.

[40] H. Senator, "Über acute polymyositis und neuromyositis," *Deutsche Medizinische Wochenschrift*, vol. 19, no. 39, pp. 933–936, 1893.

[41] G. Marinesco, "Maladies des muscles," in *Traité de Médecine et de Thérapeutique*, P. Brouardel and A. Gilbert, Eds., Baillière & Fils, Paris, France, 1902.

[42] T. D. Kinney and M. M. Maher, "Dermatomyositis: a study of five cases," *American Journal of Pathology*, vol. 16, no. 5, pp. 561–594, 1940.

[43] K. D. Barron and D. I. M. Fine, "Neuromyositis," *The Journal of Nervous and Mental Disease*, vol. 128, no. 6, pp. 497–507, 1959.

[44] W. J. McEntee and E. L. Mancall, "Neuromyositis: a reappraisal," *Neurology*, vol. 15, no. 1, pp. 69–75, 1965.

[45] K. Krampfl, B. Mohammadi, B. Buchwald et al., "IgG from patients with Guillain-Barré syndrome interact with nicotinic acetylcholine receptor channels," *Muscle and Nerve*, vol. 27, no. 4, pp. 435–441, 2003.

[46] N. F. Crum-Cianflone, "Bacterial, fungal, parasitic, and viral myositis," *Clinical Microbiology Reviews*, vol. 21, no. 3, pp. 473–494, 2008.

[47] C. Weigert, "Pathologisch-anatomischer Beitrag zur Erb'schen Krankheit (Myasthenia gravis)," *Neurologisches Zentralblatt*, vol. 20, no. 8, pp. 597–601, 1901.

[48] H. J. Oosterhuis, J. Bethlem, and T. E. Feltkamp, "Muscle pathology, thymoma, and immunological abnormalities in patients with myasthenia gravis," *Journal of Neurology Neurosurgery and Psychiatry*, vol. 31, no. 5, pp. 460–463, 1968.

[49] G. Genkins, H. Mendelow, H. J. Sobel, and K. E. Osserman, "Myasthenia gravis: analysis of thirty-one consecutive postmortem examinations," in *Myasthenia Gravis*, H. R. Viets, Ed., pp. 519–530, Thomas, Springfield, Ill, USA, 1961.

[50] H. Oosterhuis and J. Bethlem, "Neurogenic muscle involvement in myasthenia gravis. A clinical and histopathological study," *Journal of Neurology Neurosurgery and Psychiatry*, vol. 36, no. 2, pp. 244–254, 1973.

[51] A. S. Giordano and J. L. Haymond, "Myasthenia gravis: a report of two cases with necropsy," *American Journal of Clinical Patholology*, vol. 14, no. 5, pp. 253–265, 1944.

[52] H. Mendelow and G. Genkins, "Studies in myasthenia gravis: cardiac and associated pathology," *Journal of the Mount Sinai Hospital, New York*, vol. 21, no. 4, pp. 218–225, 1954.

[53] L. P. Rowland, "Prostigmine-responsiveness and the diagnosis of myasthenia gravis," *Neurology*, vol. 5, no. 9, pp. 612–623, 1955.

[54] H. O. Klein and K. J. Lennartz, "Zur syntropie von myasthenia gravis, polymyositis, myokarditis und thymom; zugleich ein beitrag zur pathogenese," *Deutsche Medizinischer Wochenschrift*, vol. 91, no. 39, pp. 1727–1730, 1966.

[55] J. S. Burke, N. M. Medline, and A. Katz, "Giant cell myocarditis and myositis. Associated with thymoma and myasthenia gravis," *Archives of Pathology*, vol. 88, no. 4, pp. 359–366, 1969.

[56] H. Suzuki, Y. Mizuno, T. Kurita, M. Tsuchiya, Y. Hosota Y, and H. Yoshimatsu, "Rare type of myositis ans myocarditis revealed in myasthenia gravis with malignant thymoma," *Saishin Igaku*, vol. 31, pp. 2417–2424, 1976.

[57] T. Namba, N. G. Brunner, and D. Grob, "Idiopathic giant cell polymyositis. Report of a case and review of the syndrome," *Archives of Neurology*, vol. 31, no. 1, pp. 27–30, 1974.

[58] M. Reznik, "Deux cas de syndrome myasthénique avec thymome, polymyosite, myocardite et thyroïdite," *Journal of the Neurological Sciences*, vol. 22, no. 3, pp. 341–351, 1974.

[59] C. Bourgeois-Droin, A. Sauvanet, F. Lemarchand, A. De Roquancourt, F. Cottenot, and C. Brocheriou, "Thymome, myasthénie, érythroblastopénie, myosite et myocardite à cellules géantes. Une observation," *La Nouvelle Presse Médicale*, vol. 10, no. 25, pp. 2097–2104, 1981.

[60] H. Tomimoto, I. Akiguchi, M. Kameyama, H. Haibara, and M. Kitaichi, "Giant cell myositis and myocarditis associated with myasthenia gravis and thymoma—an autopsy case," *Rinsho Shinkeigaku*, vol. 25, no. 6, pp. 688–693, 1985.

[61] H. Sato, E. Iwasaki, S. Nogawa et al., "A patient with giant cell myocarditis and myositis associated with thymoma and myasthenia gravis," *Rinsho Shinkeigaku*, vol. 43, no. 8, pp. 496–499, 2003.

[62] P. J. Weiller, J. M. Durand, M. A. Prince-Zucchelli et al., "L'association polymyosite, myasthénie, thymome. Un cas et revue de la littérature," *Annales de Médecine Interne*, vol. 135, no. 1, pp. 299–304, 1984.

[63] T. Kon, F. Mori, K. Tanji, Y. Miki, T. Kimura, and K. Wakabayashi, "Giant cell polymyositis and myocarditis associated with myasthenia gravis and thymoma," *Neuropathology*, vol. 33, no. 3, pp. 281–287, 2013.

[64] S. Suzuki, K. Utsugisawa, Y. Nagane, and N. Suzuki, "Three types of striational antibodies in myasthenia gravis," *Autoimmune Diseases*, vol. 2011, Article ID 740583, 7 pages, 2011.

CT Perfusion to Guide Placement of Invasive Cerebral Perfusion Monitor in Subarachnoid Hemorrhage Induced Vasospasm

Hosam Al-Jehani [1,2] Judith Marcoux,[1] Kawthar Hadhiah,[2] Faisal Alabbas,[2] Mark Angle,[1] and Jeanne Teitelbaum[1]

[1] Department of Neurology and Neurosurgery, Montreal Neurological Institute and Hospital, McGill University, Montreal, QC, Canada
[2] Department of Neurosurgery and Critical Care Medicine, King Fahad Hospital of the University, Imam Abdulrahman bin Faisal University, Al-Khobar, Saudi Arabia

Correspondence should be addressed to Hosam Al-Jehani; hosam.aljehani@gmail.com

Academic Editor: Peter Berlit

Background. Vasospasm is a challenging component of the subarachnoid hemorrhage "syndrome" that is unpredictable and very difficult to monitor using noninvasive or invasive monitoring technologies in neurocritical units. *Methods.* We describe the novel use of computerized tomography perfusion (CTP) imaging to choose proper targets for invasive cerebral blood flow monitors. *Results.* A total of 3 patients are included in this report. CTP parameters were used to generate points of interest to target using invasive cerebral monitoring of the cerebral blood flow and initiate vasodilator therapy and subsequently guide its weaning. *Conclusions.* CTP can be useful in localizing a specific anatomical target for invasive monitoring in subarachnoid hemorrhage patients suffering from vasospasm.

1. Introduction

Vasospasm is a devastating event, complicating as high as 50% of SAH with increased morbidity and mortality [1]. Most imaging modalities (such as cerebral angiogram, CT-angiogram, or transcranial Doppler) do not give continuous monitoring and therefore are typically used only if there is clinical suspicion of vasospasm. Several methods have been in use to detect vasospasm early on, prior to its clinical manifestation, including continuous transcranial Doppler (TCD) and electroencephalography (EEG) [2, 3]. More recently, invasive monitoring devices have been implemented, again in the effort to detect vasospasm early, including brain oxygen monitors and cerebral perfusion monitors [4, 5].

The major drawback of these devices is the small sampling volume, which precludes robust assessment of early changes potentially leading to vasospasm. Choosing a target has been done through standardized landmarks and insertion angles of a monitoring "bundle" in either frontal lobe depending on the seen or sometimes perceived burden of pathology. Another localizing strategy is to place the invasive cerebral monitor in the vicinity of the lesion seen on imaging in cases of focal injury with recent evidence of improvement in outcome [6]. This strategy proves less reliable and potentially futile in a dynamic disease such as SAH and vasospasm with an essentially normal brain parenchyma on CT scans until the development of vasospasm and progression to hypodensities, at which point the futility of treatment is a major concern.

Recent refinement in computed tomography perfusion (CTP) imaging led to more utilization of this technology in vasospasm [7]. Several parameters have been debated as to their ability and reliability of vasospasm detection. Of those, time-to-peak (TTP) has gained popularity as a surrogate for assessment of cerebral autoregulation, the impairment of which is thought to be conducive to vasospasm [8].

We describe a series of cases in which we used CT perfusion parameters, especially the time-to-peak, to guide localization of the Bowman Perfusion Monitor (BPM) insertion in patients suspected to have vasospasm.

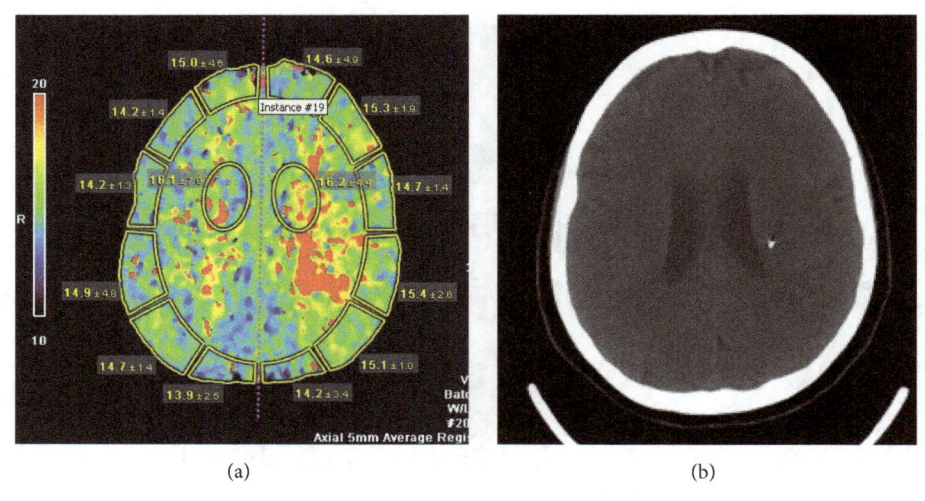

FIGURE 1: (a) prolongation of the TTP signal in the left central Rolandic white matter. (b) A plain CT scan showing the tip of the BPM in the area of the prolongation of the TTP.

2. Case Summaries

2.1. Case 1. A 34-year-old woman presented with abrupt onset headache and lethargy attributable to an acute SAH secondary to a ruptured P-1 aneurysm. She received standard therapy for SAH patients and had successful coiling of the aneurysm. On postbleeding day 4, while hemodynamically stable, she developed a new drift in the right upper extremity that progressed to grade 3/5 motor weakness with facial weakness within 30 minutes. A repeat plain CT showed no hydrocephalus. The CT perfusion showed no derangement of the cerebral blood volume (CBV) or the cerebral blood flow (CBF) with a slightly prolonged mean transit time (MTT) denoting intact brain tissue. The time-to-peak (TTP), on the other hand, was significantly prolonged in the left central Rolandic subcortical region, consistent with the clinical finding (Figure 1). A Bowman Perfusion Monitor (BPM, Hemedex, MA, USA) was inserted at the bedside, using free-hand technique aiming at the point of interest generated by the CT perfusion TTP scan. The cerebral blood flow (CBF) measured at this time was 14 cc/100 g/min, denoting severe hypoperfusion (normal level is above 25 cc/100 g/min). The patient was started on the MNH-milrinone protocol for the treatment of vasospasm [9]. Within 1 hour, the patient did not improve, necessitating endovascular vasodilator therapy, during which she received 2 mcg of milrinone over 3 minutes with immediate vasodilation of the vasospastic segment. The CBF reading improved to the 50's with the maintenance of milrinone. On 2 occasions, weaning the milrinone infusion was associated with an asymptomatic but significant drop of the measured CBF to low 20's, which delayed the weaning for 24–48 hours each time, likely related to recoil of angioplastied vessel mitigated clinically by the milrinone effect. The total monitoring period was 9 days, after which milrinone was stopped and CBF measurement ranged from 40 to 50 and the patient did not have any residual motor deficits for an additional 48 hours.

2.2. Case 2. A 46-year-old male suffered a grade 4 SAH, with clinical evidence of a rebleed prior to arrival, associated with a left frontal hematoma. Angiography showed a small blister aneurysm in the ophthalmic segment of the left internal carotid artery for which the patient was submitted to a craniotomy and clipping of the aneurysm. CTP was done postoperatively showing no asymmetry in the perfusion of the 2 cerebral hemispheres. On postadmission day 8, the patient developed new right-sided weakness; the noncontrast CT scan excluded the presence of hypodensities other than the perihematoma edema around the left frontal bleed. CT angiogram showed evidence of vasospasm in the left A1 and anterior-communicating artery with no evidence of vasospasm in the left MCA. The CTP maps showed no evidence of infarction as there was no CBF/CBV other than the artifact of the hematoma. Although subtle, there was a prolongation of the TTP map in the left central white matter, which corresponded to the patient's deficit. That point was chosen to be the target for the cerebral perfusion monitor, which was inserted using a free-hand technique. After insertion, CT scan confirmed the proper targeting of the point of interest generated by the CTP-TTP map. The initial CBF was 16 and it improved to high 30's after the milrinone protocol was instituted. The patient was weaned in due course and the follow-up CT scan demonstrated no hypodensities other than that related to the left frontal hematoma.

2.3. Case 3. A 67-year-old female suffered a grade 4 SAH from a ruptured PCOM aneurysm, which was uneventfully coiled. She had a complicated course in the NICU with a new onset atrial fibrillation and labile hypertension. She deteriorated after admission day 4 in the form of reduced level of response, but no lateralizing deficit was detected. A plain CT scan showed evidence of a new hypodensity in the right frontal region. A CTP confirmed that this hypodensity corresponded to an area of cerebral infarction by CBV/CBF maps. Interestingly, the central white matter in the right hemisphere showed prolonged TTP. We chose that as the target for the cerebral perfusion monitor. The initial CBF was 22, which improved marginally to 26 after a milrinone protocol was instituted. The trend in the first 12 hours of monitoring was that of a stable CBF reading but the brain temperature was noted to be increasing gradually from 36.6 to 38.1 without systemic fever detected by the nursing team and a stable CBF recording. This was followed after few hours by a drop of the CBF to 15 coinciding with significant worsening of the patient's level of consciousness. Another bolus of milrinone and an increased dose failed to improve the CBF, which continued to drop to as low as 6, being in the zone of frank cerebral ischemia. A new CT scan showed the development of several hypodensities bilaterally, including the area that was chosen for monitoring. Further increases of milrinone were not tolerated due to cardiac decompensation, and further escalation of therapy was deferred.

3. Discussion

Invasive cerebral monitoring of cerebral homeostatic functions is gaining popularity in the field of neurocritical care. It can provide anticipatory data in the evolution of cerebral insults prior to clinical deterioration, permitting, at least in theory, a better cerebral protection from secondary injury and improvement in outcome. One of the major concerns with these modalities of monitoring is the small sampling size within the injured or diseased brain. This and the usual placement in the frontal lobe to be as close to the known land marks of ICP monitoring insertion as possible result in a forced sampling strategy. This could be useful in a brain insult, where there is a focal lesion in or near the frontal area. On the contrary, in a dynamic or unpredictable disease such as vasospasm, choosing predetermined target might lead to missed monitoring opportunity because of lack of useful information as the deterioration might be occurring in another lobe or the other hemisphere.

Our cases illustrate the useful utilization of noninvasive CTP imaging data to generate points of interest for invasive monitoring. This combination overcomes the random field invasive monitoring, which has a great potential to reduce the accuracy of the monitoring process or missampling the "real" target area. In all 3 patients, none of the probes inserted were inserted in the frontal region, which would have been the usual target for the insertion of the monitoring bundle. In one of the patients (Case 3), if the probe had been inserted in the frontal lobe, it would have landed in an infarcted area, potentially skewing the management escalation of the patient. CTP was instrumental in detecting areas of potential derangement of cerebral autoregulation and vasospasm, which are out of the usual frontal zone of insertion of the monitoring bundle. This will allow for the ideal application of this technology in the setting of SAH, as it could detect event leading up to the clinical vasospasm, such as perturbed autoregulation, at a much earlier time frame [10]. With refinement of the technology and better understanding of its output, its advantage and clinical utility will increase. For example, the proper targeting allowed more reliable information that incurred an escalation, maintenance, and withdrawal of care in our patients. Because the potential targets would be variable based on CTP maps, free-hand insertion of invasive monitoring poses an accuracy concern. This issue can be improved and potentially resolved by the use of Neuronavigation systems abbreviated to suit the needs of "points-care" setup as in this case, the ICU.

In conclusion, utilization of data generated by noninvasive radiological imaging such as CTP would potentially increase our accuracy of targeting points of interest in monitoring for vasospasm in subarachnoid hemorrhage patients and guide their therapy.

References

[1] J. van Gijn and G. J. E. Rinkel, "Subarachnoid haemorrhage: diagnosis, causes and management," *Brain*, vol. 124, no. 2, pp. 249–278, 2001.

[2] C. M. Miller, D. Palestrant, W. I. Schievink, and M. J. Alexander, "Prolonged transcranial doppler monitoring after aneurysmal subarachnoid hemorrhage fails to adequately predict ischemic risk," *Neurocritical Care*, vol. 15, no. 3, pp. 387–392, 2011.

[3] R. Rathakrishnan, J. Gotman, F. Dubeau, and M. Angle, "Using continuous electroencephalography in the management of delayed cerebral ischemia following subarachnoid hemorrhage," *Neurocritical Care*, vol. 14, no. 2, pp. 152–161, 2011.

[4] M. Seule, C. Muroi, C. Sikorski, and E. Keller, "Monitoring of cerebral hemodynamics and oxygenation to detect delayed ischemic neurological deficit after aneurysmal subarachnoid hemorrhage," *Acta Neurochirurgica, Supplementum*, no. 115, pp. 57–61, 2013.

[5] P. Vajkoczy, P. Horn, C. Thome, E. Munch, and P. Schmiedek, "Regional cerebral blood flow monitoring in the diagnosis of delayed ischemia following aneurysmal subarachnoid hemorrhage," *Journal of Neurosurgery*, vol. 98, no. 6, pp. 1227–1234, 2003.

[6] J. Nortje and A. K. Gupta, "The role of tissue oxygen monitoring in patients with acute brain injury," *British Journal of Anaesthesia*, vol. 97, no. 1, pp. 95–106, 2006.

[7] M. Pham, A. Johnson, A. J. Bartsch et al., "CT perfusion predicts secondary cerebral infarction after aneurysmal subarachnoid hemorrhage," *Neurology*, vol. 69, no. 8, pp. 762–765, 2007.

[8] M. A. Kamp, H.-J. Heiroth, K. Beseoglu, B. Turowski, H.-J. Steiger, and D. Hänggi, "Early CT perfusion measurement after aneurysmal subarachnoid hemorrhage: A screening method to predict outcome?" *Acta Neurochirurgica, Supplementum*, no. 114, pp. 329–332, 2012.

[9] M. Lannes, J. Teitelbaum, M. del Pilar Cortés, M. Cardoso, and M. Angle, "Milrinone and homeostasis to treat cerebral vasospasm associated with subarachnoid hemorrhage: the Montreal Neurological Hospital protocol," *Neurocritical Care*, vol. 16, no. 3, pp. 354–362, 2012.

[10] H. Al-Jehani, M. Angle, J. Marcoux, and J. Teitelbaum, "Early abnormal transient hyperemic response test can predict delayed ischemic neurologic deficit in subarachnoid hemorrhage," *Critical Ultrasound Journal*, vol. 10, no. 1, 2018.

Oral High-Dose Thiamine Improves the Symptoms of Chronic Cluster Headache

Costantini Antonio ,[1,2] Tiberi Massimo,[2] Zarletti Gianpaolo,[2] Pala Maria Immacolata,[3] and Trevi Erika[2]

[1]*Università Cattolica di Roma, Largo Agostino Gemelli, Roma, Italy*
[2]*Centro Polispecialistico Giovanni Paolo I, Viterbo, Italy*
[3]*Department of Neurological Rehabilitation, The "Villa Immacolata" Clinic, Viterbo, Italy*

Correspondence should be addressed to Costantini Antonio; carapetata@libero.it

Academic Editor: Chin-Chang Huang

Cluster headache is a rare painful primary disorder occurring in either episodic or chronic patterns. Several authors found that the hypothalamus, the brain region regulating endocrine function and autonomic system, is involved in the pathophysiology of cluster headache. Some authors have found in patients affected by this disease abnormality in glucose metabolism. Considering the role of thiamine in brain function, in energetic metabolism, and in pain modulation, we treated a patient affected by cluster headache with oral high-dose thiamine. We report a 41-year-old man suffering from primary chronic cluster headache since the age of 15 years. The patient began oral therapy with high-dose thiamine in December 2016. Oral thiamine supplementation led to a dramatic improvement of the symptoms. The therapy was effective in reversing all the symptoms of the disease. Our observation suggests that a thiamine deficiency due to enzymatic abnormalities or to dysfunction of the circulation of thiamine in the intracellular space could cause a neuronal selective impairment in the centers that are involved in this disease and could have an important role in the pathogenesis of the symptoms of cluster headache.

1. Introduction

Cluster headache (CH) is a primary headache, characterized by recurrent short-lasting attacks (15 to 180 minutes) of extremely severe unilateral periorbital pain together with ipsilateral autonomic signs (lacrimation, nasal congestion, ptosis, miosis, lid edema, and redness of the eye) [1]. The precise causative mechanisms are not yet known. Several authors found that the hypothalamus, the structure regulating endocrine function and autonomic system, is involved in the pathophysiology of CH [1]. There is no therapy for CH. However, there are some effective treatments for both the acute painful attacks as well as for the prophylactic treatments. The course of the disease is unpredictable. If the CH does not have periods of regression, it can be defined as chronic cluster headache (CCH) [2, 3].

Some authors found in CH patients abnormalities of cerebral glucose brain metabolism, hypometabolism in the cerebellopontine area, perigenual anterior cingulate cortex, and prefrontal and orbitofrontal cortex during bout and out of bout [4–6]. The same authors supposed that a decreased metabolism determines a deficient top-down modulation of antinociceptive circuits in CH patients.

Recently, other authors speculated that thiamine could have an important role in relieving migraine [7]. In our previous study on the treatment of extraintestinal symptoms of ulcerative colitis we described the case of a patient who had weekly episodes of migraine type, which completely regressed with high-dose thiamine [8]. The same treatment showed effectiveness in relieving pain in fibromyalgia [9].

Thiamine-dependent processes are critical in glucose metabolism, and recent studies implicate a role of these processes in oxidative stress, protein processing, peroxisomal function, and gene expression [9]. Primary thiamine deficiency is caused by inadequate intake of thiamine. Secondary thiamine deficiency is caused by increase demand, impaired absorption, or impaired metabolism. In alcoholics, many mechanisms contribute to thiamine deficiency. Thiamine deficiency causes Beri-Beri and Wernicke-Korsakoff syndrome [10, 11].

We have been treating several patients affected by different neurodegenerative diseases, sporadic or genetic, with high-dose thiamine [12, 13]. The favorable results in motor and nonmotor symptoms we obtained thus far led us to think that the symptoms of other neurological diseases could be caused by an intracellular, focal thiamine deficiency as well. This deficiency could be linked to a dysfunction of thiamine transport or to structural enzymatic abnormalities.

We hypothesized that abnormalities of brain energy metabolism in CH could be linked to selective neuronal thiamine deficiency in the centers that are involved in this disease. Additionally, we have decided to treat with high doses of thiamine a patient affected by CCH to clarify the potential effect of thiamine in the therapy of the disease.

Written informed consent was taken from the patient. The study did not require approval by Ethic Committee as per the local retrospective observations.

2. Case Presentation

Patient is male, 41 years old, and of 95 kg weight. First attack of right periorbital headache was at the age of 15 (in 1991), some days after a motorcycle accident.

This first attack lasted about one hour; it recurred every day but at different times of the day for about one week. The severe unilateral periorbital pain was always associated with agitation and ipsilateral autonomic signs (lacrimation, nasal congestion, ptosis, lid edema, and redness of the eye). These episodes lasted a week and did not occur for some years. About three years later, at the age of 18, headache attacks reappeared with a frequency of two or three per day for 15 days. Subsequently, these attacks occurred approximately every year/a year and a half, with two attacks per day over a two-week period. No prophylactic treatment currently used (verapamil, lithium carbonate, topiramate, valproic acid, gabapentin, and baclofen) has given benefits. No therapy including oxygen, octreotide, local anesthetics, dihydroergotamine, or indomethacin was useful for the treatment of acute attacks. From the age of 20, the patient began to use Sumatriptan (only drug that was shown to be effective) in a 6 mg subcutaneous injection that, in 10 to 20 minutes, was able to stop the single attack whose pain was intolerable. However, over time, the frequency of the headache attacks intensified, until the patient was 32 years old, when the frequency of headache attacks became daily (three to four per day) and these were still treated with Sumatriptan. No other drug had ever been effective in the prevention and the treatment of individual attacks. Rarely, the headache appeared in the left head area. This situation lasted for six years, until 2013, when, following the extraction of a tooth enclosed in the right maxillary bone, headache attacks disappeared for three years. In January 2016, clusters reappeared daily (4-5 attacks), always with the same characteristics and without any headache-free period until the end of December 2016, when the patient began the treatment we proposed. During the period September–December 2016, the patient also took 75 mg of prednisone daily, orally, without any benefit. The patient's diet was free, without alcoholics.

The CH diagnosis has been confirmed by all major centers for the treatment of headache in Italy (National Institute of Neurology Carlo Besta of Milan, S. Raffaele Hospital in Milan and in Rome). The diagnosis of CH was based on clinical history, physical examination, and Nuclear Magnetic Resonance (NMR) imaging. On our first examination, the patient's clinical picture corresponded to the classification of ICHD3.

Common biochemical and haematological investigations were normal, as well as electroencephalogram, brain magnetic resonance imaging, and neurological examination. Plasma thiamine level was 64 microg/L (normal value: 28–85).

We performed the cluster headache quality of life scale (CHQ) [14]. CHQ is a rating scale assessing how much the headache influences the patient's quality of life. It is composed of 28 items and its total score ranges from 28 to 140 points (28 = cluster headache does not influence the quality of life; 140 = cluster headache influences maximally the quality of life). In addition, the patient also did the Visual Analogic Scale (VAS) test, which measures how much the person is satisfied with his/her life. This test asks the patient to express a value between 0 (completely unsatisfied) and 100 (completely satisfied) concerning his/her overall quality of life. Before starting the therapy with thiamine, the CHQ score was 107 points, and the VAS score was 40 points (see Table 1).

We started thiamine treatment with an oral dose of 250 mg in the morning. Every 3 days the dose was increased by 250 mg up to the dose of 750 mg. This procedure of increasing dosage was followed because even low doses on normal individuals or on individuals who do not need vitamin supplements may show side effects such as tachycardia, anxiety, and difficulties in falling asleep [8]. The patient repeated the neurological exam CHQ of life scale one month after the beginning of the therapy (see Table 1). The patient had a progressive improvement of the symptoms. The headache episodes decreased in frequency until they disappeared completely within 10 days. Subsequently, as sometimes the patient reported short-term episodes described as "a weight on the head," the dose was increased to one gram per day. This, however, caused the recurrence of a headache episode every morning at 4 o'clock, perfectly on time. The dose reduction to 750 mg/day caused the complete absence of headache attacks.

In March 2017, the patient had been invited to suspend the treatment to verify whether the headache attacks would reappear, but the patient refused to halt the high-dose thiamine therapy worrying that the pain and other symptoms could return. In May 2017, the patient accidentally forgot to bring the thiamine during a short vacation. Approximately 48 hours after the last dose of thiamine, he had a typical headache attack lasting about 60 minutes. The pain was strong but slightly attenuated and, therefore, tolerable compared to previous episodes. Later, the patient started a slimming diet and reduced the daily thiamine dose to 500 mg without any recurrence.

TABLE 1: *Cluster headache quality of life scale (CHQ)*. The table indicates the frequency with which cluster headache influences the events indicated in the questions below. Linkert's scale (gives a numerical value to each answer): never = 1; occasionally = 2; sometimes = 3; often = 4; always = 5. The higher the score is, the more the headache influences negatively the patient's quality of life. The scale goes from 28 (the headache does not influence the patient's life) to 140 (it influences it maximally).

	Before	After
(1) Did it avoid you leaving the house?	4	1
(2) Did it avoid making plans due to unpredictability of CH e.g. holidays?	5	1
(3) Did you feel unable to complete duties at work?	4	1
(4) Did you have difficulty in getting involved in leisure activities e.g. cinema, theatre, etc?	4	1
(5) Did you avoid crowded and noisy places e.g., public transport, pubs, etc?	5	1
(6) Did you feel that the severity of cluster headache affected your daily activities?	5	1
(7) Have you been less involved in family affairs e.g. interactions with children, planning holidays?	4	1
(8) Have you been unable to socialize/spend time with friends and family?	4	1
(9) Have you been unable to achieve your daily goals and carry out routines and chores?	4	1
(10) Did you feel less respected by others?	3	1
(11) Did you have problem with close personal relationships?	3	1
(12) Did you feel you were burden for family and friends?	3	1
(13) Did you feel self-conscious and uncomfortable about your appearance after a cluster headache attack (e.g. swelling redness of eyes and facial sweating, etc)?	4	1
(14) Did you feel that others are dismissive of your cluster headache?	3	1
(15) Did you feel aggressive?	3	1
(16) Did you feel bad about yourself, lose self-confidence or feel worthless?	2	1
(17) Did you feel like harming yourself or suicidal?	2	1
(18) Have you been irritable, impatient or less tolerant?	3	1
(19) Have you been forgetful e.g., missed appointments?	4	1
(20) Have you been unable to take care of your appearance (e.g. take a bath, put make-up on, change clothe etc)?	3	1
(21) Did you feel isolated, lonely or vulnerable?	3	1
(22) Did you find your pain is unbearable if untreated?	5	1
(23) Did you dread that the headache would not go away?	5	1
(24) Did you feel lacking in energy and constantly tired?	4	1
(25) Did you feel sleepy, worn out or less able to concentrate due to nocturnal attacks of CH?	5	1
(26) Did you have problems concentrating e.g., reading paper, watching TV, etc.?	5	1
(27) Have you been unable to think clearly?	4	1
(28) Did you feel tense or anxious?	4	1
Total score: .../140	107	28

VAS: it measures how much the person is satisfied of her/his life (0 = completely unsatisfied; 100 = completely satisfied). The score of our patient was 40 before therapy and 100 after therapy with thiamine.

3. Discussion

Our patient affected by CCH has been treated with thiamine with benefit. Several years before, the patient was diagnosed with CH from many neurology centers of excellence in Italy. The clinical features, in particular headache characteristics, duration of the attacks (lasting more than 30 minutes before the high-dose thiamine therapy), ancillary symptoms, and the absence of improvement with indomethacin treatment (typical for another type of headache, named chronic paroxysmal migraine), confirm the diagnosis of CCH.

There was also a temporal relation between thiamine supplementation and improvement of headache, and there was a temporal link between the treatment suspension and the return of the attacks. The patient had a favorable response to thiamine. These data may suggest that any abnormalities in thiamine-dependent processes could be overcome by a diffusion-mediated transport at elevated thiamine concentrations. In the presence of thiamine deficiency, the response to therapy is considered diagnostic [15]. The response of neurological symptoms to thiamine supplementation in patients with normal concentrations of plasma thiamine could be explained if referred to a form of thiamine deficiency due to structural enzymatic abnormality or to dysfunctions of the transport or the circulation of thiamine in the intracellular space [16]. A high number of recent data showed that thiamine actions are not limited only to a coenzymatic role, but even its noncoenzymatic roles are relevant, particularly in neuroprotection and, then, in neurodegenerative diseases [10, 11]. Genetic or sporadic disorders of thiamine metabolism that lead to neurological diseases can be treated with high doses of thiamine [16, 17]. The exact mechanism of thiamine responsiveness in these patients remains unknown.

Oral high-dose thiamine was effective in reversing the symptoms of CH. However, pain (and related disorders) is not a symptom of classic thiamine deficiency. In neuronal circuits that control sensory inputs, a severe dysfunction of thiamine-dependent processes could produce these dysfunctional symptoms.

There is an increasing number of reports on effects of thiamine and of its derivatives, benfotiamine and thiamine monophosphate or pyrophosphate, in modulating pain process, both in animal models and in human studies; in these reports the treatment with thiamine improved the pain relief and supported this other noncoenzymatic role of thiamine [18–20].

These clinical and experimental observations allowed supposing that symptoms featuring CCH could derive from a focal thiamine deficiency that determines a neuronal selective impairment. The administration of large amount of oral vitamin B1 increases the intracellular passive transport of the thiamine and thus the symptoms decrease when thiamine-dependent processes are led back to physiologic levels [16, 17, 21]. This effect of thiamine in neurological long-lasting diseases by reversing clinical symptoms may be probably not directly related to the regulation of glucose metabolism and suggests a neuronal dysfunction rather than a neurodegeneration.

As we write this report, the patient maintains the same clinical conditions, without any side effects. We hope that a lifelong use of high doses of thiamine in individuals affected by CH can allow keeping the attacks under control and limiting the progression of the disease. In literature, there is no mention of thiamine-related adverse effects even at high doses and for very long periods of time [12, 22]. However, we had observed that, increasing the dose to reach a better result in a patient affected by ulcerative colitis with fatigue, mild tachycardia and insomnia appeared. By reducing the dose, tachycardia reversed within a few days [8]. When the dose of thiamine is excessive for the patient's necessity, the patient may experience agitation, insomnia, and the reappearance of the neurological symptoms previously reversed, as observed during treatment of neurodegenerative diseases including Parkinson's disease, Friedreich's ataxia, and dystonia (personal data not yet published). In the case of our patient treated for CH, the increase of thiamine doses also led to the reappearance of the neurological symptoms. The mechanism that may lead to such a manifestation of previously disappeared symptoms is unclear. Previous neurological conditions were restored by reducing the vitamin dose.

In conclusion, we think that our report represents an important contribution to the issue; nonetheless, further experience is necessary to confirm the present observation.

4. Learning Points

In literature, there is no mention that thiamine deficiency could play a role in the pathogenesis of cluster disease symptoms.

The abnormalities in thiamine-dependent processes could be overcome by a diffusion-mediated transport at supernormal thiamine concentrations.

Cluster headache appears to be responsive to high-dose thiamine. Cluster headache symptoms could be substantially reduced or even canceled with a simple, inexpensive, innocuous, quick, and highly effective therapy.

Authors' Contributions

A. Costantini conceived of the study. All the authors equally collaborated in drafting and finalizing this manuscript and in reading and approving the final manuscript.

Acknowledgments

The authors thank Iara Tundo for the collaboration.

References

[1] E. Leroux and A. Ducros, "Cluster headache," *Orphanet Journal of Rare Diseases*, vol. 3, no. 1, article no. 20, 2008.

[2] M. S. Robbins, A. J. Starling, T. M. Pringsheim, W. J. Becker, and T. J. Schwedt, "Treatment of Cluster Headache: The American Headache Society Evidence-Based Guidelines," *Headache: The Journal of Head and Face Pain*, vol. 56, no. 7, pp. 1093–1106, 2016.

[3] Headache Classification Committee of the International Headache Society (IHS), "The International Classification of Headache Disorders, 3rd edition (beta version)," *Cephalalgia*, vol. 33, no. 9, pp. 629–808, 2013.

[4] R. Lodi, G. Pierangeli, and G. Tonon, "Study of hypotalamic metabolism in cluster headache by proton MR spectroscopy," *Neurology*, vol. 66, no. 8, pp. 1264–1266, 2006.

[5] A. Buture, R. Gooriah, R. Nimeri, and F. Ahmed, "Current understanding on pain mechanism in migraine and cluster headache," *Anesthesiology and Pain Medicine*, vol. 6, no. 3, Article ID e35190, 2016.

[6] T. Sprenger, K. V. Ruether, H. Boecker et al., "Altered metabolism in frontal brain circuits in cluster headache," *Cephalalgia*, vol. 27, no. 9, pp. 1033–1042, 2007.

[7] S. Prakash, A. Kumar Singh, and C. Rathore, "Chronic Migraine Responding to Intravenous Thiamine: A Report of Two Cases," *Headache: The Journal of Head and Face Pain*, vol. 56, no. 7, pp. 1204–1209, 2016.

[8] A. Costantini and M. I. Pala, "Thiamine and fatigue in inflammatory bowel diseases: An open-label pilot study," *The Journal of Alternative and Complementary Medicine*, vol. 19, no. 8, pp. 704–708, 2013.

[9] A. Costantini, M. I. Pala, S. Tundo, and P. Matteucci, "High-dose thiamine improves the symptoms of fibromyalgia," *BMJ Case Reports*, vol. 2013, no. may20 1, pp. bcr2013009019–bcr2013009019, 2013.

[10] G. Mkrtchyan, V. Aleshin, Y. Parkhomenko et al., "Molecular mechanisms of the non-coenzyme action of thiamin in brain: Biochemical, structural and pathway analysis," *Scientific Reports*, vol. 5, Article ID 12583, 2015.

[11] Y. M. Parkhomenko, A. S. Pavlova, and O. A. Mezhenskaya, "Mechanisms Responsible for the High Sensitivity of Neural Cells to Vitamin B1 Deficiency," *Neurophysiology*, vol. 48, no. 6, pp. 429–448, 2016.

[12] A. Costantini, M. I. Pala, E. Grossi et al., "Long-term treatment with high-dose thiamine in Parkinson disease: An open-label pilot study," *The Journal of Alternative and Complementary Medicine*, vol. 21, no. 12, pp. 740–747, 2015.

[13] A. Costantini, R. Giorgi, S. D'Agostino, and M. I. Pala, "High-dose thiamine improves the symptoms of Friedreich's ataxia," *BMJ Case Reports*, 2013.

[14] N. Abu Bakar, M. Torkamani, S. Tanprawate, G. Lambru, M. Matharu, and M. Jahanshahi, "The development and validation of the Cluster Headache Quality of life scale (CHQ)," *The Journal of Headache and Pain*, vol. 17, no. 1, article no. 79, 2016.

[15] S. Fauci, E. Braunwald, DL. Kasper et al., *Harrisons Principles of Internal Medicine*, Mc Graw-Hill, New York, 14th edition, 1999.

[16] S. Kono, H. Miyajima, K. Yoshida, A. Togawa, K. Shirakawa, and H. Suzuki, "Mutations in a thiamine-transporter gene and Wernicke's-like encephalopathy," *The New England Journal of Medicine*, vol. 360, no. 17, pp. 1792–1794, 2009.

[17] D. Liu, Z. Ke, and J. Luo, "Thiamine Deficiency and Neurodegeneration: the Interplay Among Oxidative Stress, Endoplasmic Reticulum Stress, and Autophagy," *Molecular Neurobiology*, vol. 54, no. 7, pp. 5440–5448, 2017.

[18] D. Onk, R. Mammadov, B. Suleyman et al., "The effect of thiamine and its metabolites on peripheral neuropathic pain Induced by cisplatin in rats," *Journal of Experimental Animal Science*.

[19] F. Alemanno, D. Ghisi, B. Westermann et al., "The use of vitamin B1 as a perineural adjuvant to middle interscalene block for postoperative analgesia after shoulder surgery," *Acta Biomedica*, vol. 87, no. 1, pp. 22–27, 2016.

[20] C. Nacitarhan, E. Minareci, and G. Sadan, "The effect of benfotiamine on mu-opioid receptor mediated antinociception in experimental diabetes," *Experimental and Clinical Endocrinology & Diabetes*, vol. 122, no. 3, pp. 173–178, 2014.

[21] D. Lonsdale, "Thiamine and magnesium deficiencies: Keys to disease," *Medical Hypotheses*, vol. 84, no. 2, pp. 129–134, 2015.

[22] H. A. Smithline, M. Donnino, and D. J. Greenblatt, "Pharmacokinetics of high-dose oral thiamine hydrochloride in healthy subjects," *BMC Clinical Pharmacology*, vol. 12, article no. 4, 2012.

Uncommon Association of Two Anatomical Variants of Cerebral Circulation: A Fetal-Type Posterior Cerebral Artery and Inferred Artery of Percheron, Complicated with Paramedian Thalamomesencephalic Stroke—Case Presentation and Literature Review

Aurelian Anghelescu [1,2]

[1]Neurorehabilitation Clinic, Teaching Emergency Hospital "Bagdasar-Arseni", Romania
[2]"Carol Davila" University of Medicine and Pharmacy, Bucharest, Romania

Correspondence should be addressed to Aurelian Anghelescu; aurelian_anghelescu@yahoo.co.uk

Academic Editor: Chin-Chang Huang

Background. The unilateral fetal variant of the posterior cerebral artery (FPCA) is characterized by the congenital absence of the P1 arterial segment. The artery of Percheron (AOP) is an uncommon vascular variant, in which a single dominant thalamoperforating arterial trunk arises from one P1 segment, bifurcates, and provides bilateral supply to the paramedian thalami and rostral midbrain. *Case Presentation*. This is a retrospective case study of a 37-year-old man with multiple lifestyle risk factors (chronic marijuana and tobacco abuse), who suffered a thalamomesencephalic stroke, rapidly worsening to comatose state. After restoration of consciousness, he clinically manifested with left paramedian midbrain syndrome. Imaging demonstrated an asymmetric paramedian thalamic infarction with mesencephalon extension, patency of the basilar, vertebral arteries, and left PCA and right-sided FPCA, respectively. Left-sided thalamoperforating arterioles were not differentiated; AOP was inferred. Neither evident clinical source of embolus nor prothrombotic states were found. Mobile cardiac telemetry and transesophageal echocardiography were not available. The diagnosis was established too late for thrombolytic treatment. Anticoagulation was indicated during the acute and subacute stages, followed by low dose of antiplatelet. *Discussion*. This uncommon cerebrovascular configuration (FPCA+AOP) might be the fourth case described in the literature. Sustained rehabilitation and abstinence from tobacco and cannabis led to favorable outcomes.

1. Background

The vascular anatomy of the posterior circulation is complex and variable. Autopsy studies and structural imaging scans have detected normal anatomical variations in the morphology of the circle of Willis (incomplete circle, asymmetrical with duplication, absence or fusion of components, and fenestrations), are present in 48–58% of the general population [1–4], and arise during fetal development.

The distinctive landmark of the fetal (origin of the) posterior cerebral artery (FPCA) refers to the precommunicating arterial segment (P1), which may be congenitally absent or markedly hypoplastic (uni- or bilaterally) [1–6]. In this fetal-type posterior circle of Willis, PCA originates directly from the ipsilateral internal carotid (ICA), with no connection with the basilar artery. Structural imaging scans demonstrated that complete agenesis of P1 and absence of the posterior communicating artery (PCoA) may be found unilaterally (in 4–26% subjects) or bilaterally (in 2–4% cases) [1, 2, 5, 6].

Studies of human cadaveric brains demonstrated four major thalamic arterial territories (anterior, paramedian, inferolateral, and posterior), with significant variations and overlaps in vascular irrigation. These territories are supplied by the polar (originating from the PCoA), paramedian/thalamoperforating arteries (TPAs), emerging from the P1 segment, thalamogeniculate (emerging from the P2 segment of the PCA), and posterior choroidal arteries [7–17].

Posterior TPAs arise from the superior, posterior, or posterosuperior surfaces of P1. Their morphological diversity and branching patterns, with multiple variations and complex courses, were subject of autopsy studies [7–17] and structural imaging scans [18–37], respectively.

These perforating arteries are of utmost importance and irrigate the posterior part of the thalamus, medial ventral thalami, the walls of the third ventricle, hypothalamus, and subthalamic–mesencephalic junctions (subthalamus, substantia nigra, red nucleus, oculomotor nucleus, trochlear nucleus, reticular formation of the midbrain, pretectum, rhomboid fossa, and the posterior part of the internal capsule) [7–17].

Artery of Percheron (AOP) is a normal, but uncommon vascular variant of the paramedian branches of the PCA in which a single dominant TPA trunk arises from one P1 segment, bifurcates, and provides bilateral supply to the paramedian thalami and the rostral midbrain [7, 8]. Occlusion of this uncommon arteriole results in a characteristic pattern of bilateral thalamic infarcts with or without mesencephalic involvement.

2. Case Presentation

This is a retrospective case study of a slim 37-year-old man exhibiting associated lifestyle risk factors (chronic marijuana and tobacco abuse, but neither alcohol excess, nor other illicit drugs) who suffered an acute thalamomesencephalic stroke, rapidly worsening to a comatose state.

Familial and personal medical history was negative for associated cardiocerebrovascular pathology or other specific risk factors.

In the evening that preceded the cerebral infarction, he submitted a large and elaborate tattoo over the left hypochondrium and abdominal (lumbar) flank and smoked a few cigarettes with cannabis.

The following morning, he experienced acute onset of dizziness, visual, speech, and gait disturbances.

He was admitted to the emergency room with walking difficulties, disturbed balance and coordination of movements, slurred speech, diplopia, confusion, and left palpebral ptosis. Neurological examination revealed right-sided severe ataxic hemiparesis, dysarthria, left palpebral ptosis and mydriasis, divergent strabismus, and fluctuating consciousness (Glasgow coma scale, GCS 10/15).

Blood tests (white blood cells count, hemoglobin, electrolytes, liver, and renal function) revealed normal results. Urine toxicology at admission was positive only for tetrahydrocannabinol; no other illicit drugs were present on tox screen. Electrocardiogram (EKG) and chest X-ray findings were normal. Clotting tests were normal [antithrombin III was 108% (>80%), homocysteine was 7.5 μmol ($\leq$ 12), lupus anticoagulant was negative, antinuclear antibodies were 0.3 UM (<0.7), C protein was 117% (70-130)].

Emergent computed tomography (CT) scan on the day of admission showed no gross abnormality and no evidence of cerebral hemorrhage or encephalitis.

In a few hours he become comatose (GCS 7/15) and was transferred to the intensive therapy unit. Intubation and ventilation support were not necessary. EKG monitoring during admission in the intensive care unit did not revealed pathological aspects.

At about 20 hours after the onset of stroke, magnetic resonance imaging (MRI) of the brain and angiography (MRA) were also performed (Figure 1). These revealed acute paramedian thalamic ischemic lesions extending to the rostral midbrain (asymmetrically, mainly on the left side). The imaging showed no evidence of cerebral venous occlusion, infiltrative neoplasm, severe infectious and inflammatory lesion, or a large embolus at the basilar tip, with stroke in the posterior circulation. MRA showed patency of the basilar and vertebral arteries, a normal appearance of the left P1 arterial segment and left PCA, and a right-sided full FPCA. Our 1.5-Tesla MRI device failed to visualize the TPAs; the left AOP was just presumed.

He recovered from a coma after 4 days and exhibited a slow, progressive evolution. Initially, he presented with severe alternating (superior) oculomotor hemiplegia (Weber syndrome), with left-sided oculomotor nerve palsy, a drooping eyelid and fixed-width pupil pointed down and out, diplopia, and dysarthria associated with contralateral severe ataxic hemiparesis.

Based on clinical and neuroimaging findings, the positive diagnosis was acute ischemic stroke in the territory of the left AOP. The clinical spectrum of the AOP infarct was outlined in the frame of a "thalamopeduncular" syndrome, associated with the typical symptoms of bilateral paramedian thalamic infarcts (confusion and coma), accompanied by with oculomotor disturbances, contralateral hemiplegia, and cerebellar ataxia.

After the acute episode, he was admitted on the neurorehabilitation department. He clinically manifested a paramedian midbrain syndrome, combining the previously described left-sided oculomotor impairment with moderate right-sided ataxic hemiparesis without hemianesthesia, tremor, dysmetria, dysarthria, and depression. Repeated EKG and blood tests and a transthoracic echocardiogram, respectively, did not reveal pathological aspects.

The diagnosis was established retrospectively, after a delay of 20 hours, too late for thrombolytic management. He initially received anticoagulant therapy (heparin for 3 weeks in the acute stroke department), followed by a novel oral anticoagulant for another 5 weeks during rehabilitation. He was discharged with small doses of aspirin, up to six months, as secondary prophylaxis. Statins were not administered, either in the acute or during the subacute stage.

He had a good evolutive trend and was discharged with a modified Rankin score (mRS) 3. Psychological evaluation emphasized a marked improvement of his masked depression and augmentation of the Mini-Mental State Examination (MMSE) score (from 23 to 29/30).

He completely changed his lifestyle, with abstinence from both tobacco and cannabis, and continued the rehabilitation program as an outpatient. He exhibited favorable outcomes, with no vascular recurrence.

Four months after the acute stroke he achieved a mRS 2 and was slightly disabled and still unable to carry out all previous activities, especially professional ones (driver). Most

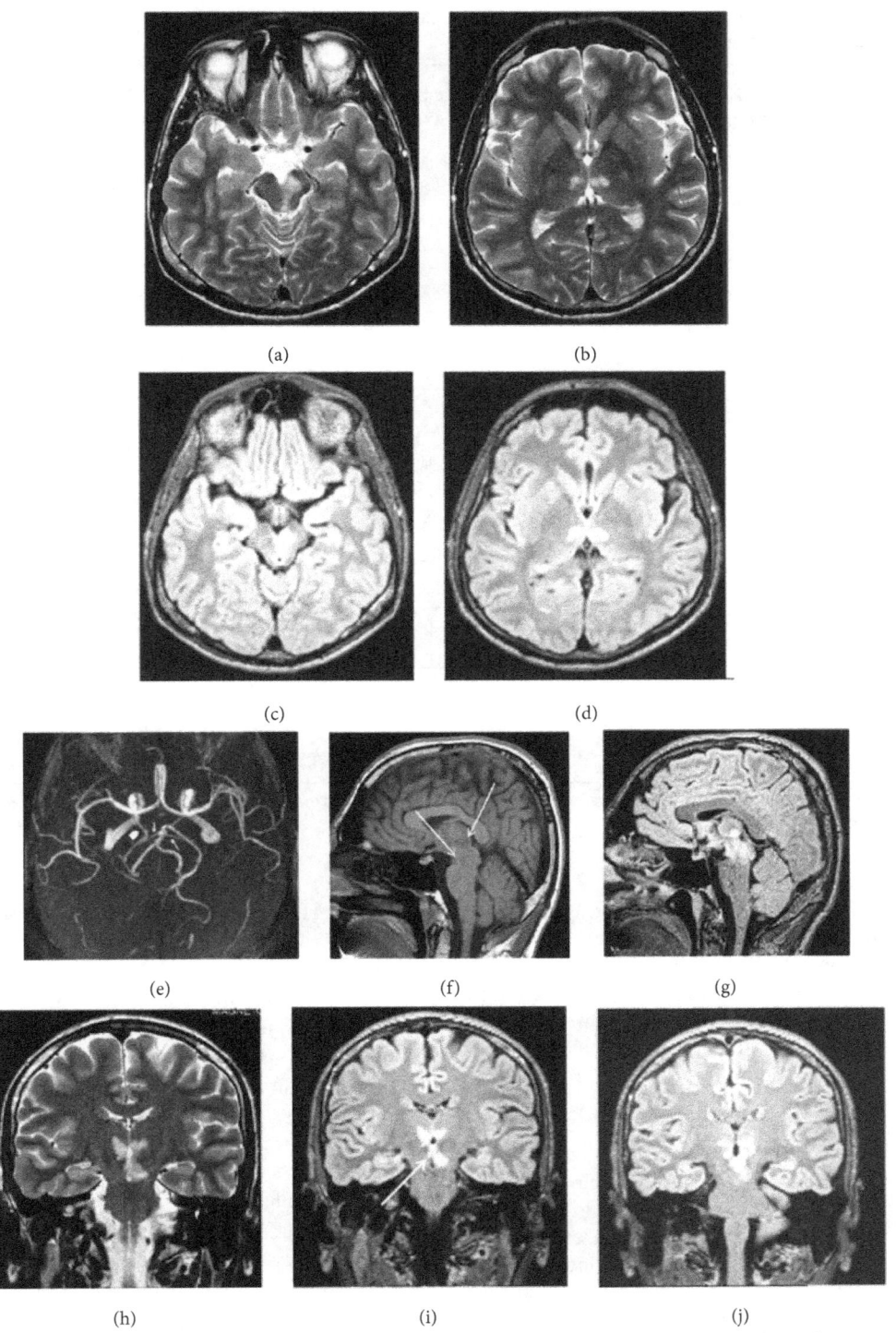

FIGURE 1: (a) Axial sections of T2-weighted images obtained 20 hours after the onset of symptoms showed areas of increased signal intensity in the left mesencephalon and (b) paramedian thalamic nuclei. (c, d) Axial brain FLAIR images. Hyperintense signals in the rostral midbrain and the paramedian thalamic suggest acute Percheron artery infarction. (c) "V-shaped" hyperintense signal along the pial surface of interpeduncular fossa in midbrain. The mesencephalon lesion extends to the periaqueductal gray matter. (e) MR angiography shows a right-sided FPCA (thick white arrow), arising directly from the ipsilateral internal carotid artery. Patency of the basilar artery and tip, left PCA, and posterior communicating artery; the thin arrows indicate the superior cerebellar arteries, with normal appearance. (f) Sagittal section, T1-weighted: showed ill-defined areas of hypodensity in the thalamopeduncular junction (white arrows). (g) Sagittal section, FLAIR: hyperintense images with the same topography. Coronal sections on T2 (h) and FLAIR images (i, j). Relatively symmetric hyperintense signals in the paramedian inferior thalami, extending (asymmetrically) into the medial and rostral mesencephalon (territory of the artery of Percheron). (i) Coronal section, FLAIR: "lambda-shaped" (Λ) hyperintense signal, adjacent to the pial layer of the interpeduncular fossa, next to the infarction zones in the thalamic–mesencephalon junction, equivalent version of the "V-shape" observed in axial sections (c). (FLAIR, fluid-attenuation inversion recovery images; FPCA, fetal posterior cerebral artery.)

TABLE 1: Summary of microvascular anatomic investigations of the posterior vascularization and reported incidence of AOP associated or not with other variants in the circle of Willis.

Author, year	Number of brain specimens	Average number of TPAs/brain	Frequency of AOP (%)	P1 segment (hypoplastic or absent)
Grochowski, Maciejewski, 2017 [9]	13	5.8	0%	Not reported
Djulejić, 2015 [10]	12-16	2.2	0%	Not reported
Griessenauer, 2013 [11]	25	Not available	12%	0% (specified)
Kocaeli, 2013 [12]	34	8.5	11,7%	Not reported
Parraga, 2011	35	6	Not reported	Not reported
Park, 2010 [13]	26 (158)	7,2	11,5%	Not reported
Kaya, 2010 [14]	14	6.8	11,7	Not reported
Pai, 2007	25	4	Not reported	Not reported
Uz, 2007 [15]	15	4	7%	Not reported
Cosson, 2003	12	7.5	Not reported	Not reported
Rassi, 1992	30	3.2	Not reported	Not reported
Caruso, 1990	50	8.2	Not reported	Not reported
Marinkovic, 1986 [16]	33	4	Not reported	Not reported
Pedroza, 1986 [17]	28	1-5	10,7%	Not reported
Lang, Bruner, 1978	50	Not available	8%	Not reported
Zeal, Rhoton, 1978	25	5.4	Not reported	Not reported
Saeki, 1977	50	8.2	8%	hypoplastic P1

AOP, artery of Percheron. Data are modified and adapted after Grochowski (2017) [9], Griessenauer (2013) [11], Kocaeli (2013) [12], and Park (2010) [13] and are chronologically arranged.

symptoms abated, except for slight visual blurring, diplopia, and residual left third cranial nerve palsy.

Favorable neurological results were consistent with repeated neuroimaging tests for control. Contrast-enhanced MR angiography remained unchanged. MRI showed no acute recurrences, but only small residual lacunae.

3. Discussion

The case reported herein depicts a peculiar association of two vascular variants of the posterior cerebral circulation: a right-sided FPCA and an inferred AOP emerging from the precommunicating segment (P1) of the left PCA, complicated with ischemic stroke, with fluctuations in consciousness [19], and reversible state of coma [20-24], in a complex chronic toxicological context, and a challenging etiopathogenic diagnosis.

Clinical findings and brain imaging have estimated Percheron infarct pattern in 0.1-2.0% first-ever acute cerebral infarctions [22, 25-27] and in 4% to 18% of all thalamic ischemic strokes [21, 27], respectively.

There is no consensus regarding the real prevalence of this uncommon artery. Percheron stated that almost one-third of human brains present this normal variant [7, 8]. Punctilious morphology studies focusing the diversity of the TPAs indicated that AOP frequency across relevant cadaveric studies performed on unselected adult brains was variable (7.0-11.7%, Table 1) [7-17].

Branching patterns of the TPAs emerging from the P1 segment have variable anatomic and radiologic aspects [7-18]. Microvascular investigations classified TPAs into five different types, schematically represented in Table 2.

In case of marked hypoplasia of a single P1 arterial segment or its complete absence (full FPCA), TPAs originate from the contralateral side and cross the midline to supply the medial aspects of both thalami and the rostral midbrain (Table 2 and Figure 2).

Since Percheron's communication in the seventies [7, 8], only isolated case reports and several short-numbered series have focused on this uncommon vascular variant and its pathology. A personal literature review based on a 1973-2018 PubMed search (key items: Percheron, stroke, P1, fetal PCA) found 76 new case reports, added to the 123 analyzed by Zapella in 2014 [24]. Considering the actual report as number two hundred (since Percheron's "description princeps"), one could consider an approximate incidence of 4,44 new cases described annually in literature.

Eleven microvascular anatomical investigations focused on TPAs were realized on unselected cadaveric specimens. Most studies did not encounter morphometric anomalies of P1 (Table 1). Kaya (2010) found different anatomical variants

TABLE 2: Variable branching patterns and origin of the TPAs, emerged unilaterally or bilaterally from the P1 arterial segment.

Type I (Park 38.5%)	
TPAs bilaterally, multiple	TPAs bilaterally, multiple
Type II (Park 26.9%)	
TPA unilateral, single	TPAs contralateral, multiple
Type III (Park 19.2%; *Percheron* 40%)	
TPA single	TPA single
Type IV (variant IIb, AOP) (Park 11.5%; *Percheron* 33%)	**Contralateral P1** segment: present/ absent (full FPCA) / hypoplastic
TPA arises unilaterally (from one P1, as a **single** unpaired trunk, AOP)	–
Type V (variant IIa) (Park 3.8%; *Percheron* 7%)	**Contralateral P1** segment: present/ absent (full FPCA)/hypoplastic
TPAs arise unilaterally (from one P1, as **multiple** branches)	–
Percheron's **variant III (C)**: an ***arterial arcade*** is bridging P1 segments of both PCAs; the perforating branches arise from this ***arterial shunt***.	

TPAs, thalamoperforating arteries. P1, proximal arterial segment of the PCA (from the top of the basilar artery, to the PCoA). IIa and IIb, arterial variants of vascularization of the thalamus and midbrain described by Percheron. In brackets Park's [13] and *Percheron's* [7, 8] data are mentioned, respectively.

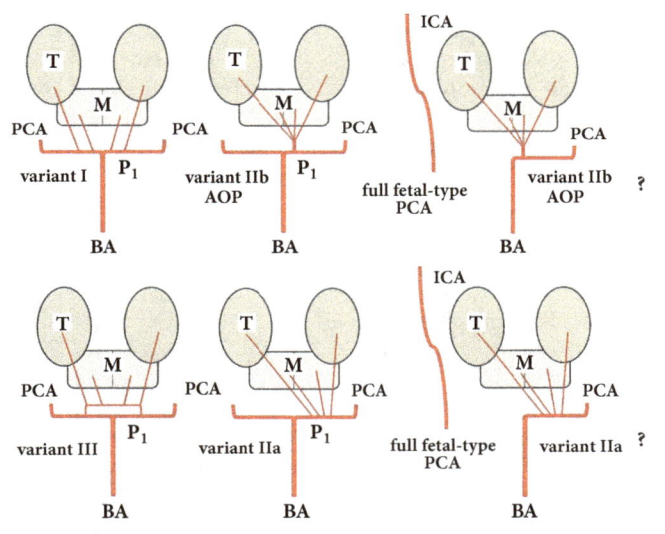

FIGURE 2: Possible variations involving paramedian perforating thalamic-mesencephalic arterial supply (according to Percheron's description) [7, 8]. **I**. The most common: many small perforating arteries arising bilaterally, from P1. **IIb**. The artery of Percheron: a single (asymmetrical) common trunk, arising from one P1 arterial segment. **IIa**. Multiple branches emerging (asymmetrically) from one P1 arterial segment. **III**. An arterial arcade is bridging the P1 segment of both PCAs, and the perforating arteries are arising from this arterial shunt. **The actual case report**: uncommon association of full fetal-type PCA (originating directly from the internal carotid artery) with Percheron's arterial variant. It was not possible to specify the particular anatomical arterial disposal (type IIb or IIa). (T, thalamus; M, mesencephalon; BA, basilar artery; PCA, posterior cerebral artery; P1, first arterial segment of the PCA; AOP, artery of Percheron; ICA, internal carotid artery.)

of the posterior circulation in 10.7% specimens, but not the association of AOP with FPCA [14].

It is difficult to visualize and demonstrate these perforating tiny vessels with conventional vascular imaging techniques. Due to their diameters (mean 0.51 mm, min. 0.125, and max. 0.8 mm [7–17]), thalamoperforating branches emerging from P1 might be imperceptible with a 1.5-Tesla MRI scanner, but a 3.0-Tesla MRA might detect them [28]. Medical imaging progress might be the explanation for the spectacular rise of new reported cases (mentioned above).

Although AOP cannot always be visualized and its presence is only presumed, failure to visualize the vascular anatomy of the perforating arteries does not exclude their presence. In our patient, MRA investigation failed to objectivity demonstrate the posterior TPAs and the ipsilateral and the cross flow to thalamus and midbrain, respectively, because AOP was occluded (or constricted), and the scanner did not exhibit ultra-performance to detect it. It was not possible to establish which of the two variants of TPAs (IIa or IIb) was "the weak link of the chain" in the etiopathogenesis of stroke (Figure 2).

Most significant case series of thalamic strokes were analyzed by Lazzaro (2010) [27], Jiménez Caballero (2010) [26], Song (2011) [29], Arauz (2014) [30], Förster (2014) [31], and Xu (2017) [32]. There were described four clinical and radiological topographic patterns of infarcts: bilateral paramedian thalamic with midbrain involvement (43%), as in the present case report; only bilateral paramedian thalamic without midbrain lesions (38%); bilateral paramedian thalamic associated with involvement of the anterior thalamus and midbrain (14%); and bilateral paramedian thalamic and anterior thalamus infarction, without midbrain involvement (5%) [27].

Matheus and Castillo (2003) [33] have proposed the following paradigm: in case of bilateral thalamic and midbrain infarctions, AOP occlusion should be considered as the main diagnosis.

Förster (2014) [31] studied a database of 600 thalamic infarcts recorded over a decade and selected 48 bilateral thalamic strokes. In 3 subjects (6.3%) he mentioned the association of AOP with FPCA. He pointed out that patients with hypoplastic/absent P1 segments were more likely to have exclusively bilateral paramedian thalamic lesions ($P < .001$).

To the best of our knowledge, the present case (uncommon vascular association of full FPCA and AOP stroke) might be the fourth one described in the literature.

The morphology and hemodynamic parameters of the perforating arteries in the interpeduncular fossa are strongly influenced by the structure of the circle of Willis [1–6, 34–36].

When an AOP is suspected, consideration should be given to the possibility of other rare anatomical variants of the posterior circulation that may be present [34].

Presence of a fetal-type PCA might also predispose to other strokes because it arises directly from the ipsilateral internal carotid artery and therefore has an established role in extensive cerebral infarction pathogenesis [1, 5, 6, 34–36]. The (full) fetal pattern of PCA hinders the subject's capacity to build leptomeningeal anastomosis interconnecting the anterior and posterior circulatory systems. By means of arterial spin labeling Barkeij Wolf (2016) [36] quantified cerebral blood flow and demonstrated interhemispheric asymmetry with decreased perfusion in the posterior circulation tributary to the unilateral FPCA.

Etiopathogenesis of this stroke was highly complex and heterogeneous and remained unclear. Extensive, but not exhaustive, investigations have been made to exclude most causes of ischemic stroke in this young adult.

Under advanced and standardized clinical workup in Germany, the detection rate of potential embolic sources was found in 54.2% of bilateral thalamic stroke [31].

The subject abused tobacco smoking, which is known to have a clear, dose-response causal link with stroke [37]. Local thrombosis could not be definitely excluded, because the MR scanner did not exhibit ultra-performance to visualize AOP, and the arteriole was either occluded or constricted.

The absence of atheromatous plaques in the posterior circulation (patency of the vertebral arteries, basilar, and left PCA) and the lack of clotting disorder have argued against an arterial embolization. No obvious clinical source of embolus such as deep venous thrombosis or paroxysmal atrial fibrillation was found.

Cardiogenic embolism could not be eliminated with certainty. In chronic marijuana users smoking can trigger cardiac tachyarrhythmias/paroxysmal atrial fibrillation [38], even with no other identifiable triggers and normal echocardiography. "Embolism not guilty" could not be asserted with certainty because the early hours of the ischemic event have remained an electrophysiopathological "terra incognita".

Transthoracic echocardiogram was negative for patent foramen ovale related stroke [28, 39, 40]. The etiological study had some weaknesses: bubble contrast echocardiography and contrast transcranial Doppler were not performed, and transesophageal echocardiography (the "golden diagnostic method") was not available. All were recommended as future investigations and mandatory for an analytical diagnostic procedure.

Knowing the traditional aphorism, "absence of evidence is not evidence of absence", analyzing the "pros and cons" mentioned below, and the fact that embolism has been criticized as the most common AOP occlusion mechanism [19, 27, 28, 38, 41], the reported case might be suspected for embolic stroke of undetermined source [42–44].

AOP infarction reflects well the aphorism: "time is brain". Sometimes, early recognition and optimal time for thrombolytic therapy could be missed. Even more, AOP stroke with delusive normal initial MRI aspects was described in literature [45].

In the diagnostic algorithm the patient underwent a cerebral CT scan (not CT angiography) as first-line imaging procedure. Due to the severity of clinical symptoms MRI was postponed, and not performed at the same time after onset of symptoms; the diagnosis was established too late to receive proper thrombolytic treatment.

A review of the literature focusing on the current therapeutic strategies in emerging AOP occlusion indicated intravenous heparin and thrombolysis with tissue plasminogen activator, as effective first-line treatment options, followed by long-term anticoagulants, whereas in nonemergent cases, without mesencephalic involvement, rehabilitation and continuous monitoring could be the option [46].

Evaluating novel oral anticoagulants versus aspirin, anticoagulants are likely to reduce recurrent brain ischemia more effectively than are antiplatelet drugs, in patients with previous suspected embolic strokes of undetermined source [42–44]. The therapeutic flow in our patient was represented by heparin, followed by a nonvitamin K anticoagulant and then a low dose of aspirin at discharge.

Presence of cognitive-behavioral disorders (memory loss, depression), possible neurological side effects, therapeutic options for polyvitamins and antioxidants (coenzyme Q10, vitamin E), and the absence of an atherosclerotic plaque to be stabilized were the arguments against statins inclusion in the therapeutic arsenal.

Cannabis-related stroke is not a myth, and cannabis consumption should be considered a risk factor for inducing ischemic stroke [40, 47–49]. The case reported a chronic marijuana and tobacco abuse, with a clear time-event related stroke after cannabis smoking (a few hours preceding the cerebral drama). The mechanism by which cannabis may cause cerebral infarction is not completely understood; a drug-induced cerebral angiopathy or a multifocal reversible cerebral vasoconstriction syndrome might be incriminated as etiopathogenetic mechanisms in predisposed chronic abusers [47–49]. In the reported case, the TPAs have not been detected and MRA did not demonstrate evidence of reversible cerebral vasospasm in the posterior circulation, so the "culprit" remained obscured.

Some short-numbered series of AOP infarcts analyzed the correlations between clinical-radiological aspects and outcomes and emphasized that associated midbrain involvement, greater infarct volume, or its hemorrhagic transformation had unfavorable outcomes [29, 30]. Arauz (2014) found that only 25% patients with bilateral paramedian thalamic and mesencephalon extension had good outcomes (mRS score ≤ 2) after a mean follow-up of 55 months [30].

The disciplined reevaluation of his lifestyle and informed decision to stop using tobacco and cannabis led to favorable outcomes. Four months after the acute stroke, the subject showed no dysarthria and motor or coordination deficits and achieved a mRS 2.

A good understanding of the clinical-radiological features of AOP infarction and standardized clinical workup in stroke units that use technology and adequate image performance are essential for early diagnosis and prompt therapeutic intervention.

Abbreviations

AOP: Artery of Percheron
CT: Computed tomography
EKG: Electrocardiogram
FLAIR: Fluid-attenuation inversion recovery images
FPCA: Fetal posterior cerebral artery
GCS: Glasgow coma scale
ICA: Internal carotid artery
MMSE: Mini-Mental State Examination
MRA: Magnetic resonance angiography
MRI: Magnetic resonance imaging
mRS: Modified Rankin scale
PCA: Posterior cerebral artery
PCoA: Posterior communicating artery
P1: Proximal arterial segment of the PCA (from the top of the basilar artery to the PCoA)
SCA: Superior cerebellar artery
TPA: Thalamoperforating artery.

References

[1] A. F. van Raamt, W. P. T. M. Mali, P. J. van Laar, and Y. van der Graaf, "The fetal variant of the circle of Willis and its influence on the cerebral collateral circulation," *Cerebrovascular Disease*, vol. 22, no. 4, pp. 217–224, 2006.

[2] S. Iqbal, "A comprehensive study of the anatomical variations of the circle of willis in adult human brains," *Journal of Clinical and Diagnostic Research*, vol. 7, no. 11, pp. 2423–2427, 2013.

[3] S. A. Gunnal, M. S. Farooqui, and R. N. Wabale, "Study of Posterior Cerebral Artery in Human Cadaveric Brain," *Anatomy Research International*, vol. 2015, Article ID 681903, 10 pages, 2015.

[4] P. Zampakis, V. Panagiotopoulos, T. Petsas, and C. Kalogeropoulou, "Common and uncommon intracranial arterial anatomic variations in multi-detector computed tomography angiography (MDCTA). What radiologists should be aware of," *Insights into Imaging*, vol. 6, no. 1, pp. 33–42, 2015.

[5] S. L. Lambert, F. J. Williams, Z. Z. Oganisyan, L. A. Branch, and E. C. Mader, "Fetal-Type Variants of the Posterior Cerebral Artery and Concurrent Infarction in the Major Arterial Territories of the Cerebral Hemisphere," *Journal of Investigative Medicine High Impact Case Reports*, vol. 4, no. 3, p. 232470961666540, 2016.

[6] A. Nouh, J. Remke, and S. Ruland, "Ischemic Posterior Circulation Stroke: A Review of Anatomy, Clinical Presentations, Diagnosis, and Current Management," *Frontiers in Neurology*, vol. 5, 2014.

[7] G. Percheron, "The anatomy of the arterial supply of the human thalamus and its use for the interpretation of the thalamic vascular pathology," *Zeitschrift für Neurologie*, vol. 205, no. 1, pp. 1–13, 1973.

[8] G. Percheron, "Arteries of the human thalamus: II. Paramedian thalamic arteries and territories from the basilar communicating artery," *Revue Neurologique*, vol. 132, no. 5, pp. 309–324, 1976.

[9] C. Grochowski and R. Maciejewski, "Diversity among posterior thalamoperforating branches originated from P1 segment: Systematic review," *Folia Morphologica (Poland)*, vol. 76, no. 3, pp. 335–339, 2017.

[10] V. Djulejić, S. Marinković, V. Milić et al., "Common features of the cerebral perforating arteries and their clinical significance," *Acta Neurochirurgica*, vol. 157, no. 8, p. 1393, 2015.

[11] C. J. Griessenauer, M. Loukas, R. S. Tubbs, and A. A. Cohen-Gadol, "The artery of Percheron: An anatomic study with potential neurosurgical and neuroendovascular importance," *British Journal of Neurosurgery*, vol. 28, no. 1, pp. 81–85, 2014.

[12] H. Kocaeli, S. Yilmazlar, T. Kuytu, and E. Korfali, "The artery of Percheron revisited: A cadaveric anatomical study," *Acta Neurochirurgica*, vol. 155, no. 3, pp. 533–539, 2013.

[13] S. Q. Park, H.-G. Bae, S.-M. Yoon, J.-J. Shim, I.-G. Yun, and S.-K. Choi, "Morphological characteristics of the thalamoperforating arteries," *Journal of Korean Neurosurgical Society*, vol. 47, no. 1, pp. 36–41, 2010.

[14] A. H. Kaya, A. Dagcinar, M. O. Ulu et al., "The perforating branches of the P1 segment of the posterior cerebral artery," *Journal of Clinical Neuroscience*, vol. 17, no. 1, pp. 80–84, 2010.

[15] A. Uz, "Variations in the origin of the thalamoperforating arteries," *Journal of Clinical Neuroscience*, vol. 14, no. 2, pp. 134–137, 2007.

[16] S. Marinkovic, M. Milisavljevic, and M. Kovacevic, "Interpeduncular perforating branches of the posterior cerebral artery. Microsurgical anatomy of their extracerebral and intracerebral segments," *World Neurosurgery*, vol. 26, no. 4, pp. 349–359, 1986.

[17] A. Pedroza, M. Dujovny, J. I. Ausman et al., "Microvascular anatomy of the interpeduncular fossa," *Journal of Neurosurgery*, vol. 64, no. 3, pp. 484–493, 1986.

[18] G. Brassier, X. Morandi, D. Fournier, S. Velut, and P. Mercier, "Origin of the perforating arteries of the interpeduncular fossa in relation to the termination of the basilar artery," *Interventional Neuroradiology*, vol. 4, no. 2, pp. 109–120, 1998.

[19] G. Raphaeli, A. Liberman, J. M. Gomori, and I. Steiner, "Acute bilateral paramedian thalamic infarcts after occlusion of the artery of Percheron," *Neurology*, vol. 66, no. 1, p. E7, 2006.

[20] M. Godani, A. Auci, T. Torri, S. Jensen, and M. Del Sette, "Coma with vertical gaze palsy: Relevance of angio-ct in acute percheron artery syndrome," *Case Reports in Neurology*, vol. 2, no. 2, pp. 74–79, 2010.

[21] A. Sandvig, S. Lundberg, and J. Neuwirth, "Artery of Percheron infarction: a case report," *Journal of Medical Case Reports*, vol. 11, no. 1, 2017.

[22] O. S. Amin, S. S. Shwani, H. M. Zangana, E. M. Hussein, and N. A. Ameen, "Bilateral infarction of paramedian thalami: a report of two cases of artery of Percheron occlusion and review of the literature," *BMJ Case Reports*, vol. 2011, no. jan18 1, pp. bcr0920103304–bcr0920103304, 2011.

[23] U. Lamot, I. Ribaric, and K. S. Popovic, "Artery of Percheron infarction: review of literature with a case report," *Radiology and Oncology*, vol. 49, no. 2, pp. 141–146, 2015.

[24] N. Zappella, S. Merceron, C. Nifle et al., "Artery of percheron infarction as an unusual cause of coma: three cases and literature review," *Neurocritical Care*, vol. 20, no. 3, pp. 494–501, 2014.

[25] E. Kumral, D. Evyapan, K. Balkir, and S. Kutluhan, "Bilateral thalamic infarction. Clinical, etiological and MRI correlates," *Acta Neurologica Scandinavica*, vol. 103, no. 1, pp. 35–42, 2001.

[26] P. E. Jiménez Caballero, "Bilateral paramedian thalamic artery infarcts: report of 10 cases," *Journal of Stroke and Cerebrovascular Diseases*, vol. 19, no. 4, pp. 283–289, 2010.

[27] N. A. Lazzaro, B. Wright, M. Castillo et al., "Artery of percheron infarction: imaging patterns and clinical spectrum," *American Journal of Neuroradiology*, vol. 31, no. 7, pp. 1283–1289, 2010.

[28] R. Itabashi, E. Mori, E. Furui, S. Sato, Y. Yazawa, and S. Fujiwara, "Bilateral thalamoperforating arteries arising from the unilateral posterior cerebral artery revealed on 3.0-tesla MR imaging," *Clinical Neurology and Neurosurgery*, vol. 114, no. 6, pp. 765–767, 2012.

[29] Y.-M. Song, "Topographic patterns of thalamic infarcts in association with stroke syndromes and aetiologies," *Journal of Neurology, Neurosurgery & Psychiatry*, vol. 82, no. 10, pp. 1083–1086, 2011.

[30] A. Arauz, H. M. Patiño-Rodríguez, J. C. Vargas-González et al., "Clinical spectrum of artery of percheron infarct: clinical-radiological correlations," *Journal of Stroke and Cerebrovascular Diseases*, vol. 23, no. 5, pp. 1083–1088, 2014.

[31] A. Förster, I. Nölte, H. Wenz et al., "Anatomical variations in the posterior part of the circle of willis and vascular pathology in bilateral thalamic infarction," *Journal of Neurogenetics*, vol. 24, no. 4, pp. 325–330, 2014.

[32] Z. Xu, L. Sun, Y. Duan, J. Zhang, M. Zhang, and X. Cai, "Assessment of Percheron infarction in images and clinical findings," *Journal of the Neurological Sciences*, vol. 383, pp. 87–92, 2017.

[33] M. G. Matheus and M. Castillo, "Imaging of Acute Bilateral Paramedian Thalamic and Mesencephalic Infarcts," *American Journal of Neuroradiology*, vol. 24, no. 10, pp. 2005–2008, 2003.

[34] J. Hendrikse, A. F. Van Raamt, Y. Van Der Graaf, W. P. T. M. Mali, and J. Van Der Grond, "Distribution of cerebral blood flow in the circle of Willis," *Radiology*, vol. 235, no. 1, pp. 184–189, 2005.

[35] C. De Monyé, D. W. J. Dippel, T. A. M. Siepman, M. L. Dijkshoorn, H. L. J. Tanghe, and A. van der Lugt, "Is a fetal origin of the posterior cerebral artery a risk factor for TIA or ischemic stroke? A study with 16-multidetector-row CT angiography," *Journal of Neurology*, vol. 255, no. 2, pp. 239–245, 2008.

[36] J. J. Barkeij Wolf, J. C. Foster-Dingley, J. E. Moonen et al., "Unilateral fetal-type circle of Willis anatomy causes right-left asymmetry in cerebral blood flow with pseudo-continuous arterial spin labeling: A limitation of arterial spin labeling-based cerebral blood flow measurements?" *Journal of Cerebral Blood Flow & Metabolism*, vol. 36, no. 9, pp. 1570–1578, 2016.

[37] D. Falkstedt, V. Wolff, P. Allebeck, T. Hemmingsson, and A.-K. Danielsson, "Cannabis, Tobacco, Alcohol Use, and the Risk of Early Stroke: A Population-Based Cohort Study of 45 000 Swedish Men," *Stroke*, vol. 48, no. 2, pp. 265–270, 2017.

[38] E. Charbonney, J.-M. Sztajzel, P.-A. Poletti, and O. Rutschmann, "Paroxysmal atrial fibrillation after recreational marijuana smoking: Another "holiday heart"?" *Swiss Medical Weekly*, vol. 135, no. 27-28, pp. 412–414, 2005.

[39] K. A. Jumean, A. Arqoub, M. A. Al Hadidi, A. Hawatmeh, and H. Shaaban, "Bilateral thalamic stroke due to occlusion of the artery of Percheron in a patient with a patent foramen ovale," *Journal of Natural Science, Biology and Medicine*, vol. 7, no. 1, pp. 109–112, 2016.

[40] J. Turner, T. Richardson, I. Kane, and S. Vundavalli, "Decreased consciousness: bilateral thalamic infarction and its relation to the artery of Percheron," *BMJ Case Reports*, vol. 2014, no. jan16 1, pp. bcr2013201848–bcr2013201848, 2014.

[41] M. A. Hawkes, J. E. Arena, C. Rollán, V. A. Pujol-Lereis, C. Romero, and S. F. Ameriso, "Bilateral paramedian thalamic infarction," *The Neurologist*, vol. 20, no. 5, pp. 89–92, 2015.

[42] R. G. Hart, L. Catanese, K. S. Perera, G. Ntaios, and S. J. Connolly, "Embolic Stroke of Undetermined Source," *Stroke*, vol. 48, no. 4, pp. 867–872, 2017.

[43] H. Diener, R. Bernstein, and R. Hart, "Secondary Stroke Prevention in Cryptogenic Stroke and Embolic Stroke of Undetermined Source (ESUS)," *Current Neurology and Neuroscience Reports*, vol. 17, no. 9, 2017.

[44] H. Kamel and J. S. Healey, "Cardioembolic Stroke," *Circulation Research*, vol. 120, no. 3, pp. 514–526, 2017.

[45] G. Cassourret, B. Prunet, F. Sbardella, J. Bordes, O. Maurin, and H. Boret, "Ischemic stroke of the artery of Percheron with normal initial MRI: A case report," *Case Reports in Medicine*, vol. 2010, 2010.

[46] X. Li, N. Agarwal, D. R. Hansberry, C. J. Prestigiacomo, and C. D. Gandhi, "Contemporary therapeutic strategies for occlusion of the artery of Percheron: a review of the literature," *Journal of NeuroInterventional Surgery*, vol. 7, no. 2, pp. 95–98, 2015.

[47] V. Wolff, J.-P. Armspach, V. Lauer et al., "Cannabis-related stroke: myth or reality?" *Stroke*, vol. 44, no. 2, pp. 558–563, 2013.

[48] D. G. Hackam, "Cannabis and stroke: systematic appraisal of case reports," *Stroke*, vol. 46, no. 3, pp. 852–856, 2015.

[49] M. Jamil, A. Zafar, S. Adeel Faizi, and I. Zawar, "Stroke from Vasospasm due to Marijuana Use: Can Cannabis Synergistically with Other Medications Trigger Cerebral Vasospasm?" *Case Reports in Neurological Medicine*, vol. 2016, Article ID 5313795, 4 pages, 2016.

Primary Sphenoidal Sinus Lymphoma with Initial Presentation as Unilateral Abducens Nerve Palsy Symptom

Xijing Mao,[1] Lifang Jin,[2] Bochi Zhu,[1] Honghua Cui,[2] Min Yao,[3] and Gang Yao[1]

[1]Department of Neurology, The Second Hospital of Jilin University, China
[2]Department of Hematology and Oncology, The Second Hospital of Jilin University, China
[3]Department of Pathology, The Second Hospital of Jilin University, China

Correspondence should be addressed to Gang Yao; yaogang0431@163.com

Academic Editor: Chin-Chang Huang

A 48-year-old man presented with 3 days of mild horizontal diplopia in the left direction, followed by the onset of headache 17 days later. A physical examination revealed isolated left abducens nerve palsy. Head computed tomography (CT) and magnetic resonance imaging (MRI) scans revealed soft-tissue density neoplasms that occupied the sphenoidal sinus and further invaded to destroy the clivus. Immunohistochemical staining of neoplasms was performed from biopsies samples. The pathological diagnosis was extranodal natural killer (NK)/T-cell lymphoma (ENKL), nasal type, associated with Epstein-Barr virus (EBV). The patient subsequently exhibited secondary symptoms (fever, night sweats), enlarged lymph nodes, renal metastases, and hemophagocytic syndrome, with clinical diagnosis stage IV of ENKL. The patient has a poor prognosis. This report is unique in two aspects: the unilateral abducens nerve palsy as the initial and isolated symptom of ENKL, and the primary sphenoidal sinus ENKL.

1. Introduction

Abducens nerve palsy is a common clinical finding in neurology practice and the etiology of the palsy is complicated. An accurate diagnosis is usually made through the cooperation of different departments, such as the ophthalmology, otolaryngology, neurology, pediatrics, pathology, and neuroimaging. The common causes of unilateral abducens nerve palsy are neoplasm and vascular disease in middle-aged people [1]. Extranodal natural killer (NK)/T-cell lymphoma (ENKL), nasal type, is the common nasal lymphoma in Asian and South America male adults [2]. The nose and maxillary sinuses are the common initial site of involvement while the sphenoidal sinuses are rarely affected. Multiple cranial nerve deficits or bilateral abducens nerve palsy associated with ENKL have been reported [3], but isolated unilateral abducens palsy is rarely reported. Herein we report a case with unilateral abducens nerve palsy as initial symptom in the primary sphenoidal sinus ENKL and investigated the clinical feature of the diagnosis and therapy.

2. Case Report

A 48-year-old man presented at the ophthalmologic outpatient department with a 3-day mild horizontal diplopia in the left direction followed by the onset of headache 17 days later. He denied nasal obstruction, epistaxis, nasal discharge, pain, hyposmia, and nasal swelling. There was no history of fever, weight loss, or nocturnal sweating. He had no history of diabetes, hypertension, or any neurological disease. On physical examination, cardiopulmonary examination was normal and neither lymphadenopathy nor hepatosplenomegaly was observed. Neuroophthalmologic examination revealed normal visual acuity, fields, and fundi. The pupils were equal and reactive to light and near stimuli. There was no ptosis, but there was limitation of movement of the left eye when he gazed to the left side. Function of the remaining cranial nerves was normal. There were no sensory or motor deficits in the upper and lower extremities; all tendon reflexes were normal. He was found to have isolated left abducens nerve palsy. Computed tomography (CT) scanning revealed soft-tissue density neoplasms filling the sphenoidal sinus

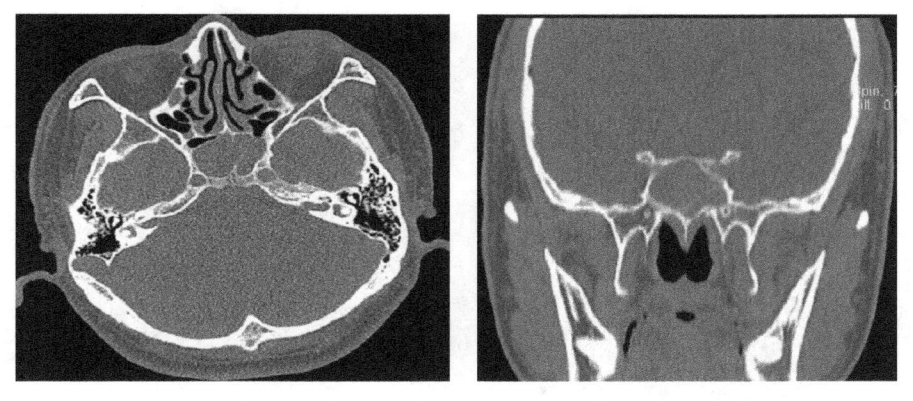

FIGURE 1: CT scan showed soft-tissue density neoplasms filling with sphenoidal sinus.

(a)

(b)

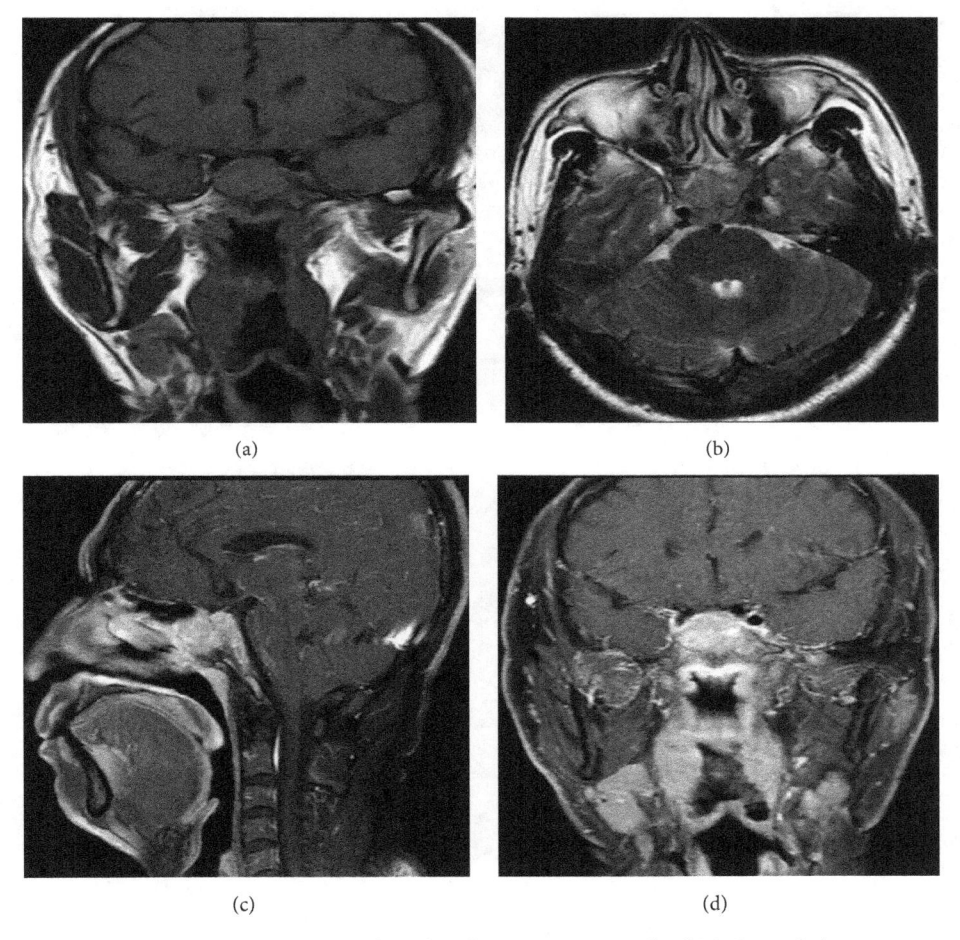

(c)

(d)

FIGURE 2: Sagittal T1-weighted magnetic resonance image (MRI) and coronary T2-weighted MRI revealed a mass occupying the sphenoidal sinus (a,b). Gadolinium-enhanced MRI demonstrated the neoplasm with homogenous soft-tissue lesion occupying the sphenoidal sinus and destroying the clivus (c,d).

(Figure 1). Magnetic resonance imaging (MRI) scanning with gadolinium injection was performed and revealed a homogeneous mass lesion (2.8cm x 2.3cm x 2.9cm) occupying the sphenoidal sinus and invading and destroying the clivus (Figure 2). Rhinoendoscopy revealed a mass at the sphenoidal sinus which was biopsied and histological examination revealed a malignant lymphoma. The immunohistochemical staining of tumor tissues showed $CD3^+$, $CD56^+$, Ki67>80%, LCA^+, $CD38^+$, and $CD20^-$ (Figure 3). The lymphoma cells were positive for EBER *in situ* hybridization. The pathological diagnosis was ENKL. Plasma EBV PCR yielded 1.18×10^6 copies/ml. Ten days later the patient had the B symptom

(a)	(b)	(c)	(d)

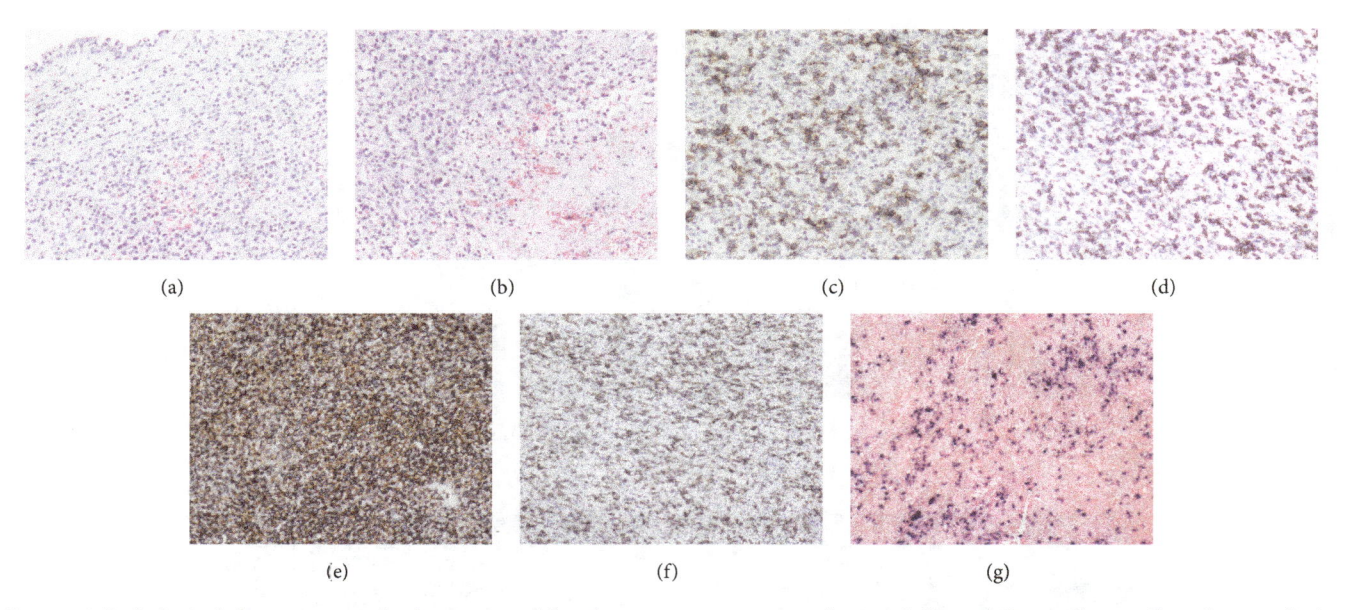

(e)	(f)	(g)

FIGURE 3: Pathological photomicrographs demonstrated that the mucosa was intact and expanded by a diffuse infiltrate of lymphoma cells (a, H&E). The mucosal lymphoid infiltrate was destructive, resulting in necrosis. The medium-to-large transformed cell nuclei had an irregular nuclear folding with granular appearance (b, H&E). Positive immunohistochemical staining was recorded for (c) CD56, (d) CD3, (e) LCA, (f) CD38, and (g) EBER *in situ* hybridization (original magnification: ×200).

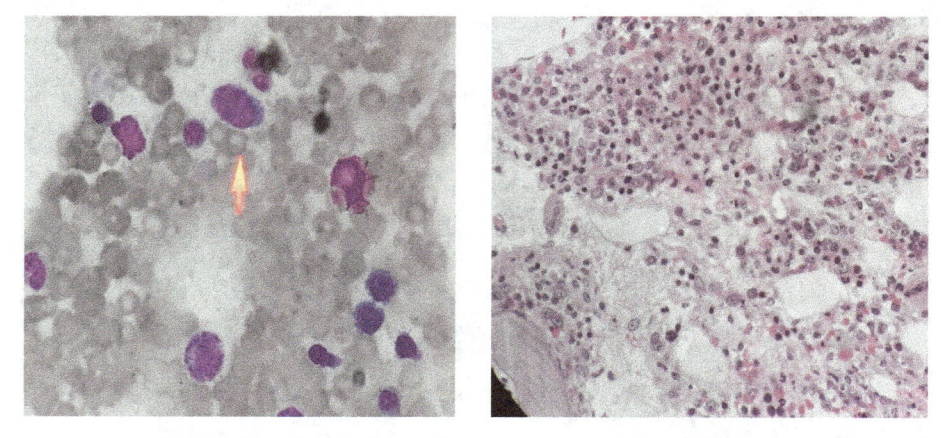

FIGURE 4: Bone marrow smear and biopsy showed active hyperplasia, immature lymphocytes accounting for 3% of heterotypic large cells with scattered distribution.

(fever, night sweats). The enlarged lymph nodes were checked in the neck, bilateral subclavian, alar, and inguinal. Contrast enhanced CT showed renal metastases. Bone marrow smear and biopsy showed active hyperplasia, immature lymphocytes accounting for 3%, and heterotypic large cells having a scattered distribution (Figure 4). Flow cytometry analysis showed lymphocytes accounting for 6.8% and suggested phenotypic abnormal NK cells in the bone marrow. Cerebrospinal fluid analysis showed glucose (2.87mmol/L) and protein content (0.22g/L) with normal cell count and no malignant cells. Blood analysis showed complete blood cell reduction. The second bone marrow biopsy suggested hemophagocytic syndrome [4]. The clinical diagnosis was stage IV of ENKL. The patient asked to be transferred to the community hospital.

3. Discussion

This report is unique in two aspects: the unilateral abducens nerve palsy as initial and isolated symptom of ENKL, and the primary sphenoidal sinus ENKL.

The abducens nerve exits the pons, runs along the bony clivus, enters the cavernous sinus through Dorello's canal, and subsequently runs through the middle of the cavernous sinus in close relation to the internal carotid artery medial to CN III, IV, and V [5, 6]. The abducens nerve is the most caudally and medially situated nerve in the sinus and is more vulnerable to pathologic lesions that involve the lateral part of the cavernous sinus. When a mass expands from the sphenoidal sinus, as in our patient, it invades the neighboring cavernous sinus and abducens nerve palsy is the common initial symptom. The incidence of cranial nerve palsy in nasopharyngeal neoplasms is 34-39% and most cases present with multiple cranial neuropathies [7, 8], but in our case only the left lateral abducens nerve was involved. Unilateral abducens nerve palsy may be caused by direct brainstem compression, intracisternal involvement, or tumor invasion of the clivus, parasellar structures, and systemic disease such as diabetes mellitus or hypertension pressure. In our case there was no evidence of brainstem and prepontine cistern involvement or compression as evidenced by gadolinium contrast MRI. The mass was confined to the sphenoidal sinus by MRI and rhinoendoscopy, compressing the left cavernous sinus and posteriorly invading the clivus, but not invading anteriorly towards the nasopharynx, so the patient experienced no nasal problem.

Epidemiological data show that the causes of unilateral abducens nerve palsy are closely related to age as trauma and tumors are common in children [9] and neoplasms and ischemia are common in middle-aged people, while high blood pressure or diabetes are common in elderly people [1, 10]. However, idiopathic isolated abducens nerve palsy comprises 26% of all patients with abducens nerve palsy, making the diagnostic plan difficult with abducens nerve palsy without other symptoms [11]. If a patient complains of diplopia caused by difficulty in abducting the muscles, a thorough workup should be performed to find the possible causes so as not to delay treatment.

ENKL is an entity of non-Hodgkin's lymphoma, mostly apparent in the nasal or paranasal area and is characterized by extensive extranodal involvement of NK or T cells [12, 13]. Susceptibility is domicile or ethnicity-related, being more common in Asia and South America than in Western Europe and North America [14]. The incidence of ENKL is 2-10% of the total number of non-Hodgkin's lymphoma, accounting for 90% of the nasal lymphoma in male adults [15]. Our patient is a 42-year-old Chinese man, presenting with initial unilateral abducens nerve palsy without nasal obstruction, nasal bleeding, and the typical progressive nasal facial damage symptoms of ENKL. CT showed soft-tissue density neoplasms filled with sphenoidal sinus, which is hard to differentiate with sphenoid sinusitis and other benign or malignant lesions. Previously reported imaging characteristics of ENKL are nasal cavity mass associated with sinus involvement, mild bone destruction with middle turbinate for CT, an equal or low T1 signal, and slightly higher T2 signals that can be enhanced with mild degree for MRI [16]. These characteristics are consistent with our ENKL case and play an important role in early diagnosis.

The diagnosis of ENKL must be based on pathologic immunohistology. The histopathology of ENKL is characterized by vascular central lesions, where the polymorphous lymphoma cells invade around small blood vessels or vascular tissue, resulting in vascular obstruction and tissue ischemia and extensive necrosis [17]. However, angiocentric growth is not always present and angiocentricity can be observed in other lymphoma types [18]. In our case the pathology revealed a medium-to-large transformed cell infiltrate in blood vessels, resulting in necrosis. These transformed cell nuclei have an irregular nuclear folding with granular appearance. The tumor cells have a $CD56^+CD3^+$ immunophenotype characteristic of NK cells.

The etiology of ENKL is unclear, but as Epstein-barr virus is detected in tumor cells in virtually all cases, ENKL is therefore regarded as an EBV-associated lymphoma [19]. ENKL is not sensitive to chemotherapy because the lymphoma cells can express P-glycoprotein [20] that mediates multidrug resistance. Involved-field radiotherapy followed by chemotherapy is regarded as a standard treatment. ENKL has a poor prognosis, which is usually worse than that associated with lymphomas at other sites in the body [15]. Multivariate analysis revealed that clinical stage, performance status, extranodal involvement, and disease type are significant and independent prognostic factors [21]. In our case the patient had many adverse prognostic factors and deteriorated very quickly following diagnosis.

To conclude, the diagnosis and treatment of unilateral abducens nerve palsy associated with ENKL are often delayed and require integration of ophthalmic, otolaryngological, neurological, and pathological assessments between clinical departments. A thorough workup should be performed including eye, ear, nose, and pharynx inspections. When adult males present with unilateral abducens nerve palsy and nasal sinuses lesions associated with sinus involvement, and imaging features of bone damage are not apparent, clinicians should be highly vigilant to rule out NK/T lymphoma. Confirmatory pathological histology, especially immunohistochemical examination, should be conducted so as to prevent the misdiagnosis of sinusitis. Radiotherapy followed by chemotherapy can improve prognosis.

References

[1] C. Elder, C. Hainline, S. L. Galetta, L. J. Balcer, and J. C. Rucker, "Isolated Abducens Nerve Palsy: Update on Evaluation and Diagnosis," *Current Neurology and Neuroscience Reports*, vol. 16, no. 8, article no. 69, 2016.

[2] E. Swerdlow, E. Campo, N. E. Harris et al., *WHO Classification of Tumours of Haematopoietic and Lymphoid Tissue*, IARC, Lyon, France, 4th edition, 2008.

[3] D. Deleu, M. Lagopoulos, M. Al Moundhry, and K. Katchy, "Isolated bilateral abducens nerve palsy in primary sphenoidal sinus non-Hodgkin lymphoma," *Acta Neurologica Belgica*, vol. 100, no. 2, pp. 103–106, 2000.

[4] S. Kojima, N. Takei, H. Mukai, Y. Hasegawa, K. Suzukawa, M. Nagata et al., "Hemophagocytic syndrome as the primary clinical symptom of Hodgkin's disease," *Annals of Hematology*, vol. 82, no. 1, pp. 53–56, 2003.

[5] S. Ambekar, A. Sonig, and A. Nanda, "Dorello's Canal and Gruber's Ligament: Historical Perspective," *Journal of Neurological Surgery Part B: Skull Base*, vol. 73, no. 06, pp. 430–433, 2012.

[6] R. S. Tubbs, V. Radcliff, M. M. Shoja et al., "Dorello canal revisited: An observation that potentially explains the frequency of abducens nerve injury after head injury," *World Neurosurgery*, vol. 77, no. 1, pp. 119–121, 2012.

[7] H. E. Rosenbaum and W. B. Seaman, "Neurologic manifestations of nasopharyngeal tumors," *Neurology*, vol. 5, no. 12, pp. 868–874, 1955.

[8] J. Turgman, J. Braham, B. Modan, and Y. Goldhammer, "Neurological complications in patients with malignant tumors of the nasopharynx," *European Neurology*, vol. 17, no. 3, pp. 149–154, 1978.

[9] M. S. Lee, S. L. Galetta, N. J. Volpe, and G. T. Liu, "Sixth nerve palsies in children," *Pediatric Neurology*, vol. 20, no. 1, pp. 49–52, 1999.

[10] T. J. Walsh, *Neuro-ophthalmology: Clinical Signs and Symptoms*, Williams & wilkins, 4th edition, 1997.

[11] C. S. Hsu, J. J. Closmann, and M. R. Baus, "Idiopathic Unilateral Cranial Nerve VI Palsy: A Case Report and Review of the Literature," *Journal of Oral and Maxillofacial Surgery*, vol. 66, no. 6, pp. 1282–1286, 2008.

[12] R. Suzuki, K. Takeuchi, K. Ohshima, and S. Nakamura, "Extranodal NK/T-cell lymphoma: Diagnosis and treatment cues," *Hematological Oncology*, vol. 26, no. 2, pp. 66–72, 2008.

[13] J. K. C. Chan, E. S. Jaffe, and E. Ralfkiaer, "Extranodal NK/T-cell lymphoma, nasal type," in *World Health Organization Classification of Tumors. Pathology and Genetics of Tumours of Haematopoietic and Lymphoid Tissues*, E. S. Jaffe, N. L. Harris, H. Stein, and J. W. Vardiman, Eds., pp. 204–207, IARC Press, Lyon, France, 2001.

[14] E. Werdlow, E. Campo, N. E. Harris et al., *WHO Classification of Tumours of Haematopoietic and Lymphoid Tissue*, IARC, Lyon, France, 4th edition, 2008.

[15] D. A. Al-Hakeem, S. Fedele, R. Carlos et al., "Extranodal NK/T-cell lymphoma, nasal type," *Oral Oncology*, vol. 43, pp. 4–14, 2007.

[16] Y. M. Park, J. H. Cho, J. Y. Cho, J. S. Huh, and J. Y. Ahn, "Non-Hodgkin's lymphoma of the sphenoid sinus presenting as isolated oculomotor nerve palsy," *World Journal of Surgical Oncology*, vol. 5, article no. 86, 2007.

[17] S. H. Swerdlow, *WHO Classification of tumours of haematopoietic and lymphoid tissues*, IARC, Lyon, France, 2008.

[18] J. K. C. Chan, V. C. Sin, K. F. Wong et al., "Nonnasal lymphoma expressing the natural killer cell marker CD56: A clinicopathologic study of 49 cases of an uncommon aggressive neoplasm," *Blood*, vol. 89, no. 12, pp. 4501–4513, 1997.

[19] L. S. Young and A. B. Rickinson, "Epstein-Barr virus: 40 Years on," *Nature Reviews Cancer*, vol. 4, no. 10, pp. 757–768, 2004.

[20] Z.-G. Xu, K. Iwatsuki, M. Ohtsuka, N. Oyama, T. Matsui, and F. Kaneko, "Polymorphism analysis of Epstein-Barr virus isolates from patients with cutaneous natural killer/T-cell lymphoproliferative disorders: A possible relation to the endemic occurrence of these diseases in Japan," *Journal of Medical Virology*, vol. 62, no. 2, pp. 239–246, 2000.

[21] R. Suzuki, J. Suzumiya, M. Yamaguchi et al., "Prognostic factors for mature natural killer (NK) cell neoplasms: aggressive NK cell leukemia and extranodal NK cell lymphoma, nasal type," *Annals of Oncology*, vol. 21, no. 5, pp. 1032–1040, 2010.

Acute Ascending Flaccid Paralysis Secondary to Multiple Trigger Factor Induced Hyperkalemia

K. H. D. Thilini Hemachandra,[1]
M. B. Kavinda Chandimal Dayasiri [id],[2] and Thamara Kannangara[1]

[1]Teaching Hospital Kandy, Kandy, Sri Lanka
[2]University Paediatrics Unit, Lady Ridgeway Hospital for Children, Colombo, Sri Lanka

Correspondence should be addressed to M. B. Kavinda Chandimal Dayasiri; kavindadayasiri@gmail.com

Academic Editor: Dominic B. Fee

Background. Acute flaccid paralysis is an uncommon, but potentially life threatening, sequel of severe hyperkalemia. Reported primary aetiologies include renal failure, Addison's disease, potassium sparing diuretics, potassium supplements, and dietary excess. Coconut water, when consumed in excess, has been reported to cause severe hyperkalemia. We report the case of acute ascending flaccid paralysis secondary to hyperkalemia induced by multiple trigger factors—king coconut water, renal failure, diabetes, metabolic acidosis, and potassium sparing diuretics. *Case Presentation.* A 78-year-old man presented with acute ascending type flaccid paralysis over five-hour duration and subsequently developed preterminal cardiac arrhythmias secondary to severe hyperkalemia (serum potassium: 7.02 mEq/L). He was on Losartan and Spironolactone for ischemic heart disease. Dietary history revealed excessive intake of king coconut water *(Cocos nucifera)* over past one week. Electrocardiogram returned to normal rhythm and serum potassium was 6.1 mEq/L within 2 hours of institution of emergency management for life threatening hyperkalemia. Neurological symptoms completely recovered within twenty-four hours without the need for dialysis. Electromyogram three days after the initial presentation revealed normal findings. *Conclusions.* The report describes a rare case of secondary hyperkalemic flaccid paralysis induced by multiple trigger factors. It is important that patients with risk factors for hyperkalemia are educated regarding avoiding excess dietary potassium. Regular follow-up of these patients is mandatory with review of medication related side effects and serum electrolytes.

1. Background

Hyperkalemia is an uncommon cause of reversible flaccid paralysis. While primary hyperkalemic paralysis is secondary to a defective sodium channel, a number of aetiologies have been reported as leading to secondary hyperkalemic paralysis. The primary aetiology could be one of renal failure [1], Addison's disease [2, 3], potassium sparing diuretics [4], potassium supplements, and dietary excess [5]. Coconut water, when consumed in excess, has been reported to cause severe hyperkalemia [6]. Recent reports suggest that patients with diabetes are at higher risk of developing hyperkalemia following ingestion of coconut water [7].

The objective of this report is to describe the case of a 78-year-old man with previously diagnosed diabetes mellitus, who presented with acute ascending type flaccid paralysis and subsequently developed preterminal cardiac arrhythmias following severe hyperkalemia. Increased dietary intake of king coconut *(Cocos nucifera)* water may have precipitated severe hyperkalemia in this patient in the presence of multiple other risk factors for hyperkalemia.

2. Case Report

A 78-year-old Sri Lankan man presented to the emergency department with acute onset upper and lower limb weakness for several-hour duration. The patient denied any limb weakness on the night prior to admission and was otherwise healthy. Upon waking up in the morning he found difficulty in getting up with weakness involving all four limbs. He was able to lift limbs but was unable to walk or dress himself. The weakness persisted and remained the same until the time of admission five hours later. Weakness was symmetrical and nonprogressive and involved all four limbs. There was no pain, numbness, or abnormal movements in limbs. Swallowing and breathing were not impaired. Urinary and faecal incontinence were absent.

Patient's past medical history consisted of type 2 diabetes, hypertension, ischemic heart disease, and systolic heart failure. Home medications included Mixtard 18 U mane and 8 U vesper, Losartan 50 mg twice daily, Nifedipine 20 mg twice daily, Spironolactone 50 mg daily, Frusemide 40 mg daily, Atorvastatin 20 mg daily, and Amiodarone 100 mg daily. Dietary history revealed that he was drinking king coconut water 2–4 servings almost every day for past one week.

He was overweight (height: 166 cm, weight: 70 kg, BMI: 25.4 kg/m^2). Xanthelasma and arcus senilis were present. He had elevated blood pressure (140/90) with cardiac apex lying in 6th intercostal space. Examination of limbs revealed symmetrical weakness with more distal involvement (proximal 4/5, distal 3/5). Limb reflexes were not impaired except for absent bilateral ankle jerks. Impaired sensation of pain and temperature was present in a glove and stocking type distribution. Joint position sensation was diminished in both upper and lower limbs. Examination of central nervous, respiratory, and gastrointestinal systems was normal.

Investigations revealed renal dysfunction (serum creatinine: 3.66 mg/dl-, eGFR: 15 ml/min, blood urea: 20.32 mmol/l, and arterial blood HCO_3^-: 12.7 meq/l). He had severe hyperkalemia (serum potassium: 7.02 mmol/l) with electrocardiogram showing tall, tented T waves and sine waves. Serum sodium was 129 meq/l. Renal ultrasound showed increased cortical echogenicity and impaired corticomedullary demarcation. Noncontrast computerized tomography of brain revealed normal findings. Electromyogram did not reveal acute radiculopathy, plexopathy, or myopathy. Nerve conduction studies revealed distal segmental axonal neuropathy suggestive of diabetic polyneuropathy.

Standard ward protocol for managing hyperkalemia was followed. Patient was initially given IV 10% calcium gluconate 10 ml over 10 minutes followed by a repeat dose. Spironolactone and Losartan were immediately withheld. He was given IV 50% Dextrose 50 ml with 10 U of Soluble Insulin. Patient was nebulized with Salbutamol 5 ml over 10 minutes and it was repeated twice. The interventions showed biochemical and electrocardiographic improvement in two hours (serum potassium: 6.1 meq/l). He was commenced on calcium resonium 15 g three times daily. Limb weakness showed rapid clinical improvement within 24 hours.

3. Discussion

Secondary hyperkalemic paralysis is characterized by vague muscle pain and ascending muscle weakness. Clinical manifestations occur only in the presence of a potential primary aetiology. Physical examination findings include absent limb reflexes and flaccid motor paralysis. Sphincter tone and sensory function are usually not deranged. Onset is usually rapid and resolves completely following correction of hyperkalemia [8].

Hyperkalemia is well recognized complication of chronic kidney disease and the patient described in this report had previously undetected chronic kidney disease secondary to diabetic nephropathy. Hyperkalemia is clinically significant since it is associated with severe complications including fatal cardiac arrhythmias [9] and seizures [10]. Paralysis is a rare complication of hyperkalemia [11].

Coconut water, which is increasingly popular as sports drink, is reportedly a cause of fatal cardiac arrhythmia following severe hyperkalemia [12]. Eight ounces of coconut water contain 600 mg of potassium [13]. King coconut (Cocos nucifera "king") is a species of coconut which is native to Sri Lanka. The recommended daily dietary intake of potassium by a person without chronic kidney disease is 4.7 g [14]. This patient had a history of short term dietary excessive intake of potassium via king coconut water and was on long term treatment with angiotensin receptor blockers and Spironolactone. Chronic kidney disease secondary to diabetic nephropathy was detected following the acute presentation. Increased dietary potassium most likely precipitated severe hyperkalemia in this patient while having other risk factors for hyperkalemia.

This presentation with ascending paralysis resembles the clinical presentation of Guillain-Barre syndrome [15]. The patient described in this report presented with rapid onset ascending type weakness over several hours without any other clinical features of Guillain-Barre syndrome. Electromyogram of this patient was normal and nerve conduction studies revealed only the long standing neuropathy. Long term hyperkalemia has been implicated as a contributing factor for neuropathy in chronic kidney disease [16]. Diabetic neuropathy is another contributing factor in this patient. Most previously reported patients had abnormal motor unit potentials in electromyograms [17] in the acute stage. This patient underwent electromyogram three days after the acute presentation since management of preterminal cardiac arrhythmias and stabilization of hyperkalemia was given priority over evaluation. Limb weakness had completely recovered by the time electromyogram was done. Electromyogram and nerve conduction velocity changes had been rapidly reversible following the correction of hyperkalemia in reported cases [18–20].

Pathophysiology and underlying genetic basis of hyperkalemic periodic paralysis are well known. There are only few case reports of secondary hyperkalemic paralysis and little is known about its underlying pathophysiology. Some reports suggest a direct influence of potassium on the muscle cell membrane/muscle fibers [15], while one report suggested a functional disturbance of the peripheral nerves [19]. Mechanism of muscle weakness and paralysis is likely due to constant and prolonged nerve membrane depolarization secondary to changes in potassium gradient and resting membrane potentials [21]. This leads to inactivation of sodium channels and impaired muscle membrane excitability. Cardiac and skeletal muscle can be adversely affected as a consequence [22].

Patients with diabetes mellitus are at a higher risk of developing hyperkalemia following ingestion of coconut water and the adverse effects are related to renal microvascular changes of diabetic nephropathy and subsequent low glomerular filtration rate. Coconut water has been found to further compromise glomerular filtration in patients with diabetic nephropathy resulting in hyperkalemia at a lower threshold [7]. Up to date there is not enough literature on recommended safe limits of daily coconut water intake for patient with comorbidities including diabetes. It is therefore important that patients with diabetes are educated regarding potential harmful effects of excessive consumption of coconut water.

The reported patient presented acute flaccid paralysis in a background of multiple trigger factors for hyperkalemia. Given the worse outcomes due to delayed treatment and complete reversibility of clinical manifestations following timely and appropriate treatment, vigilance regarding hyperkalemia is of great benefit to the patient. Further it is crucial and lifesaving that secondary hyperkalemic paralysis must be looked into while a patient is being evaluated for differential diagnosis of flaccid paralysis.

4. Conclusions

The reported patient had both preterminal cardiac rhythms and acute ascending flaccid paralysis following multiple trigger factor induced severe hyperkalemia. It is therefore crucial that patients with multiple risk factors for hyperkalemia are essentially educated regarding harmful effects of excess dietary potassium. Excessive consumption of coconut water can be detrimental in triggering off fatal hyperkalemia in these patients. Regular follow-up is mandatory with review of medication related side effects and serum electrolytes.

Authors' Contributions

K. H. D. Thilini Hemachandra carried out data collection, analysed patient data, and wrote the manuscript. M. B. Kavinda Chandimal Dayasiri carried out data collection, analysed patient data, and wrote the manuscript. Thamara Kannangara analysed data and supervised manuscript writing process.

References

[1] E. Maury, J. Lemant, J.-C. Dussaule, A. Pénicaud Védrine, and G. Offenstadt, "A reversible paralysis," *The Lancet*, vol. 360, no. 9346, p. 1660, 2002.

[2] J. J. Vilchez, A. Cabello, J. Benedito, and T. Villarroya, "Hyperkalaemic paralysis, neuropathy and persistent motor neuron discharges at rest in Addison's disease," *Journal of Neurology, Neurosurgery & Psychiatry*, vol. 43, no. 9, pp. 818–822, 1980.

[3] J. M. Sowden and D. Q. Borsey, "Hyperkalaemic periodic paralysis: A rare presentation of Addison's disease," *Postgraduate Medical Journal*, vol. 65, no. 762, pp. 238–240, 1989.

[4] D. Dutta, M. Fischler, and A. McClung, "Angiotensin converting enzyme inhibitor induced hyperkalaemic paralysis," *Postgraduate Medical Journal*, vol. 77, no. 904, pp. 114-115, 2001.

[5] M. Tamm, R. Ritz, and G. Thiel, "Der hyperkaliämische Notfall: Ursache, Diagnose und Therapie," *Schweiz Med Wochenschr*, vol. 120, pp. 1031–1036, 1990.

[6] R. N. Rees, J. Barnett, D. J. B. Marks, and M. J. George, "Coconut water-induced hyperkalaemia," *British Journal of Hospital Medicine*, vol. 73, no. 9, p. 534, 2012.

[7] M. S. Devgun, "Coconut water drink and the risk of hyperkalaemia in diabetes," *Practical Diabetes*, vol. 33, no. 3, pp. 87–89, 2016.

[8] N. S. Wilson, J. Q. Hudson, Z. Cox, T. King, and C. K. Finch, "Hyperkalemia-induced paralysis," *Pharmacotherapy*, vol. 29, no. 10, pp. 1270–1272, 2009.

[9] C. Esposito, N. Bellotti, G. Fasoli, A. Foschi, A. R. Plati, and A. Dal Canton, "Hyperkalemia-induced ECG abnormalities in patients with reduced renal function," *Clinical Nephrology*, vol. 62, no. 6, pp. 465–468, 2004.

[10] T. Sakemi, Y. Ikeda, and O. Rikitake, "Tonic convulsion associated with sinus arrest due to hyperkalemia in a chronic hemodialysis patient," *Nephron*, vol. 73, no. 2, pp. 370-371, 1996.

[11] C. Effiong, T. S. Ahuja, J. D. Wagner, P. C. Singhal, and J. Mattana, "Reversible hemiplegia as a consequence of severe hyperkalemia and cocaine abuse in a hemodialysis patient," *The American Journal of the Medical Sciences*, vol. 314, no. 6, pp. 408–410, 1997.

[12] R. N. Rees, J. Barnett, D. J. Marks, and M. J. George, "Coconut water-induced hyperkalaemia," *British Journal of Hospital Medicine*, vol. 73, no. 9, pp. 534-534, 2012.

[13] J. Hakimian, S. H. Goldbarg, C. H. Park, and T. C. Kerwin, "Death by Coconut," *Circulation: Arrhythmia and Electrophysiology*, vol. 7, no. 1, pp. 180-181, 2014.

[14] National Nutrient Database for Standard Reference, "Daily Reference Intakes - Food and Nutrition Board," 2017, http://fnic.nal.usda.gov/dietary-guidance/dietary-reference-intakes.

[15] I. R. Livingstone and W. J. K. Cumming, "Hyperkalaemic paralysis resembling Guillain-Barré syndrome," *The Lancet*, vol. 314, no. 8149, pp. 963-964, 1979.

[16] M. C. Kiernan, R. J. L. Walters, K. V. Andersen, D. Taube, N. M. F. Murray, and H. Bostock, "Nerve excitability changes in chronic renal failure indicate membrane depolarization due to hyperkalaemia," *Brain*, vol. 125, no. 6, pp. 1366–1378, 2002.

[17] V. Sitprija, R. Sribhibhadh, and C. Benyajati, "Haemodialysis in Poisoning by Sea-snake Venom," *British Medical Journal*, vol. 3, no. 5768, pp. 218-219, 1971.

[18] M. Naumann, B. Schalke, and C. Schneider, "Hyperkalaemia mimicking Guillain-Barre syndrome," *Journal of Neurology, Neurosurgery & Psychiatry*, vol. 57, no. 11, pp. 1436-1437, 1994.

[19] H. Shinotoh, T. Hattori, K. Kitano, and J. Suzuki, "Hyperkalaemic paralysis following traumatic rupture of the urinary bladder," *Journal of Neurology, Neurosurgery & Psychiatry*, vol. 48, no. 5, pp. 484-485, 1985.

[20] K. R. Naik, A. O. Saroja, and M. S. Khanpet, "Reversible electrophysiological abnormalities in acute secondary hyperkalemic paralysis," *Annals of Indian Academy of Neurology*, vol. 15, no. 4, pp. 339–343, 2012.

[21] S. Evers, A. Engelien, V. Karsch, and M. Hund, "Secondary hyperkalaemic paralysis," *Journal of Neurology, Neurosurgery & Psychiatry*, vol. 64, no. 2, pp. 249–252, 1998.

[22] Y. Mushiyakh, H. Dangaria, S. Qavi, N. Ali, J. Pannone, and D. Tompkins, "Treatment and pathogenesis of acute hyperkalemia," *Journal of Community Hospital Internal Medicine Perspectives (JCHIMP)*, vol. 1, no. 4, p. 7372, 2012.

Diagnostic Challenges of *Cryptococcus neoformans* in an Immunocompetent Individual Masquerading as Chronic Hydrocephalus

Kedar R. Mahajan,[1] Amity L. Roberts,[2] Mark T. Curtis,[2] Danielle Fortuna,[2] Robin Dharia,[1] and Lori Sheehan[1]

[1]*Department of Neurology, Thomas Jefferson University Hospital, Philadelphia, PA 19107, USA*
[2]*Department of Pathology, Anatomy and Cell Biology, Thomas Jefferson University Hospital, Philadelphia, PA 19107, USA*

Correspondence should be addressed to Kedar R. Mahajan; kedar.mahajan@jefferson.edu

Academic Editor: Isabella Laura Simone

Cryptococcus neoformans can cause disseminated meningoencephalitis and evade immunosurveillance with expression of a major virulence factor, the polysaccharide capsule. Direct diagnostic assays often rely on the presence of the cryptococcal glucuronoxylomannan capsular antigen (CrAg) or visualization of the capsule. Strain specific phenotypic traits and environmental conditions influence differences in expression that can thereby compromise detection and timely diagnosis. Immunocompetent hosts may manifest clinical signs and symptoms indolently, often expanding the differential and delaying appropriate treatment and diagnosis. We describe a 63-year-old man who presented with a progressive four-year history of ambulatory dysfunction, headache, and communicating hydrocephalus. Serial lumbar punctures (LPs) revealed elevated protein (153–300 mg/dL), hypoglycorrhachia (19–47 mg/dL), lymphocytic pleocytosis (89–95% lymphocyte, WBC 67–303 mg/dL, and RBC 34–108 mg/dL), and normal opening pressure (13–16 cm H_2O). Two different cerebrospinal fluid (CSF) CrAg assays were negative. A large volume CSF fungal culture grew unencapsulated *C. neoformans*. He was initiated on induction therapy with amphotericin B plus flucytosine and consolidation/maintenance therapy with flucytosine, but he died following discharge due to complications. Elevated levels of CSF Th1 cytokines and decreased IL6 may have affected the virulence and detection of the pathogen.

1. Introduction

Cryptococcal infections are primarily due to the following serotypes: *Cryptococcus neoformans* var. *grubii* (serotype A), *C. neoformans* var. *neoformans* (serotype D), AD haploid, and *C. gattii* (formerly *C. neoformans* var. *gattii*) (serotypes B and C) [1, 2]. Global environmental niches for *C. neoformans* var. *grubii/neoformans* are avian (pigeon) guano, soil, and decaying vegetation. *C. gattii* is found in *Eucalyptus camaldulensis*, Douglas fir trees, and surrounding soil [3, 4]. *C. neoformans* and *C. gattii* typically infect immunocompromised and immunocompetent individuals, respectively, [5, 6] and often cause significant neurologic morbidity.

C. neoformans is a spherical to oval (4–10 μm) narrow-based budding yeast that variably produces a polysaccharide capsule which can trigger complement activation and depletion, impact antibody responsiveness, and inhibit leukocyte migration and macrophage phagocytosis [7]. Capsule components include glucuronoxylomannan (GXM) which interferes with complement mediated phagocytosis [8], galactoxylomannan (GalXM), and mannoprotein [7, 9, 10]. While the main virulence factor is the capsule, others include melanin synthesis, urease and phospholipid secretion, titan cell formation, resistance to host body temperature, and surface phospholipid glucosylceramide (GlcCer) [1, 11]. Capsule formation is induced by environmental and nutritional factors (e.g., iron, carbon dioxide, glucose, amino acids, pH, and temperature [7]). Its size varies with growth conditions, increases in the host during active infection [11], and, even in the same host, variability in capsule thickness and diameter between lung and meningeal tissue has been described [8].

Diagnostics utilize CrAg for antibody based assays (sensitivity and specificity for serum): latex agglutination (LA, 97% sensitivity; 86–100% specificity [12]), enzyme immunoassay (EIA, sensitivity 94%; specificity 96% [13]), and lateral flow assay (LFA, 98.7% specificity; 100% sensitivity; IMMY package insert) 90% [4, 12, 14, 15]. Diagnosis by culture is reliable but takes time. India ink displacement around the capsule allows direct visualization of the yeast cells via light microscopy with high specificity (100%) but limited sensitivity (50%) due to dependence on both cell titer and capsule production [12].

Inhalation of desiccated yeast cells can eventually introduce the organism systemically via a hematogenous route [11], especially in immunocompromised hosts [13]. The organism can be eliminated or remain dormant in immunocompetent hosts. *Cryptococcus* can infect pulmonary, dermatologic, vascular, musculoskeletal, ophthalmologic, genitourinary, cardiac, and endocrine sites with tropism for the central nervous system (CNS) [10, 16]. *C. neoformans* transverses the blood-brain-barrier through transcytosis (internalization and transcellular transfer) and phagocytosis-mediated entry via monocytes/macrophages that are emigrating into the CNS [17]. CNS syndromes range from stroke, dementia, meningoencephalitis, abscess, subdural effusion, or spinal cord lesions [18] to recently described focal cranial neuropathies involving the optic chiasm/tracts and cranial nerves VI–VIII [19].

2. Case Report

We present the case of a 63-year-old man with progressive gait dysfunction and headache for four years. Computed tomography (CT) head revealed communicating hydrocephalus at an outside institution a year prior to our encounter (Figure 1). He had been offered, but declined, a ventriculoperitoneal shunt (VPS) given his history of frequent falls, ataxia, and dizziness. We additionally learned of his cognitive decline, urinary incontinence, chronic headache, dysarthria, and intermittent walker use. Medical comorbidities included hypertension, hyperlipidemia, and a left cerebellar stroke 3 years earlier with evidence of basal ganglia lacunar infarcts on imaging. He had a 50-pack-year history of tobacco. He was on disability at the time of admission and had most recently lived alone with a pet cockatoo in New Jersey for 6 years. Previously, he had been a truck driver and had resided in Florida for 30 years, during which he had also cleaned wastewater treatment plants. Notably on exam, he was slow to respond and dysarthric and had dysmetria with finger-to-nose and heel-to-shin testing. Gait assessment showed a normal base but severe ataxia, an inability to put feet together, and minimal retropulsion ability.

He had four serial lumbar punctures performed (Table 1), which revealed elevated protein (153–300 mg/dL), hypoglycorrhachia (19–47 mg/dL), lymphocytic pleocytosis (89–95% lymphocytes, WBC 67–303 mg/dL, and RBC 34–108 mg/dL), and normal opening pressure (13–16 cm H_2O). Gait assessment was variable after large volume lumbar punctures (LPs) with no improvement after the second LP (gait assessment not performed after first LP) and some improvement after the third LP (distance walked improved from 2 to 6 ft in 20 sec and ability to lift legs off the ground more readily) and the fourth LP (ability to get up from the chair more readily and take few steps with less assistance). Empiric treatments while the diagnosis was pending included pulse dose intravenous methylprednisolone, carbidopa/levodopa, and acetazolamide.

Direct CSF CrAg, both the Remel *Cryptococcus* Antigen LA (Thermo Scientific, Remel, Lenexa, KS) and the IMMY LFA (Immuno-Mycologics, Norman, OK), were performed on 3 of 4 LPs and were negative. Multiple direct antigen tests were utilized due to a high suspicion for cryptococcal meningitis. Fungal cultures were performed on the 1st and 4th collection of which only the 4th (high volume, 31 mL) had a light growth of *C. neoformans* on Sabouraud dextrose agar (SABs) 7 days after inoculation. The 4th collection was tested for prozone effect by both LA and LFA and remained negative. Since the initial colony type did not have typical morphology, a Remel Rapid Yeast ID panel was performed and provided an identification of *C. neoformans*. The rough colonies (Figure 2) were observed with India ink, noting an appropriate cell size but missing the capsule. Identification was confirmed by growth of dark colonies on birdseed agar (melanin production) and production of a positive reaction (pink) on rapid urea media. Additionally, matrix-assisted laser desorption/ionization time of flight mass spectrometry (MALDI-TOF-MS) (Bruker Biotyper MicroFlex, Massachusetts) confirmed the isolate identification as *C. neoformans*. Upon subculture of the original colony to SABs, the colony began reexpressing capsule (Figure 2) as noted by both the colony appearance (white and mucoid) and India ink stain of the subbed colony.

Following the positive culture, he was readmitted for induction with amphotericin B and flucytosine and consolidation/maintenance with flucytosine. He had a prolonged hospital course complicated by an epidural hematoma, deep venous thrombosis, pneumonia, and acute respiratory failure and unfortunately died due to complications.

TABLE 1: Serial lumbar punctures.

	1	2	3	4
Opening pressure, cm H_2O (mL removed)	17 (?)	13 (26)	13 (32)	16 (31)
Glucose	19	23	34	47
Protein	300	248	153	158
RBC	46, 0	54, 34	180, 13	29, 0
WBCs	235, 188	213, 303	240, 206	67, 175
% lymphocytes	60, 76	90, 88	93, 95	X, 89
Cryptoantigen	−	−	−	−
Fungal culture	−	/	/	+

1: performed during initial admission, 2: performed 8 mo later, 3: performed 2 days later, and 4: performed 6 days later. "?": volume of CSF removed during first lumbar puncture was not documented. "X": cell count for tube 1 not ordered. Pairs of data represent cell count/differential for separate tubes (typically tubes 1 and 4). Reactive (+) and nonreactive (−) cryptococcal antigen assays; fungal culture growth denoted by (+) or absence of growth (−); "/" indicates not performed.

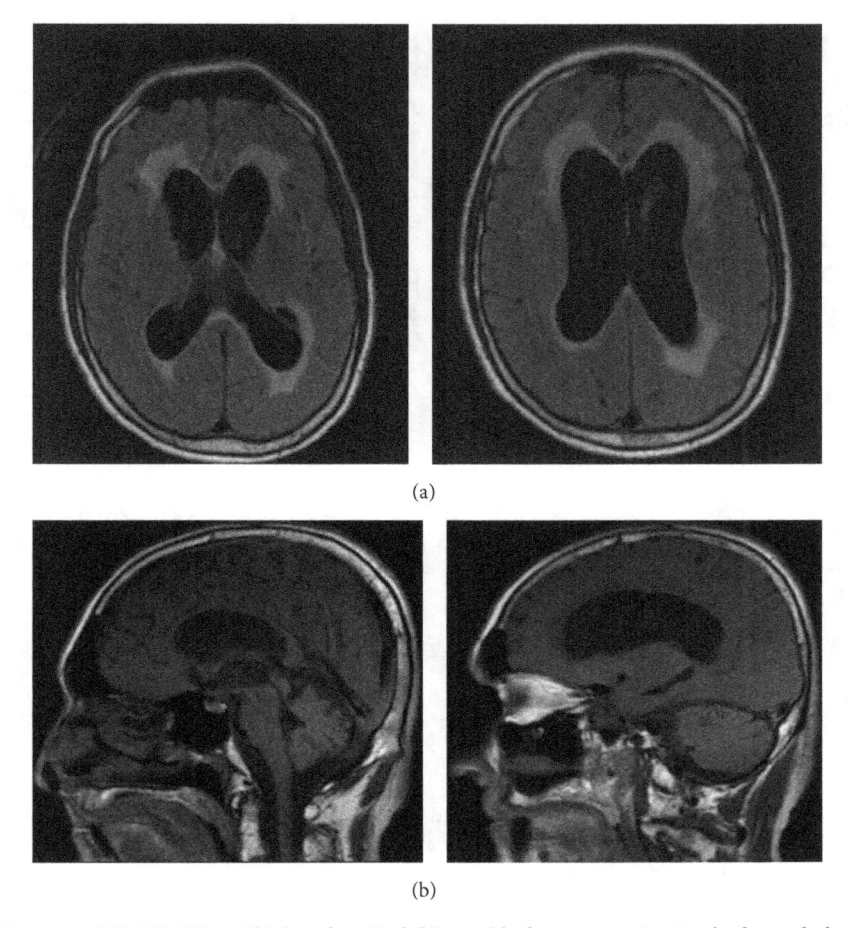

FIGURE 1: MRI FLAIR axial (a) and sagittal (b) notable for communicating hydrocephalus.

We sought to determine differences in the patient's immune response compared to individuals either without cryptococcal infection or infected with an immunocompromised state. We retrospectively compared levels of Th1 (IP10/CXCL10, IFNγ, TNFα, GRO/CXCL1, interleukin (IL)-8, and IL12p40) and Th2 (IL10 and IL6) inflammatory cytokines using a fluorescent bead-based ELISA (Luminex®) in patients with idiopathic intracranial hypertension (six noninfectious controls) and patients with cryptococcal meningoencephalitis (two HIV-positive, our immunocompetent patient, and one after cardiac transplant on immunosuppression). Although we were unable to evaluate statistical significance from inadequate sample size, Figure 3 shows relative higher levels of Th1 cytokines, higher levels of the Th2 cytokine IL10, and a lower level of IL6.

3. Discussion

We describe a case of an immunocompetent man with *Cryptococcus neoformans* meningoencephalitis that evaded detection with LA/LFA antigen based assays and one of two fungal cultures. We speculate both pathogen and host immunity that may contribute to poor detection. A low fungal CSF titer and impaired capsule production can contribute to poor detection with antigen based assays, negative staining with India ink, and fungal culture. Additionally, reluctant capsule expression until large volume culture with subculturing suggests that the inoculated strain may have been modulating capsule expression, perhaps in the presence of a competent host immune response. Host cytokine expression, with low IL6 expression, may have altered CrAg shedding. Failure to perform continued *large* volume fungal culturing at *each* lumbar puncture (fungal culture sent only with 1st and 4th LP) may represent missed opportunities.

Capsule-deficient *C. neoformans* strains can produce false-negatives on antigen assays [4]. Host mechanisms such as IL18 production can downregulate GXM, reduce fungal burden, and may contribute to a hypocapsular phenotype [20]. Reports of acapsular *C. neoformans* have been reported with pulmonary disease [21], septic arthritis [22], and meningoencephalitis [23–25].

Garber and Penar describe a young immunocompetent woman presenting with occipital headache, hydrocephalus, elevated intracranial pressure (20–30 cm H_2O), normal protein and glucose, lymphocytic pleocytosis (WBCs 15, RBCs 5, and 80% lymphs), and CSF culture revealing nonencapsulated *C. neoformans* with a negative antigen test [26]. While our patient did not have elevated intracranial pressure, he did exhibit lymphocytic pleocytosis and hydrocephalus. Del Poeta purports that the capsule is not a prerequisite

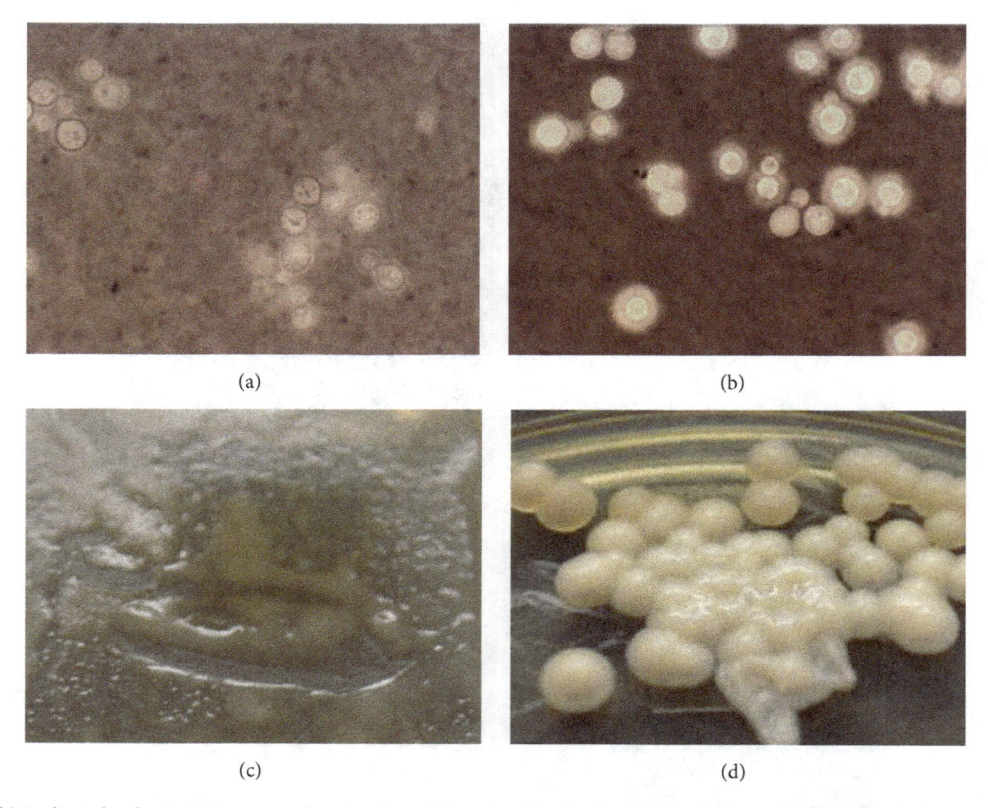

FIGURE 2: (a and b) India ink of original uncapsulated colony (a) and subbed colony (b) which produced capsule (1000x magnification). (c and d) Original colony on SABs flask; note rough colony phenotype as well as small colony formation (c). Subbed colonies, note abundant capsule production and typical large colony formation (d).

for infection based on cases of acapsular and hypocapsular strains causing disease and variation in capsular size throughout different phases of infection [27].

Aside from capsule modification, host immune responses may have perturbed detection of the CrAg in the serum and CSF by variable shedding. Boulware et al. describe "low," "intermediate," and "high" CrAg shedders normalized to fungal burden in HIV-infected *C. neoformans* patients higher shedding in increased levels of IL6/8 [28]. Lower levels of IL6 in our patient may even have modulated cryptococcal entry into the CNS as IL6 deficiency *in vivo* has been attributed to increased blood-brain-barrier permeability and higher mortality in $IL6^{-/-}$ mice and with neutralizing IL6 antibodies [29]. Because immunocompetent individuals have lower mortality and 10-fold lower serum CrAg titers [30], they likely can harbor *Cryptococcus* for longer periods without manifesting symptoms and delay diagnosis.

Elevated levels of Th1 cytokines, such as IP-10/CXCL10 secretion in response to IFN-γ, can be expected in an active infection and are associated with improved survival in *C. neoformans* meningitis [31–33]. Our immunocompetent patient had a more robust Th1 response compared with immunocompromised patients based on observed CSF levels of IFNγ, TNFα, GRO/CXCL1, IL8, and IL12p40 (Figure 3). Elevated IL10 (human cytokine synthesis inhibitory factor) in our patient, an anti-inflammatory cytokine which promotes a Th2 response, is detrimental to combating *C. neoformans* (Figure 3) and has been associated with a poorer outcome [32].

The modulation of capsule expression (early culture lack of capsule) may have been in part a function of organism response to the CNS immune state that we identified to include a robust Th1 response (elevated levels of INFγ, TNFα, GRO/CXCL1, IL8, and IL12p40) and simultaneous elevation of levels of the anti-inflammatory cytokine IL10. Low levels of IL6 may also have played a role in persistence of CNS infection in this case. Further characterization of cytokines in infections may eventually be useful in diagnosis given the observed limitations of current analytical methods.

The compilation of our patient's history, exam, lab findings, and imaging strongly suggested a fungal CNS infection that warranted repeated investigations. His indolent course made the diagnosis challenging but was consistent with the longer window from symptom onset to diagnosis in immunocompetent individuals compared with HIV-infected counterparts in a Taiwanese cohort [34]. He had subtle risk factors and exposure opportunities. Zoonotic transmission from his pet cockatoo is possible as a report with probable transmission of *C. neoformans* has been described albeit in an immunocompromised individual [35]. Additionally, *C. neoformans* has been isolated from sewage sludge to which he could be exposed while working in a wastewater treatment plant [36]. An active surveillance program found that both HIV-infected patients and control group patients who were

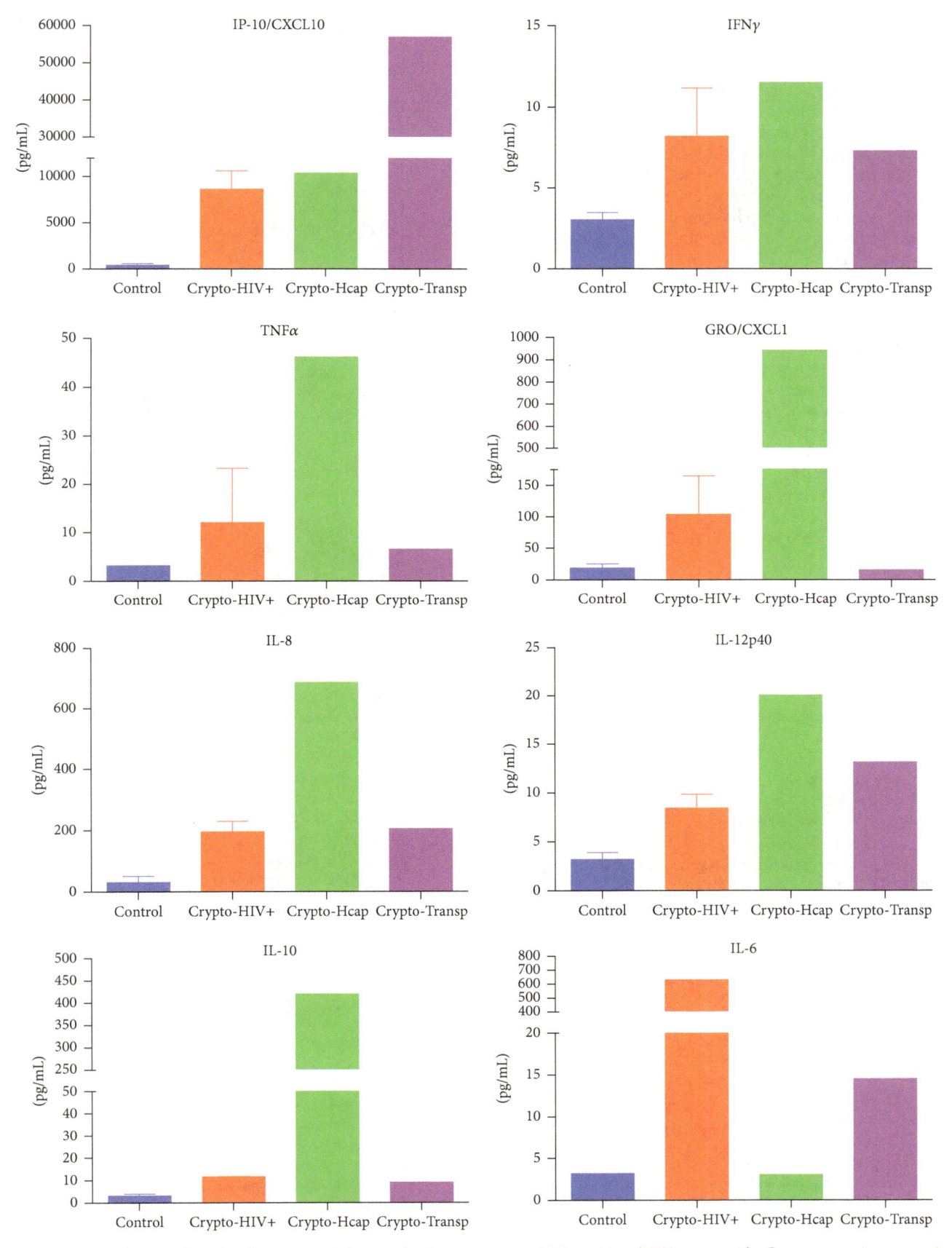

FIGURE 3: Respective cytokine levels in control ($n = 6$), *Cryptococcus* in HIV-positive (HIV+, $n = 2$), *Cryptococcus* in our patient (hypocapsular (Hcap), $n = 1$), and *Cryptococcus* after cardiac transplant (Transp, $n = 1$).

active smokers had a higher risk for cryptococcal infection [37], suggesting an increased risk with his 50-pack-year history.

Our patient's treatment was consistent with the standard of care for *C. neoformans* meningoencephalitis with antifungal therapy, serial LPs and CSF diversion for hydrocephalus, and corticosteroid therapy. Although *Cryptococcus* can produce biofilm on ventriculoatrial and ventriculoperitoneal shunts in patients previously infected with *Cryptococcus* [38], it is not contraindicated and has demonstrated improvement in cognitive impairment, gait, and papilledema in some without associated mortality or morbidity [39, 40].

We advocate an emphasis on collecting a large volume of CSF dedicated for culture at every opportunity for a lumbar puncture when a high index of suspicion exists, despite an immunocompetent host and negative antigen assays, as yeast titers are potentially low, capsule expression may be variable, and host immune response may modulate capsule expression, antigen shedding, and virulence. Since this case, our clinical microbiology department has adopted a rapid 1-hour multiplex PCR based panel for screening 14 potential bacteria, viruses, and *Cryptococcus neoformans/gattii* when considering meningitis/encephalitis (BioFire FilmArray Meningitis/Encephalitis Panel®) which may ameliorate difficulties mentioned here with traditional methods noted above.

Competing Interests

The authors do not have any competing interests to disclose.

References

[1] K. Voelz and R. C. May, "Cryptococcal interactions with the host immune system," *Eukaryotic Cell*, vol. 9, no. 6, pp. 835–846, 2010.

[2] K. Datta, K. H. Bartlett, R. Baer et al., "Spread of *Cryptococcus gattii* into Pacific Northwest Region of the United States," *Emerging Infectious Diseases*, vol. 15, no. 8, pp. 1185–1191, 2009.

[3] E. DeBess, S. R. Lockhart, N. Iqbal, and P. R. Cieslak, "Isolation of *Cryptococcus gattii* from Oregon soil and tree bark, 2010-2011," *BMC Microbiology*, vol. 14, no. 1, article 323, 2014.

[4] A. F. Gazzoni, C. B. Severo, E. F. Salles, and L. C. Severo, "Histopathology, serology and cultures in the diagnosis of cryptococcosis," *Revista do Instituto de Medicina Tropical de Sao Paulo*, vol. 51, no. 5, pp. 255–259, 2009.

[5] M. Chan, D. Lye, M. K. Win, A. Chow, and T. Barkham, "Clinical and microbiological characteristics of cryptococcosis in Singapore: predominance of *Cryptococcus neoformans* compared with *Cryptococcus gattii*," *International Journal of Infectious Diseases*, vol. 26, pp. 110–115, 2014.

[6] G. Lui, N. Lee, M. Ip et al., "Cryptococcosis in apparently immunocompetent patients," *Quarterly Journal of Medicine*, vol. 99, no. 3, pp. 143–151, 2006.

[7] O. Zaragoza and A. Casadevall, "Experimental modulation of capsule size in *Cryptococcus neoformans*," *Biological Procedures Online*, vol. 6, no. 1, pp. 10–15, 2004.

[8] S. Xie, R. Sao, A. Braun, and E. J. Bottone, "Difference in *Cryptococcus neoformans* cellular and capsule size in sequential pulmonary and meningeal infection: a postmortem study," *Diagnostic Microbiology and Infectious Disease*, vol. 73, no. 1, pp. 49–52, 2012.

[9] F. Almeida, J. M. Wolf, and A. Casadevall, "Virulence-associated enzymes of *Cryptococcus neoformans*," *Eukaryotic Cell*, vol. 14, no. 12, pp. 1173–1185, 2015.

[10] I. Bose, A. J. Reese, J. J. Ory, G. Janbon, and T. L. Doering, "A yeast under cover: the capsule of *Cryptococcus neoformans*," *Eukaryotic Cell*, vol. 2, no. 4, pp. 655–663, 2003.

[11] B. C. Haynes, M. L. Skowyra, S. J. Spencer et al., "Toward an integrated model of capsule regulation in *Cryptococcus neoformans*," *PLoS Pathogens*, vol. 7, no. 12, Article ID e1002411, 2011.

[12] R. S. Dominic, H. Prashanth, S. Shenoy, and S. Baliga, "Diagnostic value of latex agglutination in cryptococcal meningitis," *Journal of Laboratory Physicians*, vol. 1, no. 2, pp. 67–68, 2009.

[13] Y.-Y. Lin, S. Shiau, and C.-T. Fang, "Risk factors for invasive *Cryptococcus neoformans* diseases: a case-control study," *PLoS ONE*, vol. 10, no. 3, Article ID e0119090, 2015.

[14] D. R. Boulware, M. A. Rolfes, R. Rajasingham et al., "Multisite validation of cryptococcal antigen lateral flow assay and quantification by laser thermal contrast," *Emerging Infectious Diseases journal*, vol. 20, no. 1, pp. 45–53, 2014.

[15] J. E. Vidal and D. R. Boulware, "Lateral flow assay for cryptococcal antigen: an important advance to improve the continuum of hiv care and reduce cryptococcal meningitis-related mortality," *Revista do Instituto de Medicina Tropical de São Paulo*, vol. 57, supplement 19, pp. 38–45, 2015.

[16] N. Ueno and M. B. Lodoen, "From the blood to the brain: avenues of eukaryotic pathogen dissemination to the central nervous system," *Current Opinion in Microbiology*, vol. 26, pp. 53–59, 2015.

[17] J. Stie and D. Fox, "Blood-brain barrier invasion by *Cryptococcus neoformans* is enhanced by functional interactions with plasmin," *Microbiology*, vol. 158, part 1, pp. 240–258, 2012.

[18] J. N. Day, "Cryptococcal meningitis," *Practical Neurology*, vol. 4, no. 5, pp. 274–285, 2004.

[19] A. E. Merkler, N. Gaines, H. Baradaran et al., "Direct invasion of the optic nerves, chiasm, and tracts by *Cryptococcus neoformans* in an immunocompetent host," *The Neurohospitalist*, vol. 5, no. 4, pp. 217–222, 2015.

[20] H. C. Eisenman, A. Casadevall, and E. E. McClelland, "New insights on the pathogenesis of invasive *Cryptococcus neoformans* infection," *Current Infectious Disease Reports*, vol. 9, no. 6, pp. 457–464, 2007.

[21] W. S. Cheon, K.-S. Eom, B. K. Yoo et al., "A case of pulmonary cryptococcosis by capsule-deficient *Cryptococcus neoformans*," *Korean Journal of Internal Medicine*, vol. 21, no. 1, pp. 83–87, 2006.

[22] D. J. Levinson, D. C. Silcox, J. W. Rippon, and S. Thomsen, "Septic arthritis due to nonencapsulated *Cryptococcus neoformans* with coexisting sarcoidosis," *Arthritis & Rheumatism*, vol. 17, no. 6, pp. 1037–1047, 1974.

[23] I. F. Laurenson, J. D. C. Ross, and L. J. R. Milne, "Microscopy and latex antigen negative cryptococcal meningitis," *Journal of Infection*, vol. 36, no. 3, pp. 329–331, 1998.

[24] M. Kanazawa, M. Ishii, Y. Sato, K. Kitamura, H. Oshiro, and Y. Inayama, "Capsule-deficient meningeal cryptococcosis," *Acta Cytologica*, vol. 52, no. 2, pp. 266–268, 2008.

[25] Y. Sugiura, M. Homma, and T. Yamamoto, "Difficulty in diagnosing chronic meningitis caused by capsule-deficient *Cryptococcus neoformans*," *Journal of Neurology, Neurosurgery and Psychiatry*, vol. 76, no. 10, pp. 1460–1461, 2005.

[26] S. T. Garber and P. L. Penar, "Treatment of indolent, nonencapsulated cryptococcal meningitis associated with hydrocephalus," *Clinics and Practice*, vol. 2, no. 1, p. e22, 2012.

[27] M. Del Poeta, "Role of phagocytosis in the virulence of *Cryptococcus neoformans*," *Eukaryotic Cell*, vol. 3, no. 5, pp. 1067–1075, 2004.

[28] D. R. Boulware, M. von Hohenberg, M. A. Rolfes et al., "Human immune response varies by the degree of relative cryptococcal antigen shedding," *Open Forum Infectious Diseases*, vol. 3, no. 1, Article ID ofv194, 2016.

[29] X. Li, G. Liu, J. Ma, L. Zhou, Q. Zhang, and L. Gao, "Lack of IL-6 increases blood-brain barrier permeability in fungal meningitis," *Journal of Biosciences*, vol. 40, no. 1, pp. 7–12, 2015.

[30] P. G. Pappas, "Cryptococcal infections in non-HIV-infected patients," *Transactions of the American Clinical and Climatological Association*, vol. 124, pp. 61–79, 2013.

[31] E. Sionov, K. D. Mayer-Barber, Y. C. Chang et al., "Type I IFN induction via poly-ICLC protects mice against cryptococcosis," *PLoS Pathogens*, vol. 11, no. 8, Article ID e1005040, 2015.

[32] D. J. Mora, L. R. Fortunato, L. E. Andrade-Silva et al., "Cytokine profiles at admission can be related to outcome in AIDS patients with cryptococcal meningitis," *PLoS ONE*, vol. 10, no. 3, Article ID e0120297, 2015.

[33] W. C. Uicker, J. P. McCracken, and K. L. Buchanan, "Role of $CD4^+$ T cells in a protective immune response against *Cryptococcus neoformans* in the central nervous system," *Medical Mycology*, vol. 44, no. 1, pp. 1–11, 2006.

[34] C.-H. Liao, C.-Y. Chi, Y.-J. Wang et al., "Different presentations and outcomes between HIV-infected and HIV-uninfected patients with *Cryptococcal meningitis*," *Journal of Microbiology, Immunology and Infection*, vol. 45, no. 4, pp. 296–304, 2012.

[35] J. D. Nosanchuk, S. Shoham, B. C. Fries, D. S. Shapiro, S. M. Levitz, and A. Casadevall, "Evidence of zoonotic transmission of *Cryptococcus neoformans* from a pet cockatoo to an immunocompromised patient," *Annals of Internal Medicine*, vol. 132, no. 3, pp. 205–208, 2000.

[36] S. Dumontet, A. Scopa, S. Kerje, and K. Krovacek, "The importance of pathogenic organisms in sewage and sewage sludge," *Journal of the Air and Waste Management Association*, vol. 51, no. 6, pp. 848–860, 2001.

[37] R. A. Hajjeh, L. A. Conn, D. S. Stephens et al., "Cryptococcosis: population-based multistate active surveillance and risk factors in human immunodeficiency virus-infected persons. Cryptococcal Active Surveillance Group," *Journal of Infectious Diseases*, vol. 179, no. 2, pp. 449–454, 1999.

[38] M. J. Viereck, N. Chalouhi, D. I. Krieger, and K. D. Judy, "Cryptococcal ventriculoperitoneal shunt infection," *Journal of Clinical Neuroscience*, vol. 21, no. 11, pp. 2020–2021, 2014.

[39] L.-M. Tang, "Ventriculoperitoneal shunt in cryptococcal meningitis with hydrocephalus," *Surgical Neurology*, vol. 33, no. 5, pp. 314–319, 1990.

[40] M. K. Park, D. R. Hospenthal, and J. E. Bennett, "Treatment of hydrocephalus secondary to cryptococcal meningitis by use of shunting," *Clinical Infectious Diseases*, vol. 28, no. 3, pp. 629–633, 1999.

Septic Encephalopathy Characterized by Acute Encephalopathy with Biphasic Seizures and Late Reduced Diffusion and Early Nonconvulsive Status Epilepticus

Hiroshi Yamaguchi,[1] Tsukasa Tanaka,[2] Azusa Maruyama,[2] and Hiroaki Nagase[2]

[1]Department of Emergency and Critical Care Medicine, Hyogo Prefectural Kobe Children's Hospital, 1-1-1 Takakuradai, Suma-Ku, Kobe, Hyogo 654-0081, Japan
[2]Department of Neurology, Hyogo Prefectural Kobe Children's Hospital, 1-1-1 Takakuradai, Suma-Ku, Kobe, Hyogo 654-0081, Japan

Correspondence should be addressed to Hiroshi Yamaguchi; hiyamaguchi_kch@hp.pref.hyogo.jp

Academic Editor: Massimiliano Filosto

Infection, whether viral or bacterial, can result in various forms of brain dysfunction (encephalopathy). Septic encephalopathy (SE) is caused by an excessive immune reaction to infection, with clinical features including disturbed consciousness and seizures. Acute encephalopathy with biphasic seizures and late reduced diffusion (AESD) is usually accompanied by viral infection in children and is characterized by biphasic seizures and impaired consciousness. The initial neurologic symptom of AESD is typically a febrile seizure that frequently lasts longer than 30 minutes. However, the possible forms this seizure takes are unclear. For example, it is unknown if nonconvulsive status epilepticus (NCSE) could be an early seizure symptomatic of AESD. In addition, thus far no cases of combined SE and AESD have been reported. Here, we describe the first reported case of SE with AESD that notably demonstrated NCSE as an early seizure.

1. Introduction

Both bacterial and viral infections can induce forms of brain dysfunction (encephalopathy) whose symptoms frequently include seizures of one type or another. Septic encephalopathy (SE) is a brain dysfunction characterized by clinical, electrophysiological, or biochemical criteria and is considered to be primarily due to an excessive immune reaction to infection [1]. The main clinical features of SE are disturbances of consciousness, impaired cognitive function, and seizures [1]. The pathophysiology of SE is still poorly understood, although many mechanisms of its development have been proposed. These include oxidative stress, increased cytokine and proinflammatory factor levels, disturbances in cerebral circulation, injury to the brain's vascular endothelium, altered neurotransmitter levels, and bacterial endotoxins leaking through the blood-brain barrier [1]. Estimates suggest that 8–70% of the patients with diagnosed sepsis exhibit symptoms of encephalopathy [2].

Another infection-related encephalopathic disorder is acute encephalopathy with biphasic seizures and late reduced diffusion (AESD). AESD is characterized by biphasic seizures and impaired consciousness, preceded most often by viral infection. These symptoms are followed by reduced diffusion in the subcortical white matter upon magnetic resonance imaging (MRI) that is typically observed between days 3 and 9 after the clinical onset [3]. Typically, the initial neurologic symptom of AESD is a febrile seizure that usually lasts longer than 30 minutes [4, 5]. While it is possible that other types of early seizures can represent AESD, to the best of our knowledge no reports of nonconvulsive status epilepticus (NCSE) as such a seizure exist.

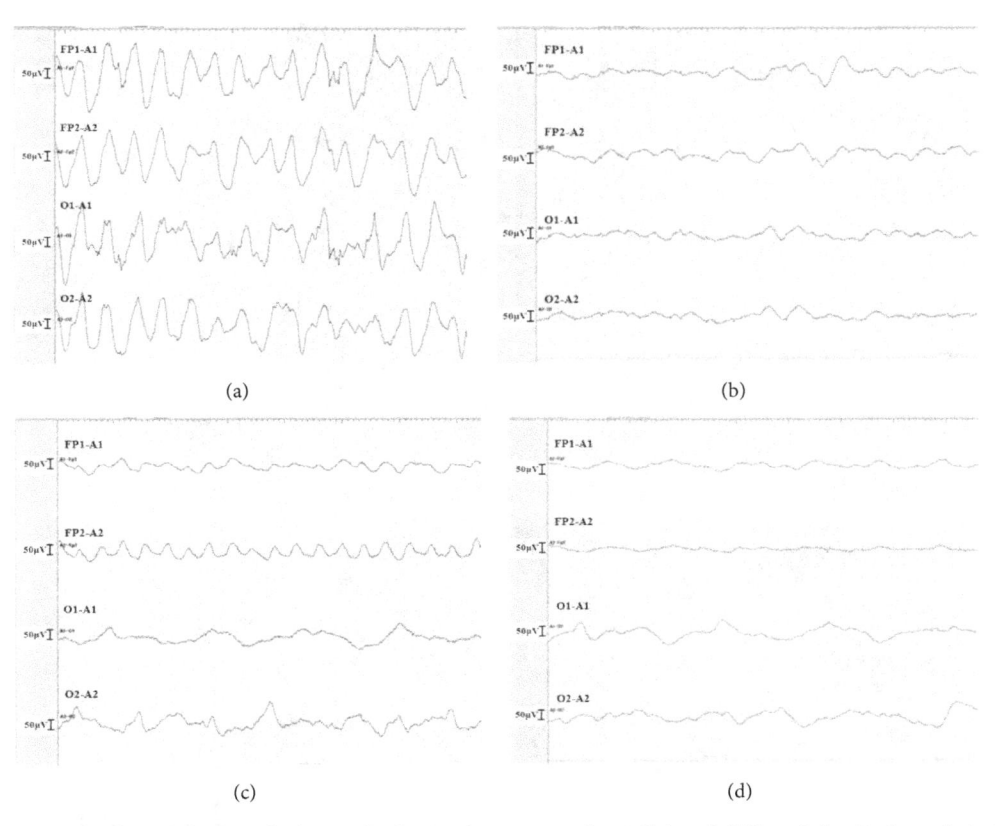

FIGURE 1: Encephalographic (EEG) findings before and after ictal events on day 1 ((a) and (b)) and day 5 after admission ((c) and (d)), respectively. EEG was digitally recorded using four channels (Fp1-A1, Fp2-A2, O1-A1, and O2-A2) according to the International 10–20 system.

To the best of our knowledge, no cases of SE in which AESD was also present have been reported. However, we report here a case of a 3-year-old Japanese boy who after *Streptococcus pneumoniae* (*S. pneumoniae*) bacteremia developed SE with both the clinical and the radiological features of AESD. Notably, this is apparently the first reported case in which NCSE represented the early seizure symptom of AESD.

2. Case Report

A 3-year-old Japanese boy was admitted to our hospital presenting with a high fever and shivering. His past medical history included congenital asplenia syndrome, an esophageal hiatal hernia after cardioplasty, and a single cardiac atrium and ventricle after a Fontan procedure. These conditions were controlled by aspirin, warfarin, diuretics, and home oxygen therapy (0.5 L/min oxygen at night). His premorbid activities of daily living (ADL) were appropriate for his age, including the ability to speak in complete sentences and the ability to walk and eat without assistance. He also had no history of hypoxic encephalopathy.

On admission, he showed disturbance of consciousness (Glasgow Coma Scale (GCS) 10 (E3, V3, and M4)). Vital signs were as follows: temperature: 40.2°C; blood pressure (BP): 80/40 mmHg; heart rate (HR): 144 bpm; respiratory rate: 56/min; and oxygen saturation: 96% (0.5 L/min oxygen).

Shortly after admission, the patient suffered a tonic-clonic convulsion for 30 seconds, which subsided without treatment. Laboratory data showed leukocytosis (white blood cell count 21,600/μL) but were otherwise normal. Cerebrospinal fluid (CSF) analysis was also normal, and a CSF culture was negative. We diagnosed him with SE and started cefotaxime (CTX; 300 mg/kg/day) for an infection of undetermined origin.

After admission, he continued to be drowsy, and, by 4 hours after admission, his mental status had deteriorated to GCS 6 (E1, V2, and M3) with mumbling. We then started electroencephalography (EEG), which revealed rhythmical, diffuse high-voltage slow activity (Figure 1(a)), which we diagnosed as NCSE. Both electrical seizures and nonconvulsive seizures such as ocular deviation continued intermittently without full recovery of consciousness, despite the administration of midazolam and fosphenytoin. The seizures were finally controlled by phenobarbital (20 mg/kg IV) ten hours after admission (Figure 1(b)). However, the NCSE, high fever (>38°C), and hemodynamic instability (systolic BP: 80–100 mmHg, HR: 150–180 bpm) continued. Treatment with volume load and vasopressor therapy (dopamine drip was up to 6 mcg/kg/min) was initiated, and within several hours the hemodynamics and urine output were restored to within normal range. Although the intermittent seizures without recovery of consciousness were suggestive of refractory status epilepticus, we were reluctant to initiate barbiturate coma

(a) DWI

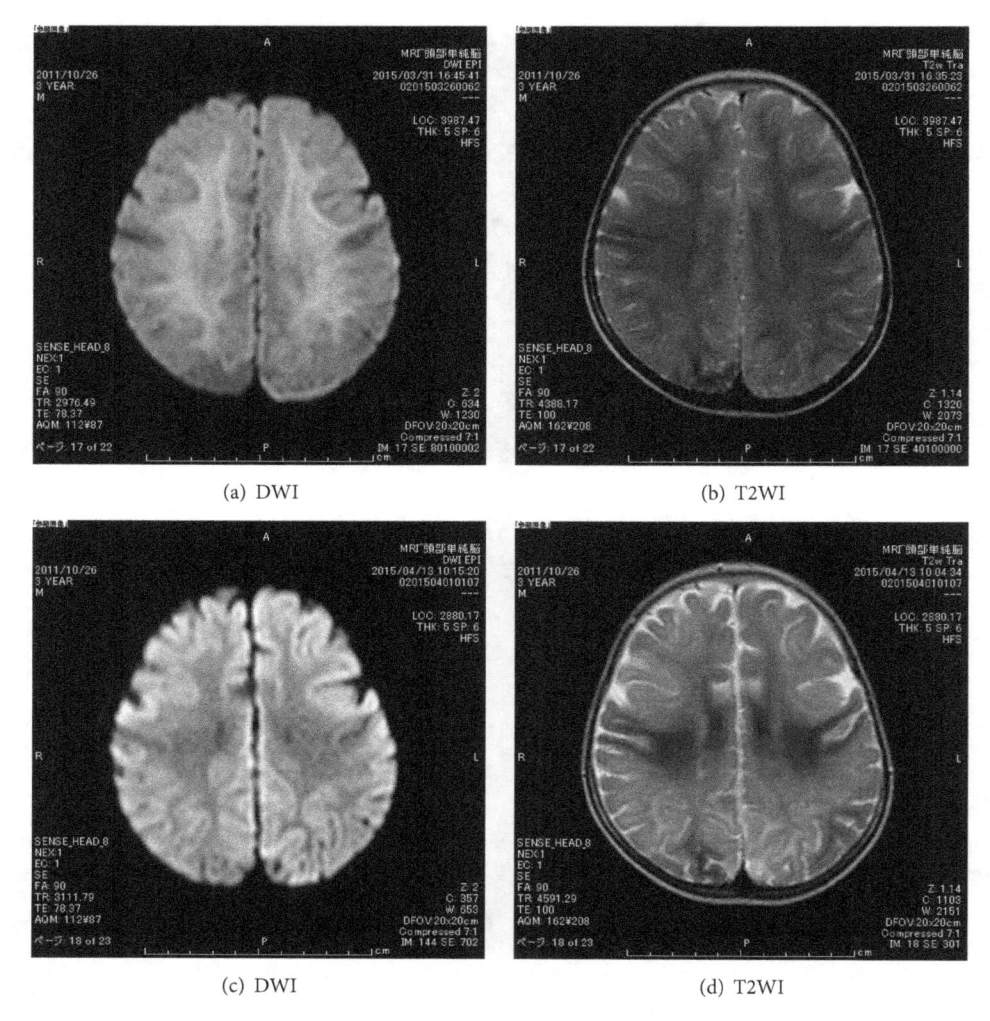

(b) T2WI

(c) DWI

(d) T2WI

Figure 2: Magnetic resonance imaging (MRI) findings. Both diffusion-weighted imaging (DWI) ((a) and (c)) and T2-weighted imaging (T2WI) ((b) and (d)) were performed. MRI performed on day 8 showed hyperintensity in the deep subcortical white matter ((a) and (b)). The hyperintensity on DWI resolved (c), but diffuse atrophy was noted.

therapy because of the hemodynamic instability. His blood culture on admission was positive for *S. pneumoniae*, so we then diagnosed him with sepsis due to *S. pneumoniae*. The next day, his hemodynamic parameters continued to improve with vasopressor therapy (dopamine drip 4.5 mcg/kg/min). At this point, neither electrical nor nonconvulsive seizures developed, so anticonvulsive therapy was discontinued. However, the patient was still drowsy, with a GCS of 6 (E1, V2, and M3).

On day 3 after admission, we discontinued vasopressor therapy. Antimicrobial susceptibility testing showed penicillin-sensitive *Streptococcus pneumoniae* (PSSP), so his antibiotics were changed to aminobenzyl penicillin (ABPC; 300 mg/kg/day), which was continued for 14 days. His altered state of consciousness also gradually improved to GCS7 (E1, V2, and M4) on day 3 and GCS9 (E2, V2, and M5) on days 4 and 5, respectively. No seizures were observed from days 3 to 5. On day 6 after admission, the patient had a brief seizure that included rolling of the eyes and apnea; an EEG showed rhythmical, right frontal-dominant slow activity (Figure 1(c)), and his mental status deteriorated again to GCS 6 (E1, V2, and M3). We restarted the treatment with fosphenytoin followed by phenobarbital. Despite these treatments, nonconvulsive and/or electrical seizures were intermittently observed without full recovery of consciousness for 12 hours. On day 7, we started high-dose phenobarbital for refractory NCSE, at daily doses of up to 20 mg/kg IV that were tapered by 50% every other day until day 12. This treatment successfully controlled the seizures (Figure 1(d)). Diffusion-weighted magnetic resonance images (DWI) taken 3 days after the second onset of seizures (day 8 after admission) revealed hyperintensity in the subcortical white matter (bright tree appearance) (Figures 2(a) and 2(b)), which subsequently resolved by day 21 after admission (Figures 2(c) and 2(d)). Thereafter, his clinical condition stabilized, including gradual recovery of consciousness (GCS 11 (E4, V2, and M5)), although he could not walk without support nor speak a meaningful word. He was finally discharged from our hospital 50 days after admission and he returned for a follow-up visit.

3. Discussion

During sepsis, the central nervous system (CNS) is one of the first organs damaged, and this clinically leads to SE. Our case of SE followed a clinical course that included biphasic seizures and worsening consciousness as has been described for AESD. Furthermore, MRI studies performed on days 8 and 21 showed the reduced diffusion characteristic of AESD. Given these similarities, we diagnosed him with SE accompanied by AESD. Viral infections such as influenza or HHV-6, or adverse effects after vaccination, have been reported as the main etiologies of AESD [5]. Although bacterial infection is a very rare cause of AESD, a case that was associated with S. pneumoniae meningoencephalitis was recently reported [6]. The most unusual aspect of our case was that the patient developed sepsis from S. pneumoniae bacteremia; however, we could not find any evidence of meningitis. Therefore, we believe the neuronal injury in this patient was not the result of bacterial circulation, but rather excitotoxicity related to the pathology of AESD [3, 5]. In fact, several mechanisms for brain injury during sepsis have been reported [1, 2], including inflammation that activates excitotoxicity and oxidative stressors which may further aggravate SE and result in neuronal dysfunction [7]. Furthermore, it is possible that the initial low BP in this patient will have led to hypoperfusion and hypoxic ischemia. However, the patient did not have significant hypotension, and his hemodynamic status was successfully controlled, so we do not believe this to be the case.

Our case also revealed NCSE as an early seizure that might lead to AESD. Though the early seizure in AESD usually lasts longer than 30 minutes [4, 5], Takanashi et al. identified some patients with AESD with brief early febrile seizures followed by secondary seizures and disturbance of consciousness on days 4 to 6 after admission [8]. It is unknown whether these patients also had nonconvulsive seizures. Here, the patient had a brief convulsive seizure, after which NCSE was identified through continuous EEG monitoring. NCSE is the diagnosis for encephalopathy caused by continuous epileptic activity on an EEG. It is a well-known cause of morbidity and mortality in critically ill neonates and adults [9, 10]. Recent prospective studies that focused on critically ill children found that NCSE is also common in critically ill children with acute encephalopathy [11, 12]. The impact of NCSE on neurological outcomes is unclear, although evidence suggests that NCSE could be an independent risk factor for hippocampal atrophy [13].

As for the second seizure, it is possible, but unlikely, that the biphasic behavior of this patient could be related to the sudden withdrawal of anticonvulsants. Sudden withdrawal of antiepileptic drugs usually appears within a few days after discontinuation of the drugs and is caused by continuous dosing of an anticonvulsant for a long period. We used anticonvulsants for the early seizures, on only the first day of admission, whereas the biphasic seizure reappeared 5 days later. In addition, the MRI results noted on day 8 are uncommonly found in situations of withdrawal of antiepileptic drugs. Therefore, the biphasic behavior of this patient is not likely to be the result of the sudden withdrawal of antiepileptic drugs.

Our case demonstrates the importance of continuous EEG monitoring for patients with disturbed consciousness even after the convulsive seizures have disappeared, particularly in cases of acute encephalopathy. In these cases, there is the possibility that the early NCSE will lead to mental deterioration and brain damage and culminate in a second seizure. In addition, our case highlights targeted temperature management and/or barbiturate coma therapy for preventing biphasic seizures and neurologic sequelae. These treatments are effective in preventing the damage caused by refractory febrile convulsive status epilepticus or acute encephalopathy [14, 15] and could likely prevent secondary seizures as well. Unfortunately, because of the hemodynamic instability, we could not perform barbiturate coma therapy as we normally would have in such a case as this.

In conclusion, we describe the first reported case of SE with clinical characteristics of AESD with NCSE as an early seizure. Further studies will be needed to determine the exact relationship between SE and AESD.

References

[1] M. Ziaja, "Septic encephalopathy," *Current Neurology and Neuroscience Reports*, vol. 13, article 383, 2013.

[2] I. M. Kafa, S. Bakirci, M. Uysal, and M. A. Kurt, "Alterations in the brain electrical activity in a rat model of sepsis-associated encephalopathy," *Brain Research*, vol. 1354, pp. 217–226, 2010.

[3] J.-I. Takanashi, "Two newly proposed infectious encephalitis/encephalopathy syndromes," *Brain and Development*, vol. 31, no. 7, pp. 521–528, 2009.

[4] M. Mizuguchi, H. Yamanouchi, T. Ichiyama, and M. Shiomi, "Acute encephalopathy associated with influenza and other viral infections," *Acta Neurologica Scandinavica*, vol. 186, no. 4, supplement, pp. 45–56, 2007.

[5] J. Takanashi, H. Oba, A. J. Barkovich et al., "Diffusion MRI abnormalities after prolonged febrile seizures with encephalopathy," *Neurology*, vol. 66, no. 9, pp. 1304–1309, 2006.

[6] S. Kuwata, H. Senzaki, Y. Urushibara et al., "A case of acute encephalopathy with biphasic seizures and late reduced diffusion associated with *Streptococcus pneumoniae* meningoencephalitis," *Brain and Development*, vol. 34, no. 6, pp. 529–532, 2012.

[7] F. Dal-Pizzol, C. D. Tomasi, and C. Ritter, "Septic encephalopathy: does inflammation drive the brain crazy?" *Revista Brasileira de Psiquiatria*, vol. 36, no. 3, pp. 251–258, 2014.

[8] J. Takanashi, M. Tsuji, K. Amemiya, H. Tada, and A. J. Barkovich, "Mild influenza encephalopathy with biphasic seizures and late reduced diffusion," *Journal of the Neurological Sciences*, vol. 256, no. 1-2, pp. 86–89, 2007.

[9] B. F. Shneker and N. B. Fountain, "Assessment of acute morbidity and mortality in nonconvulsive status epilepticus," *Neurology*, vol. 61, no. 8, pp. 1066–1073, 2003.

[10] F. Pisani, L. Sisti, and S. Seri, "A scoring system for early prognostic assessment after neonatal seizures," *Pediatrics*, vol. 124, no. 4, pp. 580–587, 2009.

[11] H. M. Greiner, K. Holland, J. L. Leach, P. S. Horn, A. D. Hershey, and D. F. Rose, "Nonconvulsive status epilepticus: the encephalopathic pediatric patient," *Pediatrics*, vol. 129, no. 3, pp. e748–e755, 2012.

[12] N. S. Abend, A. M. Gutierrez-Colina, A. A. Topjian et al., "Nonconvulsive seizures are common in critically ill children," *Neurology*, vol. 76, no. 12, pp. 1071–1077, 2011.

[13] P. M. Vespa, D. L. McArthur, Y. Xu et al., "Nonconvulsive seizures after traumatic brain injury are associated with hippocampal atrophy," *Neurology*, vol. 75, no. 9, pp. 792–798, 2010.

[14] M. Nishiyama, T. Tanaka, K. Fujita, A. Maruyama, and H. Nagase, "Targeted temperature management of acute encephalopathy without AST elevation," *Brain and Development*, vol. 37, no. 3, pp. 328–333, 2015.

[15] H. Nagase, M. Nishiyama, T. Nakagawa, K. Fujita, Y. Saji, and A. Maruyama, "Midazolam fails to prevent neurological damage in children with convulsive refractory febrile status epilepticus," *Pediatric Neurology*, vol. 51, no. 1, pp. 78–84, 2014.

High-Grade Glioma of the Ventrolateral Medulla in an Adult: Case Presentation and Discussion of Surgical Considerations

Angela Spurgeon,[1] Viet Le,[2] Sanjay Konakondla,[1] Douglas C. Miller,[3] Tamera Hopkins,[4] and N. Scott Litofsky[1]

[1]Division of Neurosurgery, University of Missouri School of Medicine, Columbia, MO 65212, USA
[2]University of Missouri School of Medicine, Columbia, MO 65212, USA
[3]Department of Pathology and Anatomical Sciences, University of Missouri School of Medicine, Columbia, MO 65212, USA
[4]Division of Hematology Oncology, University of Missouri School of Medicine, Columbia, MO 65212, USA

Correspondence should be addressed to Angela Spurgeon; spurgeona@health.missouri.edu

Academic Editor: Mehmet Turgut

Background. High-grade gliomas of the brainstem are rare in adults and are particularly rare in the anterolateral medulla. We describe an illustrative case and discuss the diagnostic and treatment issues associated with a tumor in this location, including differential diagnosis, anatomical considerations for options for surgical management, multimodality treatment, and prognosis. *Case Description.* A 69-year-old woman presented with a 3-week history of progressive right lower extremity weakness. She underwent an open biopsy via a far lateral approach with partial condylectomy, which revealed a glioblastoma. Concurrent temozolomide and radiation were completed; however, she elected to stop her chemotherapy after 5.5 weeks of treatment. She succumbed to her disease 11 months after diagnosis. *Conclusions.* Biopsy can be performed relatively safely to provide definitive diagnosis to guide treatment, but long-term prognosis is poor.

1. Introduction

Glioblastomas (GBM) account for 54% of CNS gliomas; however the incidence of glioblastoma in the brainstem is not well defined [1]. In a series of 21 patients with gliomas, Hundsberger et al. [2] found six (28.6%) brainstem glioblastomas of which two originated in the medulla. In a larger series Kesari et al. [3] had found only 3 (5.5%) glioblastomas out of 54 surgically sampled brainstem gliomas.

Due to the rarity of medullary brainstem glioblastomas, their diagnosis and management are complex and controversial. We report the case of a 69-year-old woman with a glioblastoma of the ventrolateral medulla to highlight differential diagnosis, anatomical considerations relating to options for surgical management, and multimodality treatment.

2. Case Presentation

2.1. History and Examination. A 69-year-old Caucasian woman presented to an outside hospital with a 3-week history of progressive right lower extremity weakness. An initial MRI demonstrated a 1.9 × 0.8 × 1.0 cm contrast-enhancing mass in the left ventrolateral aspect of the medulla (Figure 1). She was diagnosed with a "stroke" at the outside hospital and transferred to an inpatient rehabilitation facility. Two weeks later she developed drooling with slurred speech and was transferred to the University of Missouri Hospital and Clinic's Neurosurgery Service. Physical examination revealed a left hypoglossal nerve palsy but a right accessory nerve weakness. Motor examination demonstrated full strength on the left side, with right-sided weakness (deltoids, biceps, and triceps

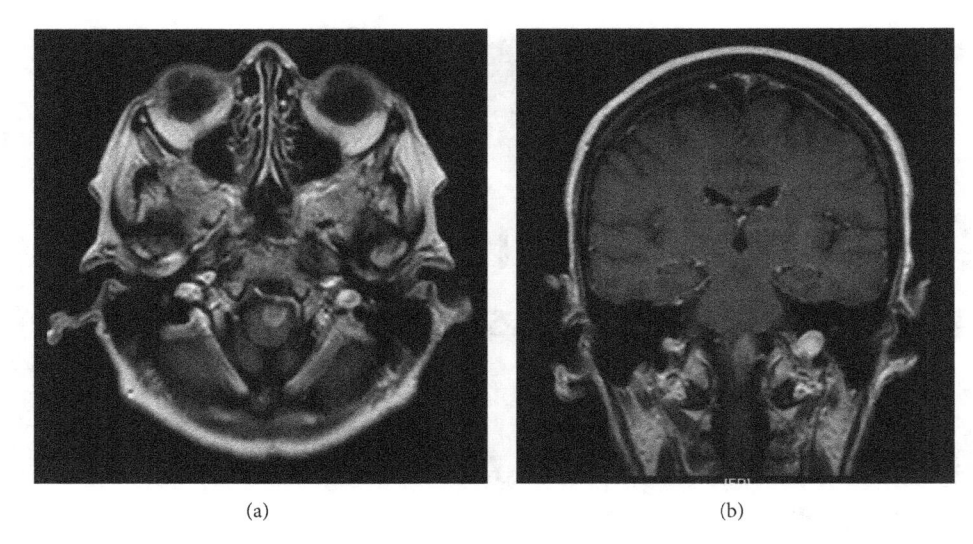

FIGURE 1: Initial brain MRI. (a) Axial T1-weighted image with gadolinium, showing the enhancing left medullary lesion. (b) Coronal T1-weighted image with gadolinium showing the same medullary lesion.

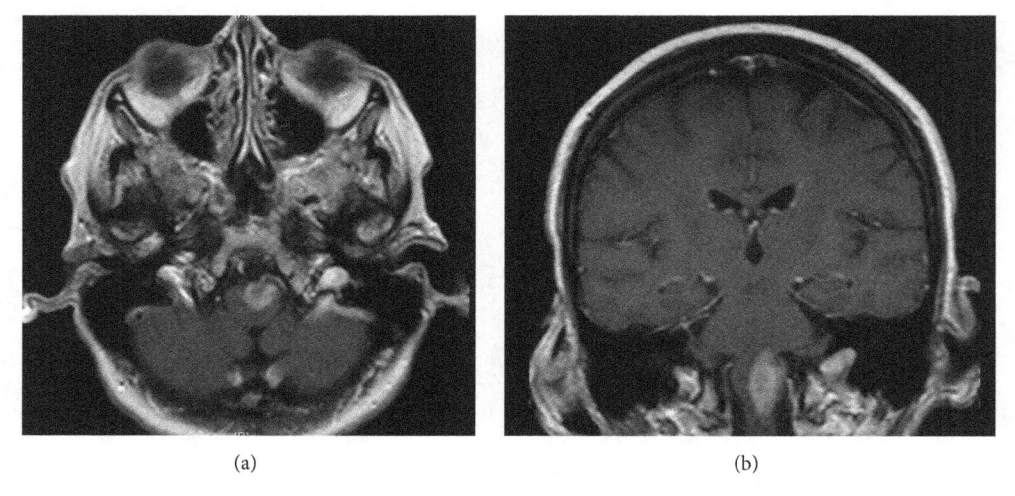

FIGURE 2: Brain MRI 2 weeks after the initial MRI. (a) Axial T1-weighted image with gadolinium, showing the enhancing left medullary lesion increased in size. (b) Coronal T1-weighted image with gadolinium showing the same medullary lesion increased in size.

4/5, grip 2/5, hip flexor and knee extensors 4/5, knee flexor, and dorsiflexion and plantar flexion 0/5).

2.2. Diagnosis. A repeat MRI revealed that the mass was larger, now $3.2 \times 1.1 \times 1.4$ cm (Figure 2). The differential diagnosis (Table 1) was quite extensive, but lymphoma and glioma were favored on the basis of history and imaging. Further metastatic workup and a lumbar puncture were negative.

Surgical intervention was planned to establish a definitive diagnosis and achieve brainstem decompression if possible. The medullary lesion was biopsied using neuronavigation with BrainLAB via a far lateral approach with partial condylectomy. Intraoperative monitoring was utilized to observe the integrity of neural pathways and included somatosensory evoked potentials (SSEPs), brainstem auditory evoked potentials (BAEPs), motor evoked potentials (MEPs), and electromyography (EMG) for the lower cranial nerves. The lesion was quite firm and rubbery but blended in with surrounding tissues. Based on an intraoperative frozen section report of high-grade glioma, the texture of the lesion, and a temporary loss of MEPs during the procedure, resection was limited. A diagnosis of glioblastoma (WHO grade IV) was subsequently confirmed by the final pathology examination (Figures 3(a)–3(d)).

2.3. Hospital Course. The patient's postsurgical course was complicated by aspiration pneumonia requiring a period of reintubation. Postoperative hoarseness led to a diagnosis of left vocal cord paralysis. Her right-sided weakness remained unchanged from her preoperative baseline. On postoperative day five, she was transferred to a hospital closer to home for continued acute care and adjuvant therapy.

(a) (b)

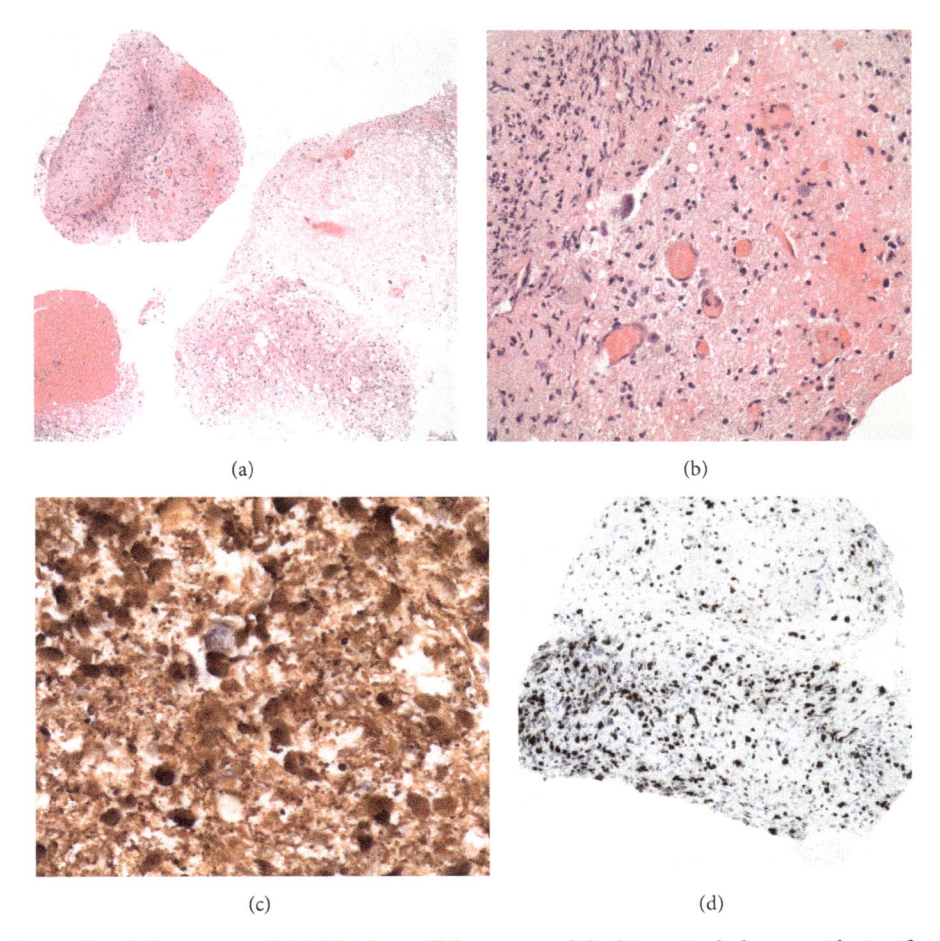

(c) (d)

FIGURE 3: Histopathology of medullary tumor. (a) Multiple small fragments of the biopsy include one with significant necrosis, one with relatively high cell density, and one with considerable hemorrhage. H&E, original magnification 100x. (b) At high magnification, this portion of the biopsy shows tumor with moderate cell density bordering necrotic tumor. H&E, original magnification 400x. (c) Many of the tumor cells have cytoplasmic GFAP immunoreactivity, establishing their astrocytomatous phenotype. Original magnification 600x. (d) A Ki67 immunostain shows a proliferative index of up to about 25%, consistent with the diagnosis of a high-grade glioma. Original magnification 200x.

2.4. Treatment. Treatment was initiated with temozolomide 100 mg/day. A concurrent course of radiation therapy (total 5600 cGy divided over 28 fractions) was completed. She achieved some improvement in lower extremity function so that she was able to stand and pivot. She was hospitalized multiple times during radiotherapy for recurrent UTIs and required pharmacologic treatment for depression. She elected to stop her chemotherapy after 5.5 weeks of daily temozolomide. Recurrent headaches 10 months after surgery prompted a repeat MRI which demonstrated disease progression (Figure 4). The patient and her family elected to proceed with palliative care. She succumbed to her disease 11 months after diagnosis.

3. Discussion

Glioblastoma of the medulla is rare; thus the ability to draw definitive conclusions from the literature can be a challenge. Most larger series combine all gliomas of the midbrain, pons, and medulla together making it difficult to draw specific conclusions with regard to GBM of the medulla. Additionally tumors of the medulla vary with regard to location (ventrolateral, ventral, diffuse, and exophytic dorsal) which affects surgical decision-making and multimodality therapies. Table 2 summarizes case reports of documented medullary adult high-grade gliomas in the literature. The remainder of the discussion will focus on the larger body of brainstem glioma literature with emphasis placed on medullary lesions as much as possible.

3.1. Clinical Features and Differential Diagnosis. The signs and symptoms of a brainstem high-grade glioma overlap with those of many other CNS diseases and are dependent on the location of the lesion. Clinical features observed at diagnosis may include gait disorders, visual disturbances, limb weakness, and cranial nerve deficits [3, 13, 14]. The differential diagnosis of a brainstem mass is extensive (Table 1) [7, 15–20].

MRI is currently an essential, noninvasive tool for evaluating brainstem lesions. While imaging characteristics can help narrow the differential diagnosis, multiple studies

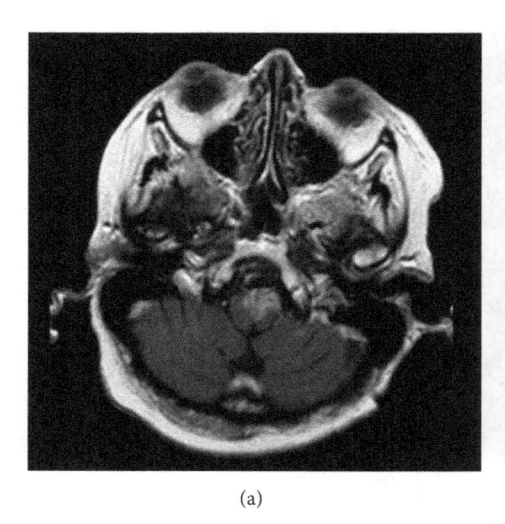

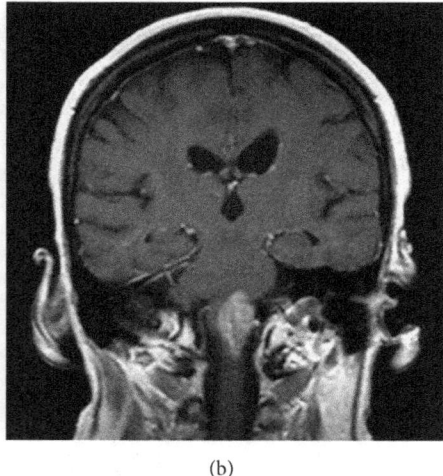

FIGURE 4: Brain MRI 10 months after surgery. (a) Axial T1-weighted image with gadolinium, showing progression of the enhancing left medullary lesion. (b) Coronal T1-weighted image with gadolinium showing the same medullary lesion.

TABLE 1: Differential diagnosis of brainstem lesions.

Category	Diseases
Inflammatory	Autoimmune encephalitis
	Bickerstaff brainstem encephalitis
	CNS vasculitis
	Demyelination (multiple sclerosis)
	Neuromyelitis optica
	Neuro-Behçet
	Neurosarcoidosis
	Sjögren's syndrome with CNS involvement
	CLIPPERS (chronic lymphocytic inflammation with pontine perivascular enhancement responsive to steroids)
Neoplastic	Glioma
	Metastatic cancer
	CNS lymphoma
	Primitive neuroectodermal tumor
	Ependymoma
	Malignant histiocytosis
Infectious	Tuberculoma
	Pyogenic abscess
Paraneoplastic	Paraneoplastic brainstem encephalitis/rhombencephalitis
Vascular	Cavernous malformation
	Hematoma
	Arteriovenous malformation
	Cavernous angioma
	Ischemic infarct

[11, 21–24] demonstrate disparity between the MRI-based diagnoses and histopathological diagnoses [11, 21–24]. Tissue confirmation to correctly diagnose and adequately treat brainstem lesions is often necessary. Our patient was eager to have a definitive diagnosis to plan for treatment and prognosis.

3.2. Anatomical Considerations in relation to Surgical Treatment. The medulla oblongata extends from the inferior pontine sulcus to the roots of C1. Anteriorly, the medulla has three longitudinal fissures. The pyramids are elevated structures on either side of the anterior median fissure and comprise the descending corticospinal tracts. The paramedian sulci, also known as the anterolateral sulci or preolivary sulci, are situated medial to the olives. The rootlets of the hypoglossal nerves exit from the preolivary sulci while the rootlets of the accessory, vagus, and glossopharyngeal nerves exit from the postolivary sulci [25].

Internal structures at this level consist of the dorsal vagus, hypoglossal, ambiguus, and inferior olivary nuclei and the nuclei of the solitary tracts. The autonomic centers participating in swallowing, respiratory, and cardiovascular functions are located in and around the reticular formation in the upper half of the dorsal medulla. The medial lemniscus originates near the caudal edge of the fourth ventricle floor and runs upward on either side of the midline, eventually coursing posterior to the pyramidal tract as it enters the pons. The pyramidal tract is found in the most anterior part of the medulla while the medial longitudinal fasciculus (MLF) runs under the posterior (ventricular) surface just lateral to the median sulcus.

Suggested safe neurosurgical entry points for open procedures into the ventrolateral medulla include the preolivary (anterolateral) sulcus located between the caudal roots of the hypoglossal and the rostral C1 rootlets [26]. Some neurosurgeons recommend this only for exophytic lesions due to its close proximity to the pyramidal tract and its decussation [27]. The postolivary sulcus, between the olive and inferior cerebellar peduncle, is ventral to the vagal and glossopharyngeal rootlets and represents another entry point.

TABLE 2: Summary of adult high-grade glioma case reports in the literature.

Reference	Year	Age	Lesion characteristics	Surgical treatment	Pathology	Multimodality therapy	Outcome
Our case	2014	69	Ventrolateral medulla	Biopsy via far lateral approach	GBM	Temozolomide and radiation	Died 11 months after diagnosis
Hundsberger et al. [2]	2014	48	Pons/medulla	Biopsy	US	US	US
		55	Medulla	Biopsy	US	US	US
Babu et al. [4]	2013	>60	Pons, MCP, medulla	US	US	US	US
Yoshikawa et al. [5]	2013	63	Ventral, diffuse medulla	None (diagnosis made at autopsy)	GBM	Temozolomide and radiation (tolerated for only 4 days)	Died 18 days after treatment
Chotai et al. [6]	2012	51	Dorsal, exophytic medulla	NTR via suboccipital approach	GBM	Temozolomide and radiation	19 months postsurgical survival
Lakhan and Harle [7]	2009	48	Diffuse, pons, medulla, cervical spine	None (diagnosis made at autopsy)	GBM	None	Died 4 weeks after presentation
Luetjens et al. [8]	2009	40	Dorsal, exophytic medulla	NTR via suboccipital approach	GBM	Temozolomide and radiation	Two years postsurgical survival
Shad et al. [9]	2005	28	Pons, medulla	Sx biopsy	AA	US	US
Kyoshima et al. [10]	2004	55	Dorsal, exophytic, medulla	GTR via suboccipital approach	GBM	Radiation for recurrence 1 year and 8 months postoperatively	Died 2 years and 3 months after surgery
Massager et al. [11]	2000	34	Medulla	US	AA	US	US
		37	Medulla	US	AA	US	US
Sahni et al. [12]	1987	24	Medulla	Sx biopsy	AA	Radiation	US
		27	Cervicomedullary junction	Sx biopsy	AA	Radiation	Died 1.5 years after surgery
		30	Medulla, 4th ventricle	Sx biopsy	AA	Radiation	US

US: unspecified.
AA: anaplastic astrocytoma.
Sx: Stereotactic.
GTR: gross total resection.
NTR: Near total resection.
MCP: middle cerebellar peduncle.

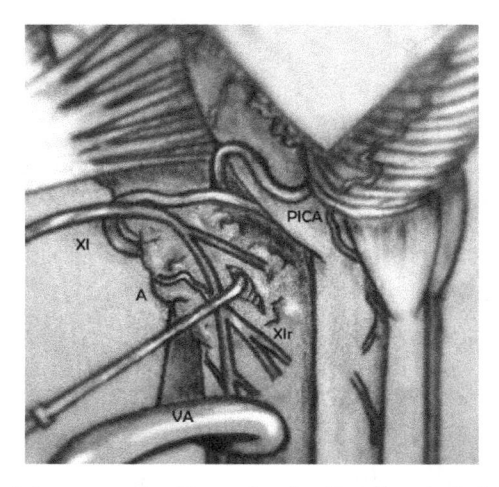

FIGURE 5: Intraoperative illustration detailing the surgical corridor from a far lateral approach. XI: cranial nerve 11; A: abnormality; VA: vertebral artery; XIr: cranial nerve 11 rootlet; PICA: posterior inferior cerebellar artery.

The nucleus ambiguus is generally encountered 0.4 cm below the postolivary sulcus [26, 28].

We opted to create a corridor between several rootlets of the accessory nerve and a bulbous region in the ventrolateral medulla near the postolivary sulcus (Figure 5). The patient's difficulty postoperatively with swallowing and her left vocal cord paralysis were likely related to infiltration of the lesion into the nucleus ambiguus. Preoperative vocal cord paralysis was not fully assessed but was likely present to some degree.

3.3. Surgical Considerations: Type of Surgery. Biopsy is recommended and allows the advantage of histopathologic diagnosis and molecular genetic analysis. Generally, stereotactic biopsies can be performed safely with high diagnostic success rates. Kickingereder et al. [29] completed a large meta-analysis of 1480 stereotactic biopsy procedures for brainstem tumors (including only 4 pure medullary tumors and 9 tumors involving both the pons and medulla). They found a diagnostic success of 96%, 7.8% overall morbidity, 1.7% permanent morbidity, and 0.9% mortality. Furthermore, subgroup analysis of biopsy trajectory, imaging modality used for biopsy planning, and tumor location failed to reveal a significant influence on outcome measures.

A number of other approaches, including ipsilateral transfrontal, contralateral transfrontal, and transcerebellar, are available for the stereotactic biopsy of medullary brainstem lesions. Each approach has advantages and disadvantages and the trajectory must be tailored to the lesion. The contralateral or ipsilateral transfrontal approaches have been shown to be effective in the biopsy of medullary lesions [12, 23, 30–32]. The tentorium may limit the accessibility of midline medullary abnormalities and the biopsy trajectory will have to be planned accordingly. The ventricular system should be avoided, not only to minimize the risk of hemorrhage, but also to prevent CSF loss and target shift. A contralateral transfrontal approach may be necessary to avoid the ventricular system when accessing laterally positioned lesions [30]. Procedures performed with only local anesthesia have been described [9, 33]. The suboccipital transcerebellar approach [32, 34] provides the shortest trajectory for accessing lesions of the lower midbrain, pons, and rostral medulla. Positioning often requires general anesthesia; however awake procedures have been described [34, 35].

Recent advances in neuroimaging, navigation technology, microsurgery, and anatomic knowledge have changed how we classify brainstem gliomas [36–39] and have helped identify surgically resectable lesions. Many studies advocate surgical resection of well-demarcated posteriorly, posterolaterally, and ventrolaterally located tumors in patients with relatively mild neurological symptoms [10, 36, 40–43].

Dey et al. [44] examined 240 patients from the Surveillance, Epidemiology and End Results (SEER) database with WHO grade III and grade IV brainstem astrocytomas. Median survival for patients who did not receive surgery was 6 months, while the median survival for patients who did undergo surgery was 9 months ($p = 0.055$).

In our patient, we considered a stereotactic biopsy but the distinct delineation and ventrolateral location of the mass guided our decision to proceed with open biopsy, anticipating the potential for decompression and thus postoperative functional improvement, which would not be possible with a stereotactic biopsy. During the case, we decided that aggressive resection was not in the patient's best interest for multiple reasons. The firm rubbery texture of the lesion contributed to a temporary loss of MEPs intraoperatively during the debulking of the lesion. Additionally, the frozen section diagnosis of high-grade glioma reduced the enthusiasm for a potentially harmful large resection. Given the infiltrative nature typical of such gliomas, aggressive resection would not be curative and carried a high risk of causing additional morbidity.

3.4. Multimodality Therapy and Prognosis. As a group, adult malignant brainstem gliomas have an overall poor prognosis with a mean overall survival ranging from 11 to 17 months [3, 13], not very different from that of cerebral examples. In general, the administration of radiotherapy and concurrent temozolomide therapy has been shown to improve survival in patients with glioblastoma and is the current standard of care [45], but this has not been rigorously examined in the small population of adults with medullary glioblastomas.

Radiochemotherapy recommendations for patients with high-grade brainstem gliomas are less clear and study cohorts are typically small. Hundsberger et al. [2] described 13 patients with high-grade brainstem gliomas (grades III and IV). Seven patients were treated with radiation and concomitant temozolomide, three patients with radiation only, and 2 patients with chemotherapy only. The median radiation dose was 5760 cGy, with doses varying widely between 4500 and 6000 cGy. Median overall survival was 11.5 months.

Primary malignant brain tumors in the elderly (age > 65 years) carry a dismal prognosis compared to younger patients [46, 47]. The optimal strategy for adjuvant therapy in the elderly population is complicated by an increase in comorbidities. Babu et al. [4] reported on seven elderly patients (age > 60 years) with brainstem gliomas (grades III and IV, 2 had pontine lesions with medullary extention). Six patients survived to receive radiation therapy (dose range 5580–6120 cGy) with concurrent temozolomide (150–400 mg/m^2 administered on days 1–5); all eventually recurred, received a variety of salvage therapies, and died. Median overall survival was 13.5 months (range 1.9–45.7 months).

Some patients may obtain clinical improvement after adjuvant therapy. In a study of 38 patients with brainstem glioma who underwent radiation treatment (mean total dose 5400 cGy), 50% experienced clinical improvement at 6 weeks [48]. Guillamo et al. [13] described only a 13% rate of clinical improvement after radiotherapy in 15 patients with grades III and IV brainstem lesions. A conservative radiotherapy dose of 5600 cGy was chosen for our patient. Approximately one month after radiation she experienced some improvement in RLE strength.

Modern evaluation and classification of gliomas are increasingly driven by molecular genetic analyses. Patients whose gliomas, even high-grade gliomas, have methylation of the promoter region of the gene for MGMT (which thereby suppresses expression of this DNA repair enzyme) have better response to radiation and alkylator chemotherapy and have longer survival. The presence in the tumor of a mutation of the IDH1 or, less commonly, IDH2 genes similarly is associated with better response to therapy and longer survival. On the other hand brainstem gliomas and other midline gliomas, mostly found in children, frequently are found to harbor mutations in the H3F3A gene (almost all the K27M mutation), and this is associated with a particularly poor prognosis and short survival. In this case the small amount of viable tumor tissue obtained for pathological analysis limited the testing done [49].

4. Conclusion

Glioblastoma of the medulla is rare. Biopsy can be performed relatively safely to provide definitive diagnosis to guide treatment, but long-term prognosis is poor.

Abbreviations

BAEPs: Brainstem auditory evoked potentials
EMG: Electromyography
CNS: Central nervous system
CSF: Cerebrospinal fluid
MRI: Magnetic resonance imaging
MLF: Medial longitudinal fasciculus
MEPs: Motor evoked potentials
SEER database: Surveillance, Epidemiology and End Results database
SSEPs: Somatosensory evoked potentials
WHO: World Health Organization.

Additional Points

(i) The differential diagnosis for lesions of the ventrolateral medulla is extensive. (ii) Biopsy can be performed safely to provide a diagnosis and guide treatment. (iii) Despite adjuvant therapy, long-term prognosis remains poor.

Competing Interests

The authors declare that they have no competing interests.

References

[1] T. A. Dolecek, J. M. Propp, N. E. Stroup, and C. Kruchko, "CBTRUS statistical report: primary brain and central nervous system tumors diagnosed in the United States in 2005-2009," *Neuro-Oncology*, vol. 14, no. 5, pp. v1–v49, 2012.

[2] T. Hundsberger, M. Tonder, A. Hottinger et al., "Clinical management and outcome of histologically verified adult brainstem gliomas in Switzerland: a retrospective analysis of 21 patients," *Journal of Neuro-Oncology*, vol. 118, no. 2, pp. 321–328, 2014.

[3] S. Kesari, R. S. Kim, V. Markos, J. Drappatz, P. Y. Wen, and A. A. Pruitt, "Prognostic factors in adult brainstem gliomas: a multicenter, retrospective analysis of 101 cases," *Journal of Neuro-Oncology*, vol. 88, no. 2, pp. 175–183, 2008.

[4] R. Babu, P. G. Kranz, I. O. Karikari, A. H. Friedman, and C. Adamson, "Clinical characteristics and treatment of malignant brainstem gliomas in elderly patients," *Journal of Clinical Neuroscience*, vol. 20, no. 10, pp. 1382–1386, 2013.

[5] A. Yoshikawa, M. Nakada, T. Watanabe et al., "Progressive adult primary glioblastoma in the medulla oblongata with an unmethylated MGMT promoter and without an IDH mutation," *Brain Tumor Pathology*, vol. 30, no. 3, pp. 175–179, 2013.

[6] S. Chotai, H. Moon, J. Kim, and T. Kwon, "Primary glioblastoma of medulla oblongata: case report and review of the literature," *Asian Journal of Neurosurgery*, vol. 7, no. 1, pp. 36–37, 2012.

[7] S. E. Lakhan and L. Harle, "Difficult diagnosis of brainstem glioblastoma multiforme in a woman: a case report and review of the literature," *Journal of Medical Case Reports*, vol. 3, article 87, 2009.

[8] G. Luetjens, M. J. Mirzayan, A. Brandis, and J. K. Krauss, "Exophytic giant cell glioblastoma of the medulla oblongata: case report," *Journal of Neurosurgery*, vol. 110, no. 3, pp. 589–593, 2009.

[9] A. Shad, A. Green, S. Bojanic, and T. Aziz, "Awake stereotactic biopsy of brain stem lesions: technique and results," *Acta Neurochirurgica*, vol. 147, no. 1, pp. 47–50, 2005.

[10] K. Kyoshima, K. Sakai, T. Goto et al., "Gross total surgical removal of malignant glioma from the medulla oblongata: report of two adult cases with reference to surgical anatomy," *Journal of Clinical Neuroscience*, vol. 11, no. 1, pp. 75–80, 2004.

[11] N. Massager, P. David, S. Goldman et al., "Combined magnetic resonance imaging- and positron emission tomography-guided stereotactic biopsy in brainstem mass lesions: diagnostic yield in a series of 30 patients," *Journal of Neurosurgery*, vol. 93, no. 6, pp. 951–957, 2000.

[12] K. S. Sahni, N. R. Ghatak, A. N. Gulati, R. T. Leshner, A. Alberico, and H. F. Young, "CT-guided stereotactic biopsies of lesions in the medulla and a case of Leigh's disease," *Applied Neurophysiology*, vol. 50, no. 1–6, pp. 203–209, 1987.

[13] J.-S. Guillamo, A. Monjour, L. Taillandier et al., "Brainstem gliomas in adults: prognostic factors and classification," *Brain*, vol. 124, no. 12, pp. 2528–2539, 2001.

[14] T. Reithmeier, A. Kuzeawu, B. Hentschel, M. Loeffler, M. Trippel, and G. Nikkhah, "Retrospective analysis of 104 histologically proven adult brainstem gliomas: clinical symptoms, therapeutic approaches and prognostic factors," *BMC Cancer*, vol. 14, article 115, 2014.

[15] C. R. Freeman and J.-P. Farmer, "Pediatric brain stem gliomas: a review," *International Journal of Radiation Oncology Biology Physics*, vol. 40, no. 2, pp. 265–271, 1998.

[16] B. M. Swinson, W. A. Friedman, and A. T. Yachnis, "Pontine atypical neurocytoma: case report," *Neurosurgery*, vol. 58, no. 5, article E990, 2006.

[17] S. N. Shenoy and A. Raja, "Cystic trochlear nerve neurinoma mimicking intrinsic brainstem tumour," *British Journal of Neurosurgery*, vol. 18, no. 2, pp. 183–186, 2004.

[18] J. A. Russell and M. D. M. Shaw, "Chronic abscess of the brain stem," *Journal of Neurology, Neurosurgery and Psychiatry*, vol. 40, no. 7, pp. 625–629, 1977.

[19] O. H. Del Brutto and A. Mosquera, "Brainstem tuberculoma mimicking glioma: the role of antituberculous drugs as a diagnostic tool," *Neurology*, vol. 52, no. 1, pp. 210–211, 1999.

[20] S. J. Pittock, J. Debruyne, K. N. Krecke et al., "Chronic lymphocytic inflammation with pontine perivascular enhancement responsive to steroids (CLIPPERS)," *Brain*, vol. 133, no. 9, pp. 2626–2634, 2010.

[21] M. Schumacher, J. Schulte-Mönting, P. Stoeter, M. Warmuth-Metz, and L. Solymosi, "Magnetic resonance imaging compared with biopsy in the diagnosis of brainstem diseases of childhood: a multicenter review," *Journal of Neurosurgery*, vol. 106, no. 2, pp. 111–119, 2007.

[22] W. Rachinger, S. Grau, M. Holtmannspötter, J. Herms, J.-C. Tonn, and F. W. Kreth, "Serial stereotactic biopsy of brainstem lesions in adults improves diagnostic accuracy compared with MRI only," *Journal of Neurology, Neurosurgery and Psychiatry*, vol. 80, no. 10, pp. 1134–1139, 2009.

[23] V. Rajshekhar and M. J. Chandy, "Computerized tomography-guided stereotactic surgery for brainstem masses: a risk-benefit analysis in 71 patients," *Journal of Neurosurgery*, vol. 82, no. 6, pp. 976–981, 1995.

[24] M. Dellaretti, N. Reyns, G. Touzet et al., "Stereotactic biopsy for brainstem tumors: comparison of transcerebellar with transfrontal approach," *Stereotactic and Functional Neurosurgery*, vol. 90, no. 2, pp. 79–83, 2012.

[25] E. H. Oldfield, P. Magistretti, and P. D. Leroux, *Youmans Neurological Surgery*, Saunders, Elsevier, Philadelphia, Pa, USA, 2011.

[26] K. Yagmurlu, A. L. Rhoton Jr., N. Tanriover, and J. Bennett, "Three-dimensional microsurgical anatomy and the safe entry zones of the brainstem," *Neurosurgery*, vol. 10, pp. 602–620, 2014.

[27] G. Cantore, P. Missori, and A. Santoro, "Cavernous angiomas of the brain stem: intra-axial anatomical pitfalls and surgical strategies," *Surgical Neurology*, vol. 52, no. 1, pp. 84–94, 1999.

[28] R. J. Recalde, E. G. Figueiredo, and E. De Oliveira, "Microsurgical anatomy of the safe entry zones on the anterolateral brainstem related to surgical approaches to cavernous malformations," *Neurosurgery*, vol. 62, no. 3, pp. 9–17, 2008.

[29] P. Kickingereder, P. Willeit, T. Simon, and M. I. Ruge, "Diagnostic value and safety of stereotactic biopsy for brainstem tumors: a systematic review and meta-analysis of 1480 cases," *Neurosurgery*, vol. 72, no. 6, pp. 873–881, 2013.

[30] E. W. Amundson, M. J. McGirt, and A. Olivi, "A contralateral, transfrontal, extraventricular approach to stereotactic brainstem biopsy procedures," *Journal of Neurosurgery*, vol. 102, no. 3, pp. 565–570, 2005.

[31] S. Blond, J. P. Lejeune, T. Dupard, M. Parent, J. Clarisse, and J. L. Christiaens, "The stereotactic approach to brain stem lesions: a follow-up of 29 cases," in *Advances in Stereotactic and Functional Neurosurgery 9*, vol. 52 of *Acta Neurochirurgica Supplementum*, pp. 75–77, Springer, Berlin, Germany, 1991.

[32] S.-Y. Chen, C.-H. Chen, M.-H. Sun, H.-T. Lee, and C.-C. Shen, "Stereotactic biopsy for brainstem lesion: comparison of approaches and reports of 10 cases," *Journal of the Chinese Medical Association*, vol. 74, no. 3, pp. 110–114, 2011.

[33] E. A. C. Pereira, T. Jegan, A. L. Green, and T. Z. Aziz, "Awake stereotactic brainstem biopsy via a contralateral, transfrontal, transventricular approach," *British Journal of Neurosurgery*, vol. 22, no. 4, pp. 599–601, 2008.

[34] N. Sanai, S. P. Wachhorst, N. M. Gupta, and M. W. McDermott, "Transcerebellar stereotactic biopsy for lesions of the brainstem and peduncles under local anesthesia," *Neurosurgery*, vol. 63, no. 3, pp. 460–466, 2008.

[35] R. Spiegelmann and W. A. Friedman, "Stereotactic suboccipital transcerebellar biopsy under local anesthesia using the Cosman-Roberts-Wells frame. Technical note," *Journal of Neurosurgery*, vol. 75, no. 3, pp. 486–488, 1991.

[36] V. Mehta, P. Chandra, P. Singh, A. Garg, and G. Rath, "Surgical considerations for 'intrinsic' brainstem gliomas: proposal of a modification in classification," *Neurology India*, vol. 57, no. 3, pp. 274–281, 2009.

[37] N. J. Fischbein, M. D. Prados, W. Wara, C. Russo, M. S. B. Edwards, and A. J. Barkovich, "Radiologic classification of brain stem tumors: correlation of magnetic resonance imaging appearance with clinical outcome," *Pediatric Neurosurgery*, vol. 24, no. 1, pp. 9–23, 1996.

[38] F. Epstein, "A staging system for brain stem gliomas," *Cancer*, vol. 56, no. 7, pp. 1804–1806, 1985.

[39] A. J. Barkovich, J. Krischer, L. E. Kun et al., "Brain stem gliomas: a classification system based on magnetic resonance imaging," *Pediatric Neurosurgery*, vol. 16, no. 2, pp. 73–83, 1990.

[40] S. Sinha, S. S. Kale, S. P. Chandra, A. Suri, V. S. Mehta, and B. S. Sharma, "Brainstem gliomas: surgical indications and technical considerations in a series of 58 cases," *British Journal of Neurosurgery*, vol. 28, no. 2, pp. 220–225, 2014.

[41] F. Epstein and J. Wisoff, "Intra-axial tumors of the cervicomedullary junction," *Journal of Neurosurgery*, vol. 67, no. 4, pp. 483–487, 1987.

[42] A. Sandri, N. Sardi, L. Genitori et al., "Diffuse and focal brain stem tumors in childhood: prognostic factors and surgical outcome: experience in a single institution," *Child's Nervous System*, vol. 22, no. 9, pp. 1127–1135, 2006.

[43] T. Sun, W. Wan, Z. Wu, J. Zhang, and L. Zhang, "Clinical outcomes and natural history of pediatric brainstem tumors: with 33 cases follow-ups," *Neurosurgical Review*, vol. 36, no. 2, pp. 311–319, 2013.

[44] M. Dey, Y. Lin, S. Melkonian, and S. Lam, "Prognostic factors and survival in primary adult high grade brainstem astrocytoma: a population based study from 1973–2008," *Journal of Clinical Neuroscience*, vol. 21, no. 8, pp. 1298–1303, 2014.

[45] R. Stupp, W. P. Mason, M. J. Van Den Bent et al., "Radiotherapy plus concomitant and adjuvant temozolomide for glioblastoma," *New England Journal of Medicine*, vol. 352, no. 10, pp. 987–996, 2005.

[46] N. H. Greig, L. G. Ries, R. Yancik, and S. I. Rapoport, "Increasing annual incidence of primary malignant brain tumors in the elderly," *Journal of the National Cancer Institute*, vol. 82, no. 20, pp. 1621–1624, 1990.

[47] A. Fleury, F. Menegoz, P. Grosclaude et al., "Descriptive epidemiology of cerebral gliomas in France," *Cancer*, vol. 79, no. 6, pp. 1195–1202, 1997.

[48] D. Schulz-Ertner, J. Debus, F. Lohr, C. Frank, A. Höss, and M. Wannenmacher, "Fractionated stereotactic conformal radiation therapy of brain stem gliomas: outcome and prognostic factors," *Radiotherapy and Oncology*, vol. 57, no. 2, pp. 215–223, 2000.

[49] L. Zhang, L. H. Chen, H. Wan et al., "Exome sequencing identifies somatic gain-of-function PPM1D mutations in brainstem gliomas," *Nature Genetics*, vol. 46, no. 7, pp. 726–730, 2014.

Progressive Multifocal Leukoencephalopathy in a Multiple Sclerosis Patient Diagnosed after Switching from Natalizumab to Fingolimod

Tim Sinnecker,[1,2,3] Jalal Othman,[1] Marc Kühl,[1] Imke Metz,[4] Thoralf Niendorf,[5,6] Annett Kunkel,[1] Friedemann Paul,[2,6,7,8] Jens Wuerfel,[2,9] and Juergen Faiss[1]

[1]*Department of Neurology, Asklepios Fachklinikum Teupitz, Teupitz, Germany*
[2]*NeuroCure Clinical Research Center, Charité-Universitätsmedizin Berlin, Berlin, Germany*
[3]*Department of Neurology, Universitätsspital Basel, Basel, Switzerland*
[4]*Department of Neuropathology, Universitätsmedizin Göttingen, Göttingen, Germany*
[5]*Berlin Ultrahigh Field Facility, Max Delbrück Center for Molecular Medicine, Berlin, Germany*
[6]*Experimental and Clinical Research Center, Charité-Universitätsmedizin Berlin and Max Delbrück Center for Molecular Medicine, Berlin, Germany*
[7]*Clinical and Experimental Multiple Sclerosis Research Center, Charité-Universitätsmedizin Berlin, Berlin, Germany*
[8]*Department of Neurology, Charité-Universitätsmedizin Berlin, Berlin, Germany*
[9]*Medical Imaging Analysis Center AG, Basel, Switzerland*

Correspondence should be addressed to Friedemann Paul; friedemann.paul@charite.de

Academic Editor: Dominic B. Fee

Background. Natalizumab- (NTZ-) associated progressive multifocal leukoencephalopathy (PML) is a severe and often disabling infectious central nervous system disease that can become evident in multiple sclerosis (MS) patients after NTZ discontinuation. Recently, novel diagnostic biomarkers for the assessment of PML risk in NTZ treated MS patients such as the anti-JC virus antibody index have been reported, and the clinical relevance of milky-way lesions detectable by MRI has been discussed. *Case Presentation and Conclusion.* We report a MS patient in whom PML was highly suspected solely based on MRI findings after switching from NTZ to fingolimod despite repeatedly negative (ultrasensitive) polymerase chain reaction (PCR) testing for JC virus DNA in cerebrospinal fluid. The PML diagnosis was histopathologically confirmed by brain biopsy. The occurrence of an immune reconstitution inflammatory syndrome (IRIS) during fingolimod therapy, elevated measures of JCV antibody indices, and the relevance of milky-way-like lesions detectable by (7 T) MRI are discussed.

1. Introduction

Progressive multifocal leukoencephalopathy (PML) is an opportunistic infection of the central nervous system (CNS) caused by JC polyomavirus (JCV) targeting oligodendrocytes and astrocytes and leading to oligodendrocyte death [1]. Symptoms are greatly variable, depending on the localisation of the infection in the brain [2]. Clinically, patients present with behavioural abnormalities, cognitive impairment, focal neurological deficits, and/or epileptic seizures. The course of the disease is often fatal or rendering the patient severely disabled [2].

PML is observed in patients with a marked immunosuppression, for instance, due to an infection with HIV or as a result of an immunosuppressive therapy after organ transplantation. It may also occur in multiple sclerosis (MS) patients treated with natalizumab (NTZ). NTZ is a monoclonal antibody directed against α4-integrin that hinders the transmigration of white blood cells through the blood vessel wall into the CNS. Risk factors of NTZ-associated PML are duration of therapy with NTZ (with a marked increase in risk after two years), use of immunosuppressants before initiation of NTZ therapy, and a positive anti-JC virus antibody status [3–7].

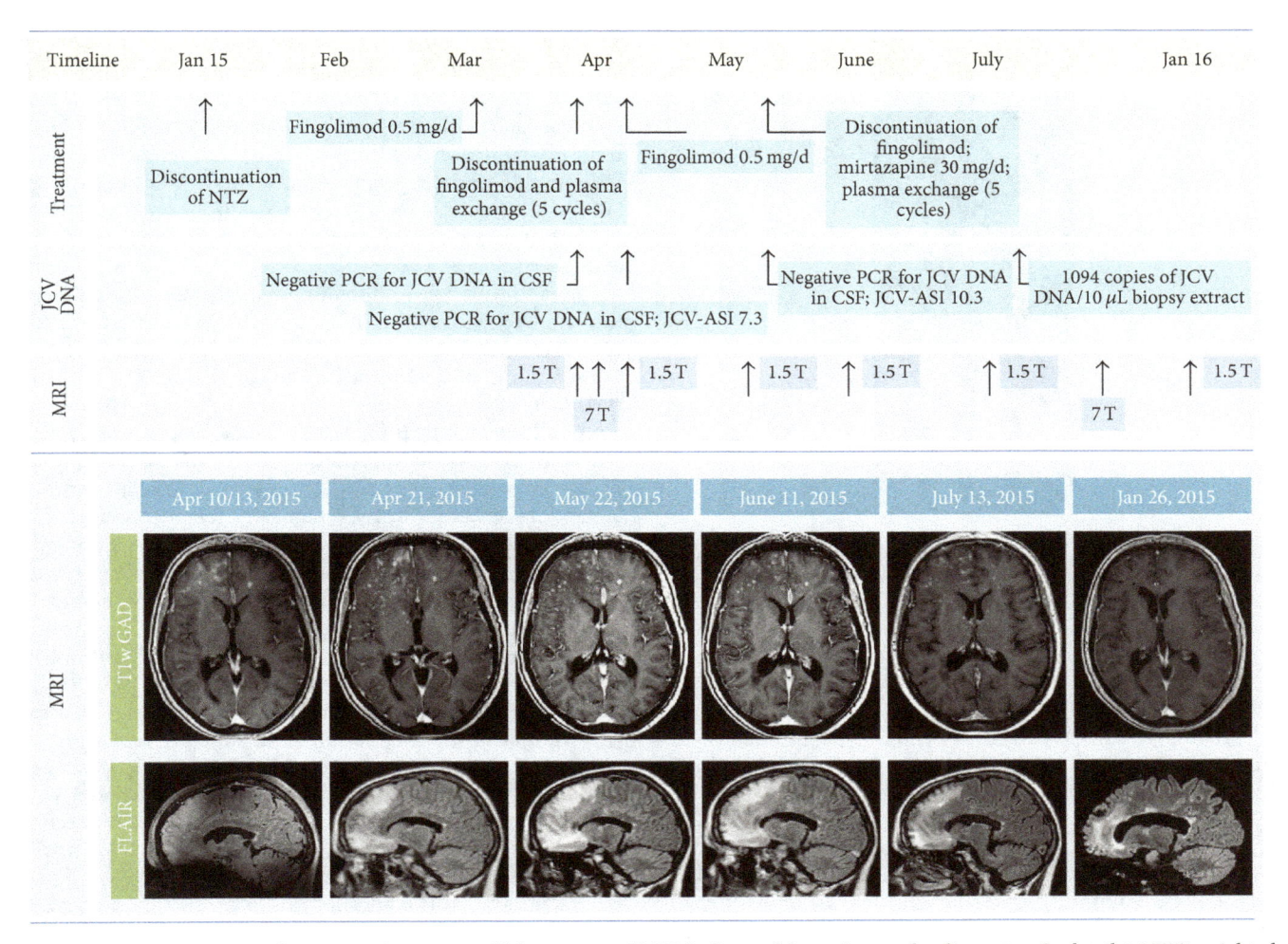

FIGURE 1: Overview. Survey of treatment decisions and laboratory and MRI findings of the patient under discussion. In detail, 1.5 T T1 weighted Gadolinium enhanced (T1W GAD) and 1.5 T fluid attenuated inversion recovery (FLAIR) images are presented.

After clinical suspicion of PML, diagnosis is established by magnetic resonance imaging (MRI) findings and PCR detection of JCV DNA in the cerebrospinal fluid (CSF) [8]. In rare cases, a brain biopsy has to be performed to diagnose PML [8].

Apart from reestablishing a competent immune response, there is no PML-specific therapy with proven efficacy [9]. In MS patients with NTZ-associated PML, plasma exchange (PLEX) or immunoadsorption (IA) is performed to accelerate NTZ clearance [10]. However, immune reconstitution inflammatory syndrome (IRIS), a condition characterized by an overwhelming inflammatory response during immune reconstitution, can develop or deteriorate during PLEX leading to clinical worsening [11].

In vitro studies postulate an infection via the serotonin receptor 5HT2a [12]. Hence, serotonin reuptake inhibitors like mirtazapine are frequently prescribed. However, along with other experimental therapeutic strategies including mefloquine or amantadine, clinical confirmation is still missing [13].

Here, we report an MS case in which PML-IRIS was diagnosed after switching from NTZ to fingolimod. Brain biopsy and advanced neuroimaging findings including ultra-high field MRI at 7 Tesla (T) are presented.

2. Case Presentation

A 48-year-old woman with relapsing-remitting MS (RRMS) was switched after 6 months of treatment with interferon-1b to NTZ in May 2008 due to ongoing clinical and paraclinical disease activity including multiple Gadolinium enhancing brain lesions detected with MRI.

At that point, the Expanded Disability Status Scale Score (EDSS) was 5.5.

We did not observe any evidence of clinical or MRI disease activity during NTZ treatment, and the EDSS subsequently decreased to 2.5.

Figure 1 chronologically summarizes all paraclinical findings including MRI results and treatment decisions.

In January 2015, NTZ was discontinued after a total of 86 infusions on the background of seroconversion to positive JCV serum antibodies (STRATIFY, Unilabs, Geneva, Switzerland), indicating an increased PML risk. Anti-JCV antibody index was not available at that time.

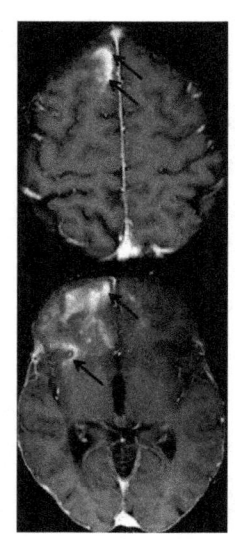

FIGURE 2: Signs of IRIS at the time of PML diagnosis. 1.5 T T1w Gadolinium enhanced MR images are presented. Extensive Gadolinium enhancement suggestive of IRIS (black arrows) was observed at the edge of confluent PML lesions.

After a wash-out period of 2 months, fingolimod was started on the 18th of March 2015. Previous brain MRI (February 2015) did not show any signs of PML.

Three weeks later (10th April 2015), routine brain MRI at 1.5 T revealed PML-suspicious bifrontal confluent lesions with (sub)cortical involvement. Moreover, multiple milky-way-like Gadolinium enhancing and T2 weighted (T2w) hyperintense punctate lesions were detected by MRI in these areas (Figure 1). In addition, perilesional contrast enhancement around confluent PML-suspicious lesions suggestive of IRIS was detectable (Figure 2). Diffusion weighted MRI did not show intralesional hyperdiffusivity nor signs of restricted diffusion at the edge of the lesions (Figure 3); both of which are considered to be typical of PML [14].

We did not observe any signs of clinical worsening, the polymerase chain reaction (PCR) testing for JCV DNA in CSF (*Institute for Virology, Heinrich Heine University, Düsseldorf, Germany*) was negative, and the lymphocyte count was only slightly decreased (0.91 G/L, reference range 1–4 G/L).

Fingolimod was immediately discontinued, and the patient underwent five cycles of plasma exchange. Ultrahigh field MRI at 7 Tesla was performed five days after discontinuation of fingolimod confirming initial 1.5 T MRI findings by detailing confluent PML-suspicious lesions with (sub)cortical involvement (Figure 4) and by delineating numerous punctate Gadolinium enhancing lesions (Figure 5, circles) on top of MS-suspicious ring-enhancing lesions (Figure 5, white arrows).

1.5 T MRI performed immediately after PLEX did not show any signs of PML progression (Figure 1), and PCR did again not reveal JCV DNA in CSF. Thus, fingolimod was reinitiated on 22th of April 2015 to prevent possible rebound effects after discontinuation of NTZ, and monthly MRIs were performed.

One month later (22th of May 2015) a control MRI at 1.5 T showed slightly enlarging FLAIR hyperintense lesions (Figure 1). Clinically, we observed a latent right-sided brachiofacial paresis and a slightly increased irritability reported by her daughter at that time; EDSS 3.0. PCR testing for JCV DNA in CSF was repeatedly negative, but JCV antibody index (JCV-ASI) was markedly increased (10.3). Retrospectively, JCV-ASI was already elevated at the time of the second CSF analysis (JCV-ASI 7.3).

As a consequence, fingolimod was again discontinued, mirtazapine 30 mg/d orally was started, and another cycle of plasma exchange was carried out. Neuropsychological examinations and electroencephalography (EEG) did not reveal any changes.

On 24th of July 2015, a stereotactic biopsy was carried out since an ultrasensitive PCR of JCV DNA (*Laboratory of Molecular Medicine and Neuroscience, National Institute of Health, Bethesda, USA*) repetitively failed to detect JCV DNA in CSF. The biopsy showed demyelinating lesions with a prominent CD8 dominated inflammatory infiltrate with numerous plasma cells (Figure 6). Although neuropathological findings were highly suggestive of IRIS in the context of PML, SV40-positive cells (JCV-infected cells) could not be detected (*Institute of Neuropathology, University of Göttingen, Germany*). JCV multiplex quantitative real-time PCR assay (JC Multiplex qPCR) of paraffin embedded brain tissue was initiated and revealed 1094 viral copies per 10 μL extract, consistent with a variant most commonly associated with PML (*Laboratory of Molecular Medicine and Neuroscience, National Institute of Health, Bethesda, USA*) [14], finally proving the PML diagnosis.

Mirtazapine was continued and glatiramer acetate treatment initiated. The patient remained clinically stable, and MRI (26th of January 2016) showed decreasing PML lesions without any signs of Gadolinium enhancement (Figure 1, EDSS 3.0).

3. Discussion

We report a case of subclinical simultaneous PML-IRIS that was diagnosed after switching from NTZ to fingolimod. Initially, PML was suspected exclusively on the basis of MRI findings despite repeatedly negative (ultrasensitive) PCR testing for JCV DNA in CSF. The diagnosis was further complicated by the absence of PML-characteristic changes in diffusivity as investigated by diffusion weighted MRI. Finally, PML was confirmed via brain biopsy.

Along with other reports in the literature [15, 16], this case thus underlines the need of additional sensitive biomarkers for an earlier diagnosis of PML. In fact, PCR testing for JCV DNA in CSF is limited in sensitivity even when using ultrasensitive PCR assays that can detect up to 10 copies of JCV DNA per milliliter CSF [8, 16]. Notwithstanding these efforts, such highly sensitive assays are not broadly available, and the clinical relevance of very low measures of JCV DNA copies is still under discussion [17].

Recently, the JCV antibody index was introduced as a novel biomarker that potentially can help to better distinguish between NTZ-associated PML and non-PML MS patients [4,

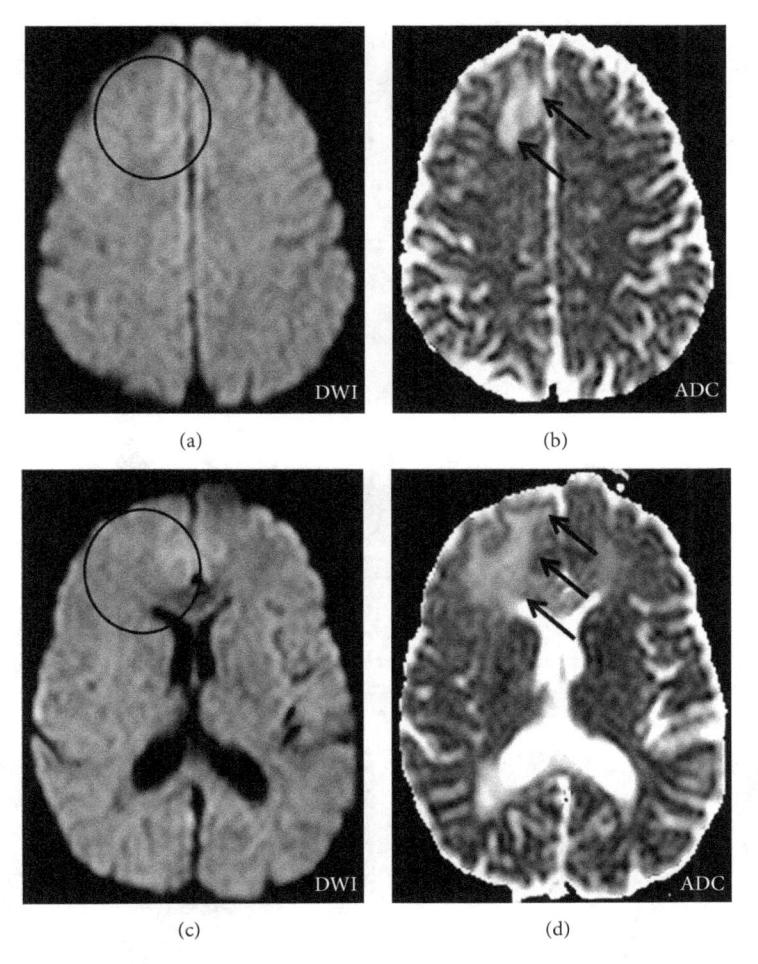

FIGURE 3: No signs of abnormal diffusion. Diffusion weighted MRI at 1.5 T ((a) and (c)) did reveal neither signs of central hyperdiffusibility (circles) nor signs of restricted diffusion (circles) at the edge of PML lesions (black arrows, (b) and (d)). Both of which were reported to be characteristic for PML lesions.

16]. Indeed, the JCV antibody index was markedly increased in our case and continued to rise during PML expansion. Other PML cases of elevated JCV antibody indices despite repeatedly negative PCR testing for JCV DNA in CSF have been reported [15, 16].

Furthermore, the presented case also highlights the importance of a stringent clinical and paraclinical follow-up of MS patients before and after discontinuing NTZ since PML(-IRIS) was previously described after NTZ discontinuation [18] and while switching from NTZ to another immunomodulatory therapy. As reported previously, IRIS may even occur during fingolimod-associated lymphopenia [19, 20]. Indeed, marginally decreased blood lymphocyte counts and signs of IRIS were detectable at the time of first PML-suspicious MRI lesions in our case.

In addition to this extensive laboratory and clinical workup, we performed highly resolving ultrahigh field MRI at 7 T. In general, 7 T MRI benefits from an increased signal-to-noise ratio, a high spatial resolution, and enhanced susceptibility effects. Thus, 7 T MRI has improved the detection and morphological characterization of neuroinflammatory brain lesions [21–23]. Most importantly, a small venous vessel is often detectable within the center of MS lesions by using gradient echo MR techniques at 7 T [24–28], facilitating the distinction to other CNS diseases such as neuromyelitis optica [29, 30] and Susac syndrome [31].

Recently, 7 T MRI revealed contrast-enhancing milky-way-like lesions that expanded into more typical PML lesions over time in a single case of simultaneous PML, IRIS, and an ongoing MS disease activity [32]. In contrast to MS lesions, a small central vessel was not commonly detectable within these lesions [32].

In general, the mechanisms of contrast enhancement in NTZ-associated PML are not fully understood. Contrast enhancement is a correlate of blood-brain-barrier (BBB) breakdown [11, 13, 33–35]. However, JCV-infected lymphocytes may also cross the intact BBB to infect oligodendrocytes [36, 37]. In other words, BBB breakdown is not a prerequisite of PML development. In HIV, indeed, PML is frequently characterized by little or no inflammatory signs and absence of BBB breakdown [38]. Thus, patchy areas of peripheral contrast enhancement at the edge of HIV-PML lesions are commonly considered as a sign of IRIS but not a PML imaging feature [38, 39]. Following this assumption,

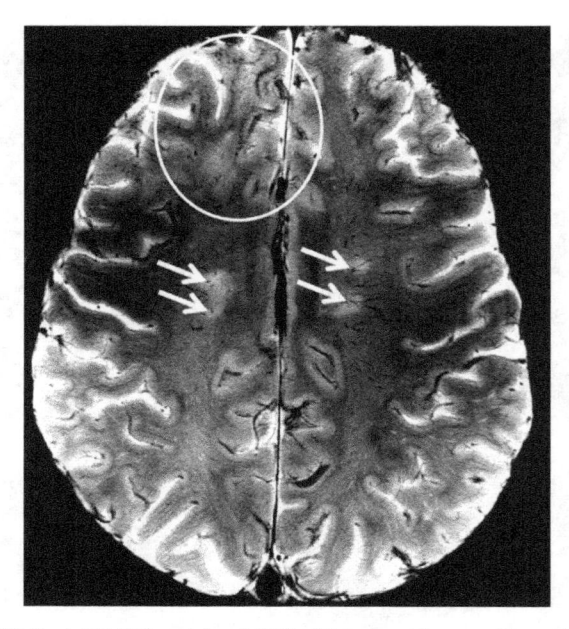

FIGURE 4: 7 T T2* weighted imaging in PML. A 7 T T2* weighted (T2*w) image with a spatial resolution of (0.2 × 0.2) mm is shown. Please note the difference in lesion morphology between periventricular oval MS lesions that are centered on a small venous vessel (arrows) and confluent PML lesions (circle) that also involve U-fibers and subcortical areas.

(a)

(b)

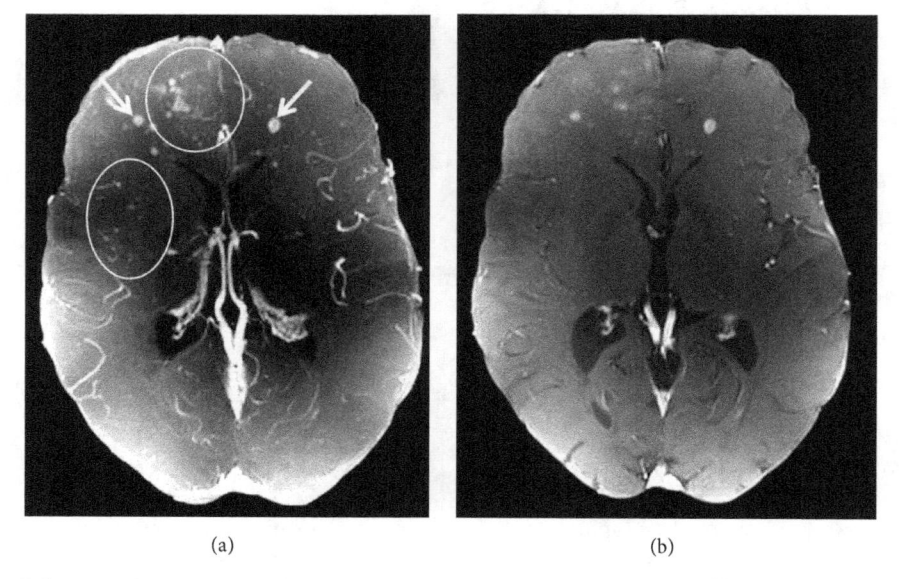

FIGURE 5: Patterns of Gadolinium enhancement on 7 T VIBE images. A maximum intensity projection map of a 7 T T1 weighted Gadolinium enhanced volumetric interpolated brain examination ((a), VIBE) and an exemplary VIBE image (b) are displayed. PML-suspicious punctate Gadolinium enhancing lesions are clearly visible (circles). Ring-enhancing lesions (e.g., arrows) suggestive of MS lesions are delineated.

recent PML studies have interpreted any kind of contrast enhancement in or around PML lesions as a sign of IRIS [11]. However, it is not known whether this also holds true for NTZ-associated PML, where the immune response is present and thus different compared to HIV. In a recent report, no histopathological features of IRIS were present in a bioptical probe of NTZ-associated PML, despite perilesional contrast enhancement on MRI. The authors concluded that, up to date, IRIS remains a histopathological diagnosis [40]. In our case, histopathology revealed prominent CD8 dominated inflammatory infiltrates with numerous plasma cells highly suggestive of IRIS, although clinical worsening, that usually accompanies IRIS, was absent.

In addition to patchy contrast enhancement at the edges of PML lesions, punctate contrast-enhancing lesions have been described [35, 41–43]. The clinical relevance of such small punctate lesion is, however, still a matter of discussion: On the one hand, milky-way-like punctate lesions were

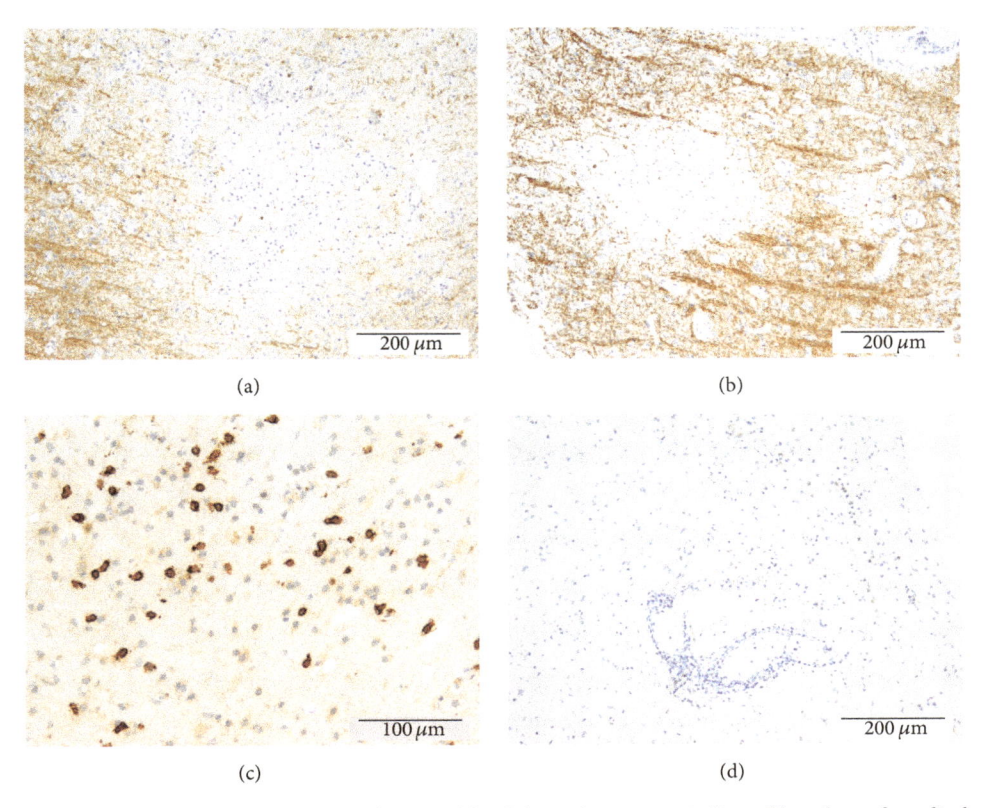

FIGURE 6: Neuropathological findings. Histology revealed areas of focal demyelination as indicated by a loss of myelin basic protein (a) and proteolipid protein (b). Despite the presence of prominent CD8 dominated inflammatory infiltrates (c), SV40-positive cells (JCV-infected cells, (d)) could not be detected.

associated with an overwhelming immunoreaction, namely, IRIS, against JCV [43]. Methylprednisolone pulse therapy would be beneficial in such a situation. On the other hand, it was hypothesized that these lesions represent areas of active JCV replication that is probably adequately recognized by the immune system [41]. In such a scenario, glucocorticoid induced immunosuppression might be harmful. In alignment with this hypothesis, we have previously described clinical worsening and increasing JCV DNA copies in CSF in a NTZ-PML case with punctate lesions during methylprednisolone pulse therapy [32].

Interestingly, there are some differences in the clinical presentation and MRI finding between the "current" PML case presented here and the previous one [32]. In detail, we observed fewer milky-way-like lesions and the expansion of confluent lesions over time was more limited in the "current" case. Of note, the "current" patient only received plasma exchange, and she was not treated with methylprednisolone. Which of all these factors has primarily influenced the overall better clinical outcome of the presented patient remains unknown, but it emphasizes the need of systematic (ultra)high field MRI studies to address these questions.

Disclosure

Tim Sinnecker's current address is as follows: Department of Neurology, Universitätsspital Basel, Basel, Switzerland.

Competing Interests

The authors declare that they have no competing interests.

Authors' Contributions

Tim Sinnecker, Jalal Othman, Marc Kühl, Jens Wuerfel, and Juergen Faiss are equally contributing first and senior authors.

References

[1] S. M. Richardson-Burns, B. K. Kleinschmidt-DeMasters, R. L. DeBiasi, and K. L. Tyler, "Progressive multifocal leukoencephalopathy and apoptosis of infected oligodendrocytes in the central nervous system of patients with and without AIDS," *Archives of Neurology*, vol. 59, no. 12, pp. 1930–1936, 2002.

[2] P. Vermersch, L. Kappos, R. Gold et al., "Clinical outcomes of natalizumab-associated progressive multifocal leukoencephalopathy," *Neurology*, vol. 76, no. 20, pp. 1697–1704, 2011.

[3] G. Bloomgren, S. Richman, C. Hotermans et al., "Risk of natalizumab-associated progressive multifocal leukoencephalopathy," *The New England Journal of Medicine*, vol. 366, no. 20, pp. 1870–1880, 2012.

[4] N. Schwab, T. Schneider-Hohendorf, B. Pignolet et al., "Therapy with natalizumab is associated with high JCV seroconversion and rising JCV index values," *Neurology - Neuroimmunology Neuroinflammation*, vol. 3, no. 1, p. e195, 2016.

[5] M. Meira, C. Sievers, F. Hoffmann et al., "Natalizumab-induced POU2AF1/Spi-B upregulation," *Neurology—Neuroimmunology Neuroinflammation*, vol. 3, article e223, 2016.

[6] E. O. Major and A. Nath, "A link between long-term natalizumab dosing in MS and PML: putting the puzzle together," *Neurology-Neuroimmunology Neuroinflammation*, vol. 3, no. 3, article e235, 2016.

[7] A. Javed and A. T. Reder, "Rising JCV-Ab index during natalizumab therapy for MS: inauspicious for a highly efficacious drug," *Neurology: Neuroimmunology & Neuroinflammation*, vol. 3, no. 1, article e199, 2016.

[8] J. R. Berger, A. J. Aksamit, D. B. Clifford et al., "PML diagnostic criteria: consensus statement from the AAN neuroinfectious disease section," *Neurology*, vol. 80, no. 15, pp. 1430–1438, 2013.

[9] R. A. Du Pasquier, M. J. Kuroda, Y. Zheng, J. Jean-Jacques, N. L. Letvin, and I. J. Koralnik, "A prospective study demonstrates an association between JC virus-specific cytotoxic T lymphocytes and the early control of progressive multifocal leukoencephalopathy," *Brain: A Journal of Neurology*, vol. 127, no. 9, pp. 1970–1978, 2004.

[10] B. O. Khatri, S. Man, G. Giovannoni et al., "Effect of plasma exchange in accelerating natalizumab clearance and restoring leukocyte function," *Neurology*, vol. 72, no. 5, pp. 402–409, 2009.

[11] I. L. Tan, J. C. McArthur, D. B. Clifford, E. O. Major, and A. Nath, "Immune reconstitution inflammatory syndrome in natalizumab-associated PML," *Neurology*, vol. 77, no. 11, pp. 1061–1067, 2011.

[12] G. F. Elphick, W. Querbes, J. A. Jordan et al., "The human polyomavirus, JCV, uses serotonin receptors to infect cells," *Science*, vol. 306, no. 5700, pp. 1380–1383, 2004.

[13] D. B. Clifford, A. DeLuca, D. M. Simpson, G. Arendt, G. Giovannoni, and A. Nath, "Natalizumab-associated progressive multifocal leukoencephalopathy in patients with multiple sclerosis: lessons from 28 cases," *The Lancet Neurology*, vol. 9, no. 4, pp. 438–446, 2010.

[14] J. Hodel, O. Outteryck, C. Dubron et al., "Asymptomatic progressive multifocal leukoencephalopathy associated with natalizumab: diagnostic precision with MR imaging," *Radiology*, vol. 278, no. 3, pp. 863–872, 2016.

[15] J. Kuhle, R. Gosert, R. Bühler et al., "Management and outcome of CSF-JC virus PCR-negative PML in a natalizumabtreated patient with MS," *Neurology*, vol. 77, no. 23, pp. 2010–2016, 2011.

[16] C. Warnke, G. von Geldern, P. Markwerth et al., "Cerebrospinal fluid JC virus antibody index for diagnosis of natalizumab-associated progressive multifocal leukoencephalopathy," *Annals of Neurology*, vol. 76, no. 6, pp. 792–801, 2014.

[17] E. Iacobaeus, C. Ryschkewitsch, M. Gravell et al., "Analysis of cerebrospinal fluid and cerebrospinal fluid cells from patients with multiple sclerosis for detection of JC virus DNA," *Multiple Sclerosis*, vol. 15, no. 1, pp. 28–35, 2009.

[18] S. Gheuens, D. R. Smith, X. Wang, D. C. Alsop, R. E. Lenkinski, and I. J. Koralnik, "Simultaneous PML-IRIS after discontinuation of natalizumab in a patient with MS," *Neurology*, vol. 78, no. 18, pp. 1390–1393, 2012.

[19] J. Killestein, A. Vennegoor, A. E. L. van Golde, R. L. J. H. Bourez, M. L. B. Wijlens, and M. P. Wattjes, "PML-IRIS during fingolimod diagnosed after natalizumab discontinuation," *Case Reports in Neurological Medicine*, vol. 2014, Article ID 307872, 4 pages, 2014.

[20] Z. Calic, C. Cappelen-Smith, S. J. Hodgkinson, A. McDougall, R. Cuganesan, and B. J. Brew, "Treatment of progressive multifocal leukoencephalopathy-immune reconstitution inflammatory syndrome with intravenous immunoglobulin in a patient with multiple sclerosis treated with fingolimod after discontinuation of natalizumab," *Journal of Clinical Neuroscience*, vol. 22, no. 3, pp. 598–600, 2015.

[21] T. Sinnecker, J. Kuchling, P. Dusek et al., "Ultrahigh field MRI in clinical neuroimmunology: a potential contribution to improved diagnostics and personalised disease management," *EPMA Journal*, vol. 6, article 16, 2015.

[22] T. Sinnecker, P. Mittelstaedt, J. Dörr et al., "Multiple sclerosis lesions and irreversible brain tissue damage: a comparative ultrahigh-field strength magnetic resonance imaging study," *Archives of Neurology*, vol. 69, no. 6, pp. 739–745, 2012.

[23] J. Kuchling, C. Ramien, I. Bozin et al., "Identical lesion morphology in primary progressive and relapsing-remitting MS -an ultrahigh field MRI study," *Multiple Sclerosis Journal*, vol. 20, no. 14, pp. 1866–1871, 2014.

[24] I. Bozin, Y. Ge, J. Kuchling et al., "Magnetic resonance phase alterations in multiple sclerosis patients with short and long disease duration," *PLoS ONE*, vol. 10, no. 7, Article ID e0128386, 2015.

[25] K. Müller, J. Kuchling, J. Dörr et al., "Detailing intra-lesional venous lumen shrinking in multiple sclerosis investigated by sflair mri at 7-t," *Journal of Neurology*, vol. 261, no. 1, pp. 2032–2036, 2014.

[26] T. Sinnecker, I. Bozin, J. Dörr et al., "Periventricular venous density in multiple sclerosis is inversely associated with T2 lesion count: a 7 Tesla MRI Study," *Multiple Sclerosis Journal*, vol. 19, no. 3, pp. 316–325, 2013.

[27] M. Blaabjerg, K. Ruprecht, T. Sinnecker et al., "Widespread inflammation in CLIPPERS syndrome indicated by autopsy and ultra-high-field 7T MRI," *Neurology-Neuroimmunology Neuroinflammation*, vol. 3, no. 3, article e226, 2016.

[28] T. Sinnecker, S. Schumacher, K. Mueller et al., "MRI phase changes in multiple sclerosis vs neuromyelitis optica lesions at 7T," *Neurology Neuroimmunology Neuroinflammation*, vol. 3, no. 4, article e259, 2016.

[29] T. Sinnecker, J. Dörr, C. F. Pfueller et al., "Distinct lesion morphology at 7-T MRI differentiates neuromyelitis optica from multiple sclerosis," *Neurology*, vol. 79, no. 7, pp. 708–714, 2012.

[30] I. Kister, J. Herbert, Y. Zhou, and Y. Ge, "Ultrahigh-field MR (7 T) imaging of brain lesions in neuromyelitis optica," *Multiple Sclerosis International*, vol. 2013, Article ID 398259, 7 pages, 2013.

[31] J. Wuerfel, T. Sinnecker, E. B. Ringelstein et al., "Lesion morphology at 7 Tesla MRI differentiates Susac syndrome from multiple sclerosis," *Multiple Sclerosis Journal*, vol. 18, no. 11, pp. 1592–1599, 2012.

[32] T. Sinnecker, J. Othman, M. Kühl et al., "7T MRI in natalizumab-associated PML and ongoing MS disease activity: a case study," *Neurology: Neuroimmunology & Neuroinflammation*, vol. 2, no. 6, article e171, 2015.

[33] M. P. Wattjes, M. T. Wijburg, A. Vennegoor et al., "MRI characteristics of early PML-IRIS after natalizumab treatment in patients with MS," *Journal of Neurology, Neurosurgery & Psychiatry*, vol. 87, no. 8, pp. 879–884, 2016.

[34] M. P. Wattjes, N. D. Richert, J. Killestein et al., "The chameleon of neuroinflammation: magnetic resonance imaging characteristics of natalizumab-associated progressive multifocal

leukoencephalopathy," *Multiple Sclerosis Journal*, vol. 19, no. 14, pp. 1826–1840, 2013.

[35] J. Hodel, C. Darchis, O. Outteryck et al., "Punctate pattern: a promising imaging marker for the diagnosis of natalizumab-associated PML," *Neurology*, vol. 86, no. 16, pp. 1516–1523, 2016.

[36] B. F. Sabath and E. O. Major, "Traffic of JC virus from sites of initial infection to the brain: the path to progressive multifocal leukoencephalopathy," *Journal of Infectious Diseases*, vol. 186, no. 2, pp. S180–S186, 2002.

[37] A. S. Saribaş, A. Özdemir, C. Lam, and M. Safak, "JC virus-induced progressive multifocal leukoencephalopathy," *Future Virology*, vol. 5, no. 3, pp. 313–323, 2010.

[38] A. K. Bag, J. K. Curé, P. R. Chapman, G. H. Roberson, and R. Shah, "JC virus infection of the brain," *American Journal of Neuroradiology*, vol. 31, no. 9, pp. 1564–1576, 2010.

[39] K. Tan, R. Roda, L. Ostrow, J. McArthur, and A. Nath, "PML-IRIS in patients with HIV infection: clinical manifestations and treatment with steroids," *Neurology*, vol. 72, no. 17, pp. 1458–1464, 2009.

[40] I. Metz, E.-W. Radue, A. Oterino et al., "Pathology of immune reconstitution inflammatory syndrome in multiple sclerosis with natalizumab-associated progressive multifocal leukoencephalopathy," *Acta Neuropathologica*, vol. 123, no. 2, pp. 235–245, 2012.

[41] M. P. Wattjes, L. Verhoeff, W. Zentjens et al., "Punctate lesion pattern suggestive of perivascular inflammation in acute natalizumab-associated progressive multifocal leukoencephalopathy: productive JC virus infection or preclinical PML-IRIS manifestation?" *Journal of Neurology, Neurosurgery and Psychiatry*, vol. 84, no. 10, pp. 1176–1177, 2013.

[42] M. P. Wattjes, A. Vennegoor, M. D. Steenwijk et al., "MRI pattern in asymptomatic natalizumab-associated PML," *Journal of Neurology, Neurosurgery & Psychiatry*, vol. 86, no. 7, pp. 793–798, 2015.

[43] T. A. Yousry, D. Pelletier, D. Cadavid et al., "Magnetic resonance imaging pattern in natalizumab-associated progressive multifocal leukoencephalopathy," *Annals of Neurology*, vol. 72, no. 5, pp. 779–787, 2012.

Alzheimer's Dementia due to Suspected CTE from Subconcussive Head Impact

Shauna H. Yuan [iD][1] and Sonya G. Wang[2]

[1]*Department of Neurosciences, University of California, San Diego, La Jolla, CA 92093, USA*
[2]*Department of Neurology, University of Minnesota, Minneapolis, MN 55455, USA*

Correspondence should be addressed to Shauna H. Yuan; shyuan@ucsd.edu

Academic Editor: Samuel T. Gontkovsky

Chronic traumatic encephalopathy (CTE) has been receiving increasing attention due to press coverage of professional football players. The devastating sequelae of CTE compel us to aim for early diagnosis and treatment. However, by current standards, CTE is challenging to diagnose. Clear clinical diagnostic criteria for CTE have not been established. Only recently, pathological diagnostic criteria have been recognized, but postmortem diagnosis is too late. Reliable biomarkers are not available. By imaging criteria, cavum septum pellucidum has been the only consistent identifiable MRI finding. Because of the imprecise nature of diagnosis based on clinical suspicion, physicians must become cognizant of the broad spectrum of presentations of CTE. With this awareness, appropriate workup can be initiated. CTE can present with early symptoms of emotional changes or late symptoms with memory decline and dementia. Here we present an unusual case of a patient with Alzheimer's disease secondary to suspected CTE that stems from subconcussive head impacts presenting with severe memory and MRI changes. Clinicians should be aware of this presentation and consider CTE in their differential diagnoses while undergoing workup of memory disorders.

1. Introduction

Chronic traumatic encephalopathy (CTE) is the long-term consequence of brain injury, due to repetitive brain trauma. It is associated with collision sport athletes, military personnel, domestic violence, and head banging behavior. The incidence for concussion is high, affecting between 1.6 and 3.8 million people per year [1, 2]. The prevalence for CTE is less clear; however, a recent study suggests that up to 87% of the brains from former football players displayed CTE pathology [3].

CTE was first described as "punch drunk" syndrome in retired boxers [4]. Later it was clinically labelled "dementia pugilistica" or "boxer's dementia" [1, 5]. Patients can present with behavioral, motor, and cognitive symptoms. Behavioral manifestations are frequently seen earlier in the disease, including symptoms of depression, emotional lability, apathy, aggression, suicidality, and apathy. Spasticity, tremor, ataxia, dysarthria, and incoordination are associated motor symptoms. Cognitively, patients develop impaired attention and concentration, memory deficits, and dementia. Clinical diagnostic criteria based on the numerous manifestations aforementioned have been proposed for research purposes only [6–8] and overall are extremely vague. Definitive diagnosis of CTE is by examination of the postmortem tissue. Diagnostic criteria on tissue pathology include a dot-like distribution of phosphorylated tau aggregated in neurons, astrocytes, and cell processes in perivascular spaces within the depth of the cortical sulci [9]. Phosphorylated tau aggregates in cortical layers II and III and hippocampal CA2 and CA4 regions are supportive of diagnosis of CTE. TDP43 and amyloid plaques can be associated with CTE.

There is no reliable biomarker for CTE. Imaging of CTE shows numerous varied findings, with only cavum septum pellucidum being a consistent finding. In a study of boxers, brain MRI showed hippocampal atrophy and cavum septum pellucidum, periventricular white matter changes, and cortical atrophy [10, 11]. Studies involving Diffusion Tensor Imaging (DTI) have shown abnormalities in the deep white matter and cortical gray matter in boxers [12, 13]. Cerebral perfusion studies in boxers have shown increased abnormalities in the boxer group in multiple regions scattered throughout the cortex compared to control [14]. FDG-PET imaging shows decreased uptake bilaterally in the posterior cingulate cortex, parietooccipital and frontal lobes, and cerebellum in boxers [6]. PET tracers such as THK5317, THK5351, AV1451, PBB3, and [F-18] FDDNP can be utilized to trace tau deposition; however the usage is still experimental and the efficacy of using these to diagnose CTE still needs to be evaluated [7, 8, 15, 16].

Emerging evidence shows that repetitive subconcussive head impacts correlate best with CTE [17–19], suggesting that subconcussive head injuries are harmful. Subconcussion is defined by impact to the head, which causes brain changes similar to concussion, without the acute clinical symptoms [20]. Thus, CTE can be missed as a diagnosis since patients and families do not typically recall these subtler events without loss of consciousness. Studies have shown that subconcussive impact leads to brain changes [21]. Cognitive, functional, and biochemical changes occur in the brains of contact sport players, without a clearly diagnosed concussion [22–24]. Neuropathologically confirmed CTE cases all had previous history of repetitive brain trauma [25]. Repetitive brain trauma leads to neurodegenerative diseases, such as Parkinson's disease, frontotemporal lobar degeneration (FTLD), and Alzheimer's dementia [26, 27].

Currently management of CTE is symptomatic treatment of the neuropsychiatric or cognitive symptoms. Because many of the patients present at a younger age, while they are still working, diagnosis of CTE is critical for treatment, counseling, and prognosticating. Unless physicians consider CTE in their differential diagnosis, these younger patients cannot obtain their necessary early treatment interventions. In addition, the proper diagnosis is particularly important for caregivers as they will require guidance in terms of planning and coping with this devastating disease.

Increasing the awareness of these clinical presentations for the clinicians is key to facilitating the appropriate workup and management. Here we present a case of presumed CTE with a former football player, who suffered from repetitive subconcussive brain impact. He presented with severe memory, cognitive deficits, and significant MRI changes and thus was diagnosed with Alzheimer's disease secondary to suspected CTE.

2. Case Presentation

Patient was a 54-year-old right-handed male, former professional football player. He first developed memory problems at the age of 46. Initially, he seemed more forgetful. The onset and the progression of the short-term memory problem were gradual over about eight years. He always did his own finances in the past. However at the age of 46, he started spending money more irrationally and was not paying the bills on-time. He repeated questions, sometimes even just a few minutes later. He had trouble learning new information. He could not manage his own calendar. He has become dependent on the GPS to get around. Patient had become less social. He did not

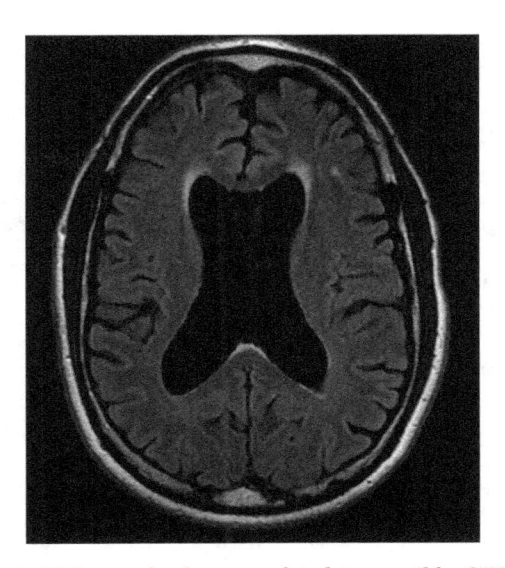

FIGURE 1: **MRI reveals changes related to possible CTE.** Axial image reveals both cortical and subcortical atrophy, enlarged lateral and third ventricle, and cavum septum pellucidum.

have depressed mood; however, he had become more irritable and more easily angered. He had no behavioral issues. His activities of daily living (ADLs) were intact.

Patient started playing football when he was age 7 or 8. He played football in high school and college and then professionally. He played football for total of 23 years. Although he never lost consciousness, he experienced brief moment of flashes. This type of head injury averaged 3-4 times per game. There is no family history of dementia.

His mini-mental status exam (MMSE) was 24/30, and the clinical dementia rating (CDR) was 1. On neuropsychological testing, he had significant impaired verbal and nonverbal learning, recall, and recognition with rapid forgetting (more than two standard deviations). Patient's MRI showed cortical and subcortical atrophy, enlarged ventricles, and cavum septum pellucidum (Figure 1). The hippocampal volume was below 5 percentile and the inferior lateral ventricle volume was greater than 95 percentile. His diagnosis was major neurocognitive disorder, likely Alzheimer's disease due to CTE.

3. Discussion

This case was diagnosed as early onset Alzheimer's dementia with presumed CTE, for insidious gradual onset of memory impairment. Findings in the neuropsychological testing are consistent with AD. However, history of playing professional football and no other risk factors for AD suggest that CTE is the underlying cause of his memory impairment and MRI findings. Because there are no established clinical diagnostic guidelines for CTE, the diagnosis for CTE can only be proposed. Patient had low hippocampal volume, which fits the profile for AD [28]. The history of subconcussive head impact and the presence of cavum septum pellucidum are supportive of CTE. AD pathology may coexist with CTE; therefore, it is important for clinicians to recognize that these two conditions can overlap. In neuropathological study, amyloid plaque coexists in 50% of CTE pathology [29]; therefore, beta-amyloid deposition is possibly induced by CTE pathology.

In contrast to early presentation of neuropsychological symptoms [30], this patient presented with memory changes and cognitive impairment later in life that developed into dementia. This presentation is consistent with the current understanding that neuropsychological symptoms of early and cognitive impairment/dementia occur late in the course of CTE [31]. The degree of ventricular enlargement was significantly large for his age, consistent with advanced stage of CTE [32].

The anatomical distribution of hyperphosphorylated tau deposition suggests possible breakdown of blood brain barrier and inflammatory response during traumatic brain injury. Phosphorylated tau appearance later in disease in area other than the perisulcal space suggests that possible tau propagation. Mechanism for CTE has been proposed to involve three stages of pathological changes, including an acute/subacute state, followed by chronic/static state and then neurodegeneration [33].

In conclusion, we suggest that the clinicians should be aware of subconcussion contributing to CTE. They should include CTE in their differential diagnosis when evaluating patients with memory impairment and dementia and recognize that Alzheimer's and CTE can coexist.

References

[1] J. A. N. Corsellis, C. J. Bruton, and D. Freeman-Browne, "The aftermath of boxing," *Psychological Medicine*, vol. 3, no. 3, pp. 270–303, 1973.

[2] J. A. Langlois, W. Rutland-Brown, and M. M. Wald, "The epidemiology and impact of traumatic brain injury: a brief overview," *The Journal of Head Trauma Rehabilitation*, vol. 21, no. 5, pp. 375–378, 2006.

[3] J. Mez, D. H. Daneshvar, P. T. Kiernan, B. Abdolmohammadi, V. E. Alvarez, B. R. Huber et al., "Clinicopathological Evaluation of Chronic Traumatic Encephalopathy in Players of American Football," *The Journal of the American Medical Association*, vol. 318, no. 4, pp. 360–370, 2017.

[4] H. S. Martland, "Punch drunk," *Journal of the American Medical Association*, vol. 91, no. 15, pp. 1103–1107, 1928.

[5] J. Millspaugh, "Dementia pugilistica," *US Naval Med Bull*, vol. 35, no. 297, p. e303, 1937.

[6] F. A. Provenzano, B. Jordan, R. S. Tikofsky, C. Saxena, R. L. Van Heertum, and M. Ichise, "F-18 FDG PET imaging of chronic traumatic brain injury in boxers: A statistical parametric analysis," *Nuclear Medicine Communications*, vol. 31, no. 11, pp. 952–957, 2010.

[7] J. R. Barrio, G. W. Small, K.-P. Wong et al., "In vivo characterization of chronic traumatic encephalopathy using [F-18]FDDNP PET brain imaging," *Proceedings of the National Academy of Sciences of the United States of America*, vol. 112, no. 16, pp. E2039–E2047, 2015.

[8] B. Omalu, G. W. Small, J. Bailes et al., "Postmortem Autopsy-Confirmation of Antemortem [F-18]FDDNP-PET Scans in a Football Player With Chronic Traumatic Encephalopathy," *Neurosurgery*, vol. 82, no. 2, pp. 237–246, 2018.

[9] A. C. McKee, N. J. Cairns, D. W. Dickson et al., "The first NINDS/NIBIB consensus meeting to define neuropathological criteria for the diagnosis of chronic traumatic encephalopathy," *Acta Neuropathologica*, vol. 131, no. 1, pp. 75–86, 2016.

[10] H. S. Levin, S. C. Lippold, A. Goldman et al., "Neurobehavioral functioning and magnetic resonance imaging findings in young boxers," *Journal of Neurosurgery*, vol. 67, no. 5, pp. 657–667, 1987.

[11] W. W. Orrison Jr., E. H. Hanson, T. Alamo et al., "Traumatic brain injury: A review and high-field MRI findings in 100 unarmed combatants using a literature-based checklist approach," *Journal of Neurotrauma*, vol. 26, no. 5, pp. 689–701, 2009.

[12] M. H. Chappell, A. M. Uluğ, L. Zhang et al., "Distribution of microstructural damage in the brains of professional boxers: A diffusion MRI study," *Journal of Magnetic Resonance Imaging*, vol. 24, no. 3, pp. 537–542, 2006.

[13] L. Zhang, L. A. Heier, R. D. Zimmerman, B. Jordan, and A. M. Ulug, "Diffusion anisotropy changes in the brains of professional boxers," *AJNR Am J Neuroradiol*, vol. 27, no. 9, 2000.

[14] P. M. Kemp, A. S. Houston, M. A. MacLeod, and R. J. Pethybridge, "Cerebral perfusion and psychometric testing in military amateur boxers and controls," *Journal of Neurology, Neurosurgery & Psychiatry*, vol. 59, no. 4, pp. 368–374, 1995.

[15] L. Saint-Aubert, L. Lemoine, K. Chiotis, A. Leuzy, E. Rodriguez-Vieitez, and A. Nordberg, "Tau PET imaging: present and future directions," *Molecular Neurodegeneration*, vol. 12, no. 1, article no. 19, 2017.

[16] G. W. Small, V. Kepe, P. Siddarth et al., "PET scanning of brain tau in retired national football league players: Preliminary findings," *The American Journal of Geriatric Psychiatry*, vol. 21, no. 2, pp. 138–144, 2013.

[17] C. M. Baugh, J. M. Stamm, D. O. Riley et al., "Chronic traumatic encephalopathy: Neurodegeneration following repetitive concussive and subconcussive brain trauma," *Brain Imaging and Behavior*, vol. 6, no. 2, pp. 244–254, 2012.

[18] P. H. Montenigro, C. M. Baugh, D. H. Daneshvar et al., "Clinical subtypes of chronic traumatic encephalopathy: literature review and proposed research diagnostic criteria for traumatic encephalopathy syndrome," *Alzheimer's Research & Therapy*, vol. 6, no. 5-8, article no. 68, 2014.

[19] A. C. McKee, R. C. Cantu, C. J. Nowinski et al., "Chronic traumatic encephalopathy in athletes: progressive tauopathy after repetitive head injury," *Journal of Neuropathology & Experimental Neurology*, vol. 68, no. 7, pp. 709–735, 2009.

[20] J. E. Bailes, A. L. Petraglia, B. I. Omalu, E. Nauman, and T. Talavage, "Role of subconcussion in repetitive mild traumatic brain injury," *Journal of Neurosurgery*, vol. 119, no. 5, pp. 1235–1245, 2013.

[21] I. K. Koerte, B. Ertl-Wagner, M. Reiser, R. Zafonte, and M. E. Shenton, "White matter integrity in the brains of professional soccer players without a symptomatic concussion," *Journal of the American Medical Association*, vol. 308, no. 18, pp. 1859–1861, 2012.

[22] T. M. Talavage, E. A. Nauman, E. L. Breedlove et al., "Functionally-detected cognitive impairment in high school football players without clinically-diagnosed concussion," *Journal of Neurotrauma*, vol. 31, no. 4, pp. 327–338, 2014.

[23] M. R. Zhang, S. D. Red, A. H. Lin, S. S. Patel, and A. B. Sereno, "Evidence of Cognitive Dysfunction after Soccer Playing with Ball Heading Using a Novel Tablet-Based Approach," *PLoS ONE*, vol. 8, no. 2, Article ID e57364, 2013.

[24] E. L. Breedlove, M. Robinson, T. M. Talavage et al., "Biomechanical correlates of symptomatic and asymptomatic neurophysiological impairment in high school football," *Journal of Biomechanics*, vol. 45, no. 7, pp. 1265–1272, 2012.

[25] R. A. Stern, D. O. Riley, D. H. Daneshvar, C. J. Nowinski, R. C. Cantu, and A. C. McKee, "Long-term Consequences of Repetitive Brain Trauma: Chronic Traumatic Encephalopathy," *PM&R : The Journal of Injury, Function, and Rehabilitation*, vol. 3, no. 10, pp. S460–S467, 2011.

[26] L.-N. Hazrati, M. C. Tartaglia, P. Diamandis et al., "Absence of chronic traumatic encephalopathy in retired football players with multiple concussions and neurological symptomatology," *Frontiers in Human Neuroscience*, vol. 7, no. MAY, 2013.

[27] M. C. Tartaglia, L.-N. Hazrati, K. D. Davis et al., "Chronic traumatic encephalopathy and other neurodegenerative proteinopathies," *Frontiers in Human Neuroscience*, vol. 8, 2014.

[28] B. Dubois, H. H. Feldman, C. Jacova et al., "Advancing research diagnostic criteria for Alzheimer's disease: the IWG-2 criteria," *The Lancet Neurology*, vol. 13, no. 6, pp. 614–629, 2014.

[29] T. D. Stein, P. H. Montenigro, V. E. Alvarez et al., "Beta-amyloid deposition in chronic traumatic encephalopathy," *Acta Neuropathologica*, vol. 130, no. 1, pp. 21–34, 2015.

[30] S. H. Yuan and S. G. Wang, "Emotional Lability as a Unique Presenting Sign of Suspected Chronic Traumatic Encephalopathy," *Case Reports in Neurological Medicine*, vol. 2018, 4 pages, 2018.

[31] B. D. Jordan, "The clinical spectrum of sport-related traumatic brain injury," *Nature Reviews Neurology*, vol. 9, no. 4, pp. 222–230, 2013.

[32] A. C. McKee, T. D. Stein, P. T. Kiernan, and V. E. Alvarez, "The neuropathology of chronic traumatic encephalopathy," *Brain Pathology*, vol. 25, no. 3, pp. 350–364, 2015.

[33] I. K. Koerte, A. P. Lin, A. Willems et al., "A review of neuroimaging findings in repetitive brain trauma," *Brain Pathology*, vol. 25, no. 3, pp. 318–349, 2015.

Clival Ectopic Pituitary Adenoma Mimicking a Chordoma: Case Report and Review of the Literature

Constantine L. Karras,[1] Isaac Josh Abecassis,[2] Zachary A. Abecassis,[3] Joseph G. Adel,[3,4] Esther N. Bit-Ivan,[5] Rakesh K. Chandra,[6] and Bernard R. Bendok[3,4]

[1]The Ohio State University College of Medicine, Columbus, OH 43212, USA
[2]Department of Neurological Surgery, University of Washington, Seattle, WA 98122, USA
[3]Feinberg School of Medicine, Northwestern University, Chicago, IL 60611, USA
[4]Department of Neurological Surgery, Northwestern University, Chicago, IL, USA
[5]Department of Pathology, Feinberg School of Medicine, Northwestern University, Chicago, IL 60611, USA
[6]Department of Otolaryngology, Feinberg School of Medicine, Northwestern University, Chicago, IL 60611, USA

Correspondence should be addressed to Isaac Josh Abecassis; abecassi@uw.edu

Academic Editor: Mehmet Turgut

Background. Purely ectopic pituitary adenomas are exceedingly rare. Here we report on a patient that presented with an incidental clival mass thought to be a chordoma. Endonasal resection, tumor pathology, and endocrinology workup revealed a prolactinoma. *Case Presentation.* A 41-year-old male presented with an incidental clival lesion presumed to be a chordoma. On MRI it involved the entire clivus, extended laterally to the petroclival junction, and invaded the cavernous sinuses bilaterally, encasing both internal carotid arteries, without direct extension into the sella. Intraoperatively, it was clear that the tumor originated from the clivus and that the sellar dura was completely intact. Frozen-section pathology was consistent with a pituitary adenoma. Immunostaining was positive for synaptophysin and prolactin with a low Ki-67 index, suggestive of a prolactinoma. Additional immunohistochemical stains seen in chordomas (EMA, S100, and Brachyury) and other metastatic tumors were negative. A postoperative endocrine workup revealed an elevated serum prolactin of 881.3 ng/mL (normal < 20). *Conclusions.* In conclusion, it is crucial to maintain an extensive differential diagnosis when evaluating a patient with a clival lesion. Ectopic clival pituitary adenomas, although rare, may warrant an endocrinological workup preoperatively as the majority may respond to medical treatment.

1. Introduction

Pituitary adenomas are the most common cause of a sellar or parasellar mass, comprising about 10 to 15 percent of all intracranial tumors [1, 2]. It is well documented that pituitary adenomas have the capacity to invade adjacent and nearby structures, most commonly the sphenoid sinus [3]. Less commonly, pituitary adenomas may also involve the cavernous sinus, suprasellar region, nasopharynx, and rarely the clivus [4]. Purely ectopic pituitary adenomas are extremely unusual and must be confirmed via imaging and intraoperative visualization to be completely separate from an intact pituitary gland and the sella turcica. Here we report on a patient that presented with an incidental clival mass thought to be a chordoma. Endonasal resection, pathology of the tumor, and endocrinology workup revealed a purely ectopic prolactin-secreting pituitary adenoma.

2. Case Report

Our patient was a 41-year-old right-handed male who presented with an incidental clival lesion, originally presumed to be a chordoma. Subjectively, the patient reported no neurological complaints. The patient's medical history was significant only for chronic neck and lower back pain and there were no noteworthy findings on physical examination,

(a)   (b)

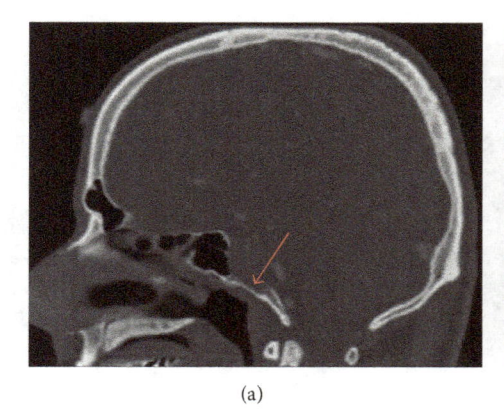

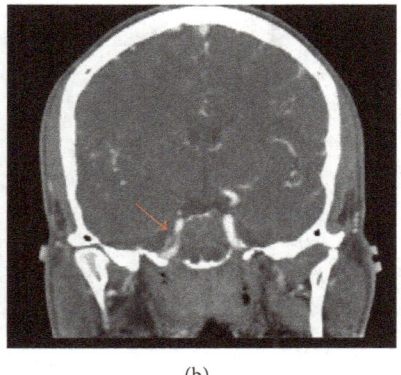

FIGURE 1: Preoperative computed tomography angiogram (CTA) scan, sagittal bone window (a) and coronal vascular window (b) sections, showing poorly vascularized clival mass that erodes the clivus (a) and encases the right internal carotid artery (b).

which included a thorough neurological exam. His complete blood count, chemistry panel, and metabolic panel were all normal.

Repeat magnetic resonance imaging (MRI) revealed an enhancing lesion measuring 1.7 × 2.6 × 3.2 cm that involved the entire clivus, extended laterally to the petroclival junction, and invaded the cavernous sinuses bilaterally with further encasement of the internal carotid arteries (ICAs) bilaterally, without direct extension into the sella (Figures 1(a)-1(b) and 2(a)-2(c)). This lesion was stable in comparison to outside hospital images. The case was discussed at an interdisciplinary brain tumor meeting and, ultimately, the patient was advised to undergo surgical resection via an endoscopic endonasal approach. Intraoperatively, it was very clear that the tumor originated from the clivus and that the sellar dura was completely intact. The frozen-section pathology surprisingly was consistent with a pituitary adenoma. Accordingly, a decision was made perioperatively to proceed with only partial resection due to the potential for medical management of most functional adenomas postoperatively and the risks associated with complete resection given the complex distribution of the lesion. The patient had no complications and was discharged home on postoperative day 2.

Postoperative imaging revealed expected residual enhancing lesions along the petroclival junctions bilaterally and on the right cavernous sinus near the right ICA (Figures 3(a) and 3(b)). Immunostaining of the tumor tissue demonstrated an epithelial neoplasm that stained positive for synaptophysin and prolactin with a low Ki-67 index (Figures 4(a)-4(d)), suggestive of a prolactin-secreting pituitary adenoma. Additional immunohistochemical stains seen in chordomas (EMA, S100, and Brachyury) and other metastatic tumors were negative. A postoperative endocrine workup (Table 1) revealed an elevated serum prolactin of 881.3 ng/mL (normal male < 20 ng/mL). The patient was referred to an endocrinologist and began dopamine agonist (cabergoline) therapy given his prolactin level and residual tumor. He has since been followed up for over 1 year with monthly visits. His most recent prolactin level (11 months postoperatively)

TABLE 1: Patient's endocrinological lab values.

	Patient	Reference range
Free T4 (ng/dL)	0.7	0.7–1.5
TSH (μIU/mL)	2.58	0.4–4.0
Prolactin (ng/mL)	881.3	2.6–13.1
FSH (mIU/mL)	3	1.0–8.0 (Men)
LH (mIU/mL)	3.1	2.0–12.0 (Men)
Cortisol, 2PM (μg/dL)	6.8	0–25
Total testosterone (ng/dL)	290	250–1100
Free testosterone (pg/mL)	58.4	35–155

T4 = thyroxine hormone.
TSH = thyroid stimulating hormone.
FSH = follicle stimulating hormone.
LH = luteinizing hormone.

was 20.6 ng/mL; his lowest level was 15.2 ng/mL, collected 6 months postoperatively. He remains neurologically intact.

3. Discussion

Clival tumors are generally rare, comprising 1% of all intracranial neoplasms. The differential diagnosis for a clival lesion is vast, including chordoma most commonly (40%), meningioma, chondrosarcoma, astrocytoma, craniopharyngioma, germ cell tumor, non-Hodgkin's lymphoma, melanoma, metastatic carcinoma, and rarely pituitary adenoma [4]. Our patient was presumed to have a chordoma based on the radiographic characteristics and the tumor location. Clival chordomas are typically managed with gross total resection with proton beam therapy. There has been one previous report of an ectopic pituitary adenoma thought to be a chordoma [12] and vice versa [4].

Ectopic pituitary adenomas are thought to arise from residual cells along the migration tract of the pharyngeal pituitary as it travels from Rathke's pouch to the sella turcica. The anterior portion of the pituitary initially develops as a pharyngeal outpouching of epithelial ectoderm, known as Rathke's pouch. Around week 8 of gestation, a portion

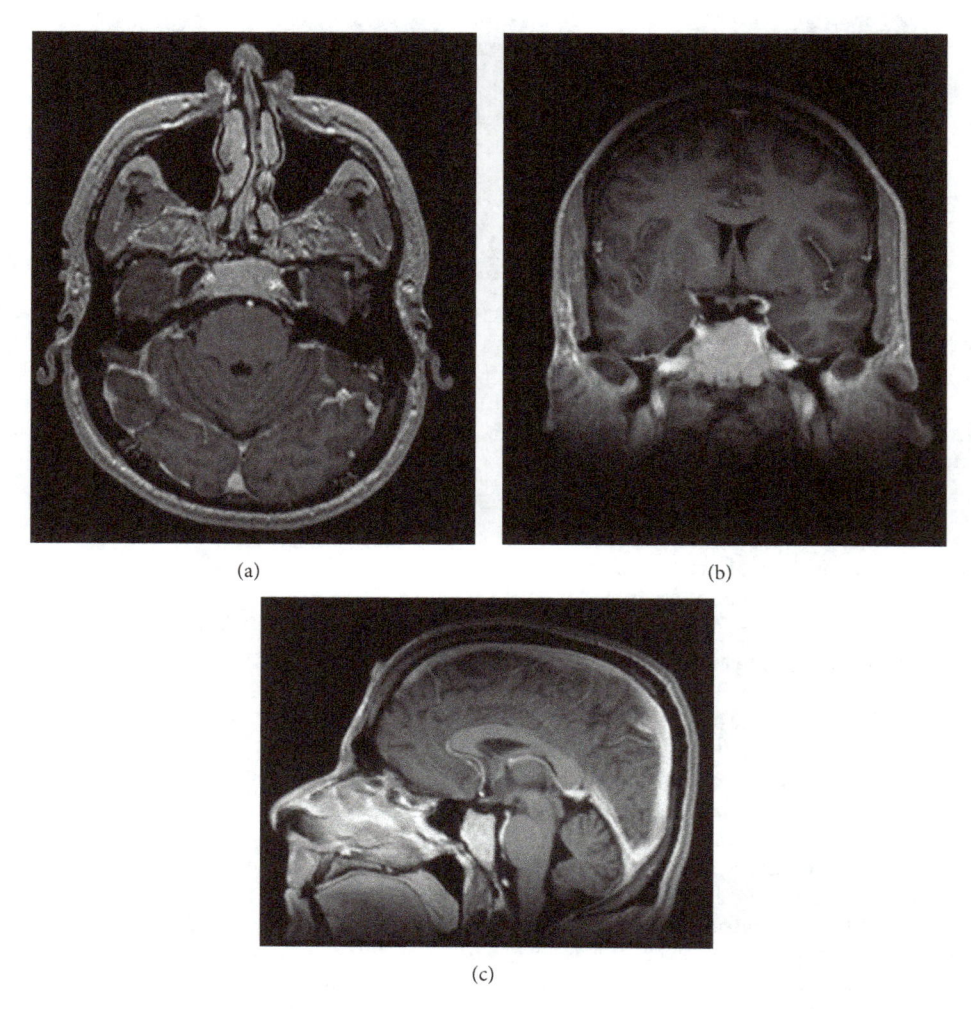

FIGURE 2: Preoperative magnetic resonance imaging, with contrast, axial (a), coronal (b), and sagittal (c) sections, demonstrating contrast enhancing, clival tumor.

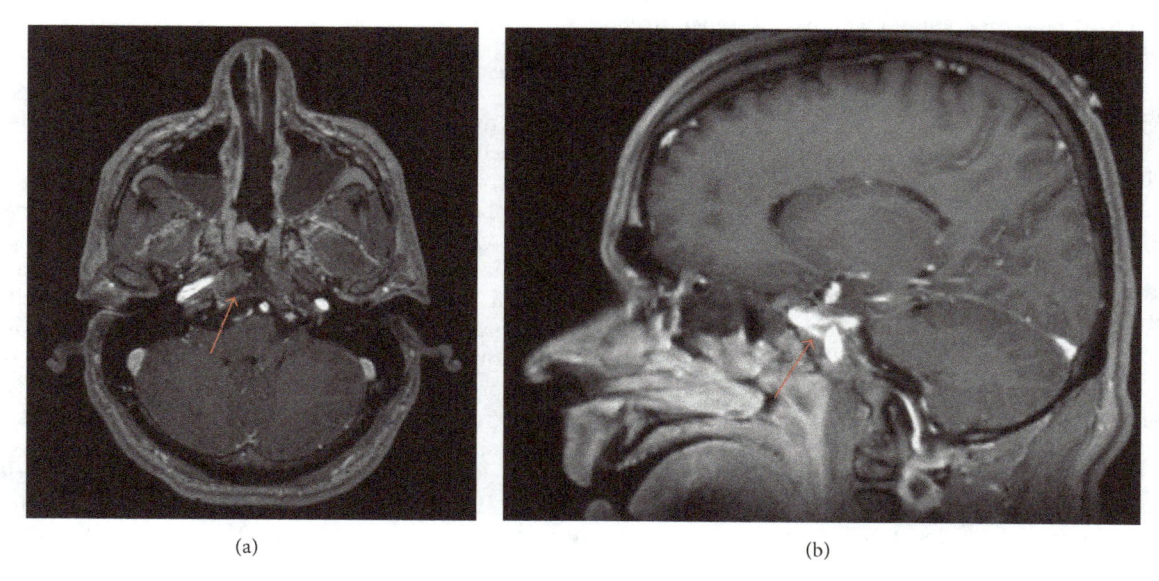

FIGURE 3: Postoperative magnetic resonance imaging, with contrast, axial (a) and sagittal (b) sections, demonstrating a small amount of residual tumor.

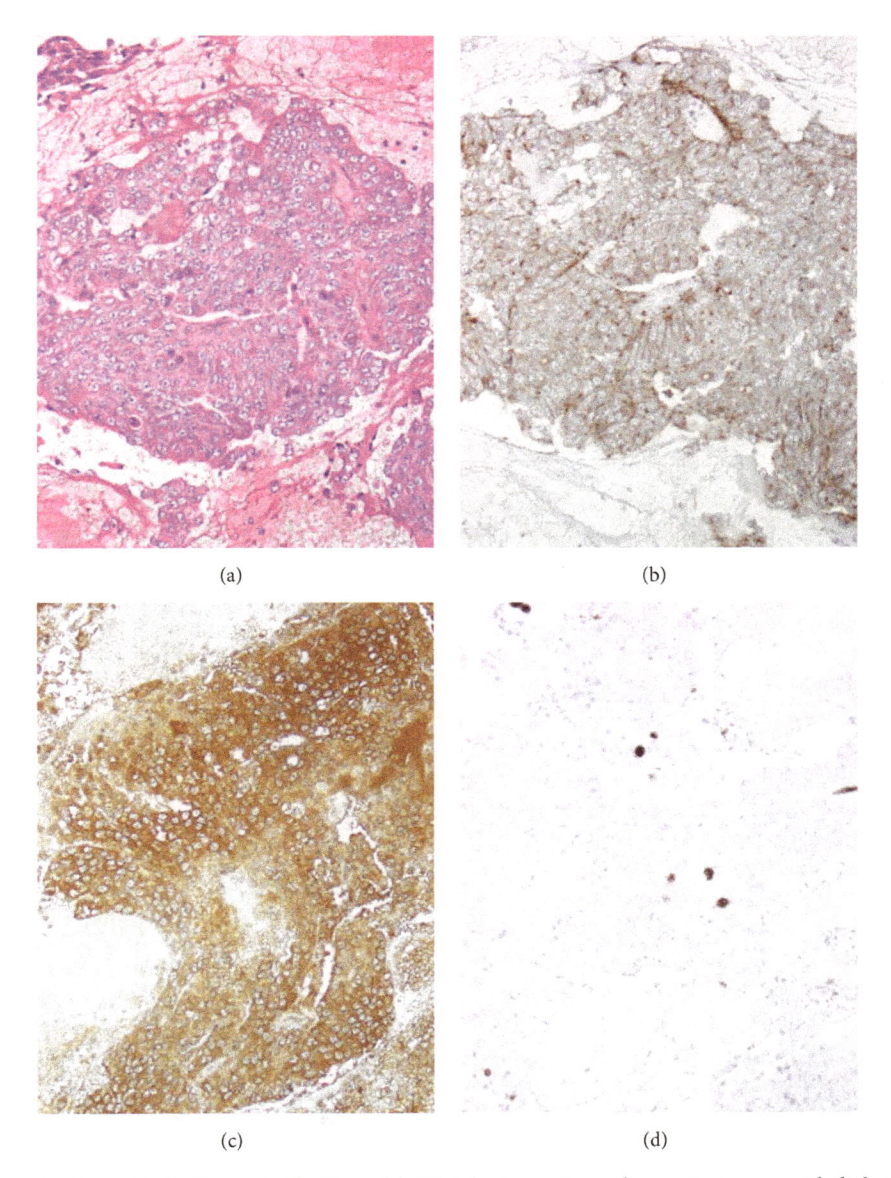

FIGURE 4: Pathologic evaluation, all at 20x magnification. (a) Histologic sections demonstrate an epithelial neoplasm composed of monomorphic cells with increased nuclear to cytoplasmic ratios and prominent nucleoli. (b) Immunohistochemical staining positive for synaptophysin. (c) Prolactin diffusely and strongly labels the neoplastic cells. (d) The proliferation index is approximately 2% on Ki-67 staining.

separates and migrates through the craniopharyngeal canal into the sella, forming the anterior portion of the pituitary, from which most pituitary adenomas arise [9, 16]. Ectopically deposited cells can rarely develop into adenomas anywhere along this tract, though. There have been over 100 descriptions of ectopic pituitary adenomas in the literature, most originating in the sphenoid sinus [17]. The first reported, in 1901, was an ectopic pituitary adenoma [10] located in the sphenoid sinus that presented with acromegaly. However, purely ectopic clival pituitary adenomas—that is, tumors that originate in the clivus with no involvement of the pituitary gland—are exceedingly rare.

We encountered 16 prior reported cases of clival ectopic pituitary adenomas (Table 2) [4–9, 11–14, 17–21]. They seem to be fairly equally distributed between genders (9 males, 8 females) and the median age at presentation was 50 years old.

Like pituitary adenomas, ectopic tissue can be categorized by size as either a macroadenoma (>1 cm) or microadenoma (<1 cm). The tumor can be further classified as functional (65% of nonectopic adenomas) or nonfunctional based on whether or not the cell type is hormone-secreting. Prolactin-secreting pituitary adenomas (nonectopic) are the most common and comprise 48% of all functional adenomas [22]. Occasionally, pituitary adenomas can lack the cardinal features found on light microscopy and immunohistochemical staining that were present in our case. Electron microscopy of these tumors may aid in further classification of the cell type based on appearance of the nucleus, cytoplasm, organelles

TABLE 2: Prior reported cases of ectopic pituitary adenomas located in the clivus.

(a)

Authors	Patient age and gender	Immunostaining	Initial presentation
Ortiz-Suarez and Erickson, 1975 [11]	15 F	ACTH	Obesity, irregular menstrual cycles, increased facial hair, episodic headaches, and facial numbness
Shenker et al., 1986 [21]	49 M	Prolactin	Worsening renal failure, hypercalcemia, duodenal ulcer, parathyroid hyperplasia, fatigue, muscle pains, vomiting, and impotence
Anand et al., 1993 [18]	58 F	ACTH	Nasal obstruction, blurred vision, anosmia, and headache
Mount et al., 1993 [20]	71 M	Prolactin	Aphasia and R hemiplegia
Arnesen and Scheithauer, 1994 [7]	40 M	Prolactin	Bloody, mucoid nasal discharge, and nasal obstruction
Kikuchi et al., 1994 [12]	49 F	Null cell	Headaches, nausea, and vomiting after neck injury; incidentally discovered
Wong et al., 1995 [4]	67 M	Null cell	Unknown
De Witte et al., 1998 [19]	47 F	Prolactin	Headache
Hori et al., 1999 [17]	63 M	Null cell	Visual disturbances
Ballaux et al., 1999 [14]	80 F	Prolactin	Minor headache and transient amnesia
Sakakibara et al., 2002 [6]	70 F	Prolactin	Progressive L sided exophthalmos
Bhatoe et al., 2007 [5]	35 F	GH	Dull generalized headache, acral enlargement, weight gain, and coarsening facial features
Rocque et al., 2009 [9]	20 M	Prolactin	Bilateral gynecomastia and galactorrhea
Appel et al., 2012 [8]	50 F	GH/prolactin	Daily headaches, impaired concentration, fatigue, generalized muscle/joint pain, and acromegalic facial features
Mudd et al., 2012 [14]	78 M	Null cell	Acute onset blurred vision, apoplexy
Narese et al., 2015 [4]	65 M	Prolactin	Right ptosis, eyelid edema, and headache
This paper	41 M	Prolactin	Incidental imaging due to chronic neck and lower back pain

(b)

Focal neurological findings	Imaging	Abnormal preoperative labs (ng/mL)	Treatment	Follow-up; outcomes
Oculomotor and trigeminal nerve palsies	Skull XR: mottling, sclerosis of sella turcica, and lesser wing of sphenoid. CT: normal. Carotid angiogram: medial displacement of ICA	None	Right transfrontal craniotomy + 5000 Rads	1 year; returned to baseline
None	Skull XR: enlarged sella, CT: partially empty sella, destroyed sella floor, and mass at base of sella with invasion into sphenoid sinus	PRL = 1900	Endonasal transsphenoidal resection + cabergoline	1 year; no recurrence, impotence resolved
L eye inferior medial quadrant visual field defect	MRI: 3 × 3 cm, midline homogenous mass filling posterior nasopharynx and clivus	None	Total resection via open-door maxillotomy approach + 4550 Rads over 25	1 year; complete resolution of symptoms
Unknown	CT/MRI: L frontotemporal hematoma, meningioma, expansile density with invasion into sphenoid bone and clivus, and encasing ICAs	None	Endonasal transsphenoidal biopsy only + radiation	No improvement, transferred to receive supportive care
Unknown	MRI: tumor eroding through skull base into the clivus extending into sphenoid sinus, cavernous sinus, and surrounding ICA	Unknown	Partial endonasal transsphenoidal resection	Unknown

(b) Continued.

Focal neurological findings	Imaging	Abnormal preoperative labs (ng/mL)	Treatment	Follow-up; outcomes
None	Skull XR: normal size sella, slight erosion of floor CT/MRI: large enhancing mass in sphenoid sinus invading sphenoid wing and clivus	None	Partial resection via sublabial transnasal approach + 50 Gy radiation/6 wks	Unclear; "under careful observation"
Unknown	MRI: clival destruction	PRL = 7	Unknown	Unknown
None	CT/MRI: clival lesion, destruction of bone	None (Post-op PRL = 34,000)	Endonasal transsphenoidal partial resection + bromocriptine	4 months; normalization of lab values
Bitemporal hemianopsia	CT: lesion in extradural sella-clivus region	Unknown	Transfacial surgery	Unknown
None	CT: tumor at clivus with surrounding bony destruction. MRI: enhancing mass with cystic component, invading sphenoid sinus	PRL = 2519.8	Cabergoline only	6 months; resolution of lab values and symptoms
Exophthalmos with external ocular movement disorders and decreased visual acuity on L	CT: bony destruction of clivus, sphenoid sinus, and medial aspect of middle cranial fossa, MRI: abnormal enhancement in sphenoid sinus	PRL = 645.7	Endonasal transsphenoidal resection + Bromocriptine therapy	1 year f/u; resolution of visual symptoms
Unknown	Skull radiograph: normal, MRI: clival mass connected to intrasellar lesion	GH = 30.6	Endonasal transsphenoidal resection	1 year; normalization of lab values
None	MRI: 13 mm erosive mass in clivus with focal area of bony erosion	PRL = 178	Endonasal transsphenoidal total resection	6 months; complete resolution of symptoms
None	MRI: 2 mm hypointense lesion on pituitary gland. Clival lesion discovered incidentally during surgery	IGF-1 = 937, PRL = 26	Endoscopic transsphenoidal; clival mass encountered and resected, pituitary unremarkable	3 months; normalization of lab values, no report on clinical status
L CN 6 palsy	MRI: lytic lesion of left clivus, compression of cavernous sinuses, clival mass, and normal sella	None	Endoscopic transsphenoidal resection	2.5 years; resolution of CN6 palsy and no recurrence
None	MRI: large tumor at height of clivus, partial destruction of surrounding bone structure	Unknown	Endoscopic transsphenoidal resection	Unknown
None	MRI: enhancing lesion in clivus with extension into cavernous sinuses and encasement of the ICAs	PRL = 881.3	Endoscopic transsphenoidal; subtotal resection and dopamine antagonist	1 year; no symptoms

F = female.
M = male.
GH = growth hormone.
PRL = prolactin.
ACTH = adrenocorticotropic hormone.
IGF-1 = insulin-like growth factor-1.
MRI = magnetic resonance imaging.
CT = computed tomography.
XR = X-ray.
ICAs = internal carotid arteries.
L = left.
CN = cranial nerve.

(including rough endoplasmic reticulum and Golgi apparatus), and granule morphology [7].

Analysis of Table 2 reveals that 10/17 clival ectopic pituitary tumors described were prolactinomas, 2/17 secreted ACTH, 2/17 secreted GH, and only 4/17 were nonfunctional—one tumor secreted both prolactin and GH [8]. Some (especially nonfunctional tumors) presented asymptomatically or with focal neurological deficits (5/17 cases) due to compression of nearby structures. The most common theme among patient presentations in the literature review was "frequent headache" in the period leading up to diagnosis. Pituitary adenomas often classically present with bitemporal hemianopsia, but ectopic adenomas typically do not unless they happen to involve the optic chiasm. One case presented as pituitary apoplexy—tumor infarction or hemorrhage resulting in a constellation of symptoms that may include headache, visual deficits, ophthalmoplegia, or altered mental status [13]. Most of these findings are nonspecific, however, and cannot distinguish a pituitary adenoma from other lesions such as a chordoma.

Fortunately, a surprising 76% (13/17) of reported cases were functional adenomas, permitting a possible preoperative diagnosis based on history, physical exam, and basic labs alone. ACTH-secreting adenomas may present with Cushing's syndrome (moon facies, truncal obesity, abdominal striae, hirsutism, etc.), characterized by hypercortisolism and an abnormal dexamethasone suppression test. GH-secreting adenomas may manifest as acromegaly in adults, which presents with enlargement of the extremities, coarse facies (frontal bossing, prognathism), carpal tunnel syndrome, diabetes, or cardiomyopathy—labs would reveal elevated IGF-1 (insulin-like growth factor) and a failed oral glucose tolerance test. Prolactinomas, which comprised the majority of cases (10/17), may present with gynecomastia, erectile dysfunction, decreased libido, galactorrhea, amenorrhea (in females), and an elevated prolactin level. Of note, after a more focused history following our postoperative diagnosis of prolactinoma, it was discovered retrospectively that our patient had actually had a significant drop in libido throughout the previous 7-8 years.

Our case was unique in that it was the first reported clival ectopic pituitary adenoma that invaded both cavernous sinuses and the internal carotid arteries, making it the most aggressive tumor of all reported cases—this is unusual for adenomas, as they typically are quite less infiltrative. This is why it was originally confused for a chordoma, but it is particularly important to maintain pituitary adenomas on the differential for sphenoidal or clival lesions because the diagnosis can have significant implications on the management of the tumor. For example, dopamine agonists (cabergoline, bromocriptine) and somatostatin analogs (octreotide, lanreotide) or GH antagonists (pegvisomant) are first-line therapy for prolactinomas and GH-secreting adenomas, respectively, depending on the clinical symptoms and anatomical distribution of the tumor. They may be used as monotherapy or as adjunctive treatment for tumor shrinkage. With 76% (13/17) of reported clival ectopic adenomas being hormone-secreting and 85% (11/13) of these being susceptible to medical management (GH- or prolactin-secreting), a significant opportunity exists for more conservative management if the diagnosis can be made preoperatively rather than retrospectively based on histology. This is especially useful for more aggressive tumors (such as our patient's, which invaded the cavernous sinus), where a complete resection may carry significant risk of bleeding and morbidity. Adjunctive pharmacotherapy can also potentially delay or even eliminate the need for surgery, especially in elderly individuals or in those with significant medical comorbidities and relative contraindications to surgery.

A common theme among reported cases, including ours, was that the correct diagnosis was made histologically rather than preoperatively. Management could have been drastically altered in most of these cases had a more focused, thorough history and physical exam alone occurred.

4. Conclusions

In conclusion, it is important to maintain an extensive differential diagnosis when evaluating a patient with a clival lesion. Ectopic clival pituitary adenomas, although rare, warrant consideration as the majority respond to pharmacotherapy [14] and thus are managed much differently than lesions such as chordomas. The diagnosis can easily be screened for with a focused history and physical exam directed toward symptoms of the most common types (prolactin-, GH-, and ACTH-secreting adenomas), which make up the majority (76%) of reported clival ectopic adenomas. If the history and physical exam yield a positive screen, a preoperative endocrinological workup is necessary to confirm the diagnosis.

References

[1] P. J. Pernicone and B. W. Scheithauer, "Invasive pituitary adenomas and pituitary carcinomas," in *Surgical Pathology of the Pituitary Gland*, R. V. Lloyd, Ed., pp. 121–136, WB Saunders, Philadelphia, Pa, USA, 1993.

[2] T. Terada, K. Kovacs, L. Stefaneanu, and E. Horvath, "Incidence, pathology, and recurrence of pituitary adenomas: study of 647 unselected surgical cases," *Endocrine Pathology*, vol. 6, no. 4, pp. 301–310, 1995.

[3] F. Tovi, M. Hirsch, M. Sacks, and A. Leiberman, "Ectopic pituitary adenoma of the sphenoid sinus: report of a case and review of the literature," *Head and Neck*, vol. 12, no. 3, pp. 264–268, 1990.

[4] K. Wong, J. Raisanen, S. L. Taylor, M. W. McDermott, C. B. Wilson, and P. H. Gutin, "Pituitary adenoma as an unsuspected clival tumor," *The American Journal of Surgical Pathology*, vol. 19, no. 8, pp. 900–903, 1995.

[5] H. S. Bhatoe, N. Kotwal, and S. Badwal, "Clival pituitary adenoma with acromegaly: case report and review of literature," *Skull Base*, vol. 17, no. 4, pp. 265–268, 2007.

[6] Y. Sakakibara, H. Sekino, Y. Taguchi, and M. Tadokoro, "Unilateral exophthalmos caused by a prolactin producing ectopic pituitary adenoma: case report," *Neurological Surgery*, vol. 30, no. 6, pp. 623–628, 2002.

[7] M. Arnesen and B. W. Scheithauer, "Aggressive small cell tumor of the skull base," *Ultrastructural Pathology*, vol. 18, no. 1-2, pp. 191–197, 1994.

[8] J. G. Appel, M. Bergsneider, H. Vinters, N. Salamon, M. B. Wang, and A. P. Heaney, "Acromegaly due to an ectopic pituitary adenoma in the clivus: case report and review of literature," *Pituitary*, vol. 15, supplement 1, pp. S53–S56, 2012.

[9] B. G. Rocque, K. A. G. Herold, M. S. Salamat, Y. Shenker, and J. S. Kuo, "Symptomatic hyperprolactinemia from an ectopic pituitary adenoma located in the clivus," *Endocrine Practice*, vol. 15, no. 2, pp. 143–148, 2009.

[10] J. Erdheim, "Über einen hypophysentumor von ungewöhnlichem," *Beiträge zur Pathologischen Anatomie und zur Allgemeinen Pathologie*, vol. 46, pp. 233–240, 1909.

[11] H. Ortiz-Suarez and D. L. Erickson, "Pituitary adenomas of adolescents," *Journal of Neurosurgery*, vol. 43, no. 4, pp. 437–439, 1975.

[12] K. Kikuchi, M. Kowada, J. Sasaki, and M. Sageshima, "Large pituitary adenoma of the sphenoid sinus and the nasopharynx: report of a case with ultrastructural evaluations," *Surgical Neurology*, vol. 42, no. 4, pp. 330–334, 1994.

[13] P. A. Mudd, S. Hohensee, K. O. Lillehei, T. T. Kingdom, and B. K. Kleinschmidt-DeMasters, "Ectopic pituitary adenoma of the clivus presenting with apoplexy: case report and review of the literature," *Clinical Neuropathology*, vol. 31, no. 1, pp. 24–30, 2012.

[14] D. Ballaux, J. Verhelst, B. Pickut, P. P. De Deyn, and C. Mahler, "Ectopic macroprolactinoma mimicking a chordoma: a case report," *Endocrine-Related Cancer*, vol. 6, no. 1, pp. 117–122, 1999.

[15] D. Narese, V. Virzì, G. Virzì et al., "Ectopic prolactinoma in the clivus: a case report," *La Clinica Terapeutica*, vol. 166, no. 4, pp. 176–178, 2015.

[16] W. J. Hamilton, J. D. Boyd, and H. W. Mossman, "Prenatal development of form and function," in *Human Embryology*, Heffer and Sons Ltd, pp. 345–346, Cambridge, UK, 1945.

[17] A. Hori, D. Schmidt, and E. Rickels, "Pharyngeal pituitary: development, malformation, and tumorigenesis," *Acta Neuropathologica*, vol. 98, no. 3, pp. 262–272, 1999.

[18] V. K. Anand, C. M. Osborne, and H. L. Harkey III, "Infiltrative clival pituitary adenoma of ectopic origin," *Otolaryngology—Head and Neck Surgery*, vol. 108, no. 2, pp. 178–183, 1993.

[19] O. De Witte, N. Massager, I. Salmon, S. Meyer, G. Dooms, and J. Brotchi, "Ectopic prolactinoma in the clivus," *Acta Chirurgica Belgica*, vol. 98, no. 1, pp. 10–13, 1998.

[20] S. L. Mount, D. J. Taatjes, and T. D. Trainer, "Ultrastructural study of a pituitary adenoma (prolactinoma) within the clivus bone using immunoelectron microscopy," *Ultrastructural Pathology*, vol. 17, no. 6, pp. 637–642, 1993.

[21] Y. Shenker, R. V. Lloyd, L. Weatherbee, F. K. Port, R. J. Grekin, and A. L. Barkan, "Ectopic prolactinoma in a patient with hyperparathyroidism and abnormal sellar radiography," *Journal of Clinical Endocrinology and Metabolism*, vol. 62, no. 5, pp. 1065–1069, 1986.

[22] B. M. Biller, B. Swearingen, N. T. Zervas, and A. Klibanski, "A decade of the massachusetts general hospital neuroendocrine clinical center," *The Journal of Clinical Endocrinology & Metabolism*, vol. 82, no. 6, pp. 1668–1674, 1997.

Friedreich's Ataxia: Clinical Presentation of a Compound Heterozygote Child with a Rare Nonsense Mutation and Comparison with Previously Published Cases

Vamshi K. Rao [1,2] Christine J. DiDonato,[2,3] and Paul D. Larsen[4]

[1]Division of Neurology, Ann & Robert H. Lurie Children's Hospital of Chicago, Chicago, IL 60611, USA
[2]Department of Pediatrics, Feinberg School of Medicine, Northwestern University, Chicago, IL 60611, USA
[3]Human Molecular Genetics Program, Ann & Robert H. Lurie Children's Hospital, Stanley Manne Research Institute, Chicago, IL 60611, USA
[4]Division of Neurology, Department of Pediatrics, University of Nebraska Medical Center and Children's Hospital and Medical Center, Omaha, NE, USA

Correspondence should be addressed to Vamshi K. Rao; vrao@luriechildrens.org

Academic Editor: Dominic B. Fee

Friedreich's ataxia is a neurodegenerative disorder associated with a GAA trinucleotide repeat expansion in intron 1 of the frataxin (FXN) gene. It is the most common autosomal recessive cerebellar ataxia, with a mean age of onset at 16 years. Nearly 95-98% of patients are homozygous for a 90-1300 GAA repeat expansion with only 2-5% demonstrating compound heterozygosity. Compound heterozygous individuals have a repeat expansion in one allele and a point mutation/deletion/insertion in the other. Compound heterozygosity and point mutations are very rare causes of Friedreich's ataxia and nonsense mutations are a further rarity among point mutations. We report a rare compound heterozygous Friedreich's ataxia patient who was found to have one expanded GAA FXN allele and a nonsense point mutation in the other. We summarize the four previously published cases of nonsense mutations and compare the phenotype to that of our patient. We compared clinical information from our patient with other nonsense FXN mutations reported in the literature. This nonsense mutation, to our knowledge, has only been described once previously; interestingly the individual was also of Cuban ancestry. A comparison with previously published cases of nonsense mutations demonstrates some common clinical characteristics.

1. Introduction

Friedrich's ataxia is the most common inherited ataxia with an estimated prevalence of 1 in 30,000-50,000 and a carrier frequency of 1 in 90-110 in the Caucasian population [1, 2]. It is characterized typically by progressive gait and limb ataxia, loss of deep tendon reflexes, and dysarthria. Additional features can include hypertrophic cardiomyopathy [3], diabetes [4], scoliosis, distal wasting, optic atrophy, and sensorineural deafness [5, 6].

The mutation causing Friedrich's ataxia was mapped to chromosome 9 by Chamberlain et al. in 1988 [7]. Subsequently in 1995 Montermini et al. [8] isolated the critical region on 9q13 and in 1996 Campuzano et al. [9] demonstrated the intronic GAA triplet repeat expansion that is associated with the disease.

The identification of the gene led to a phenotypic characterization of the disease. The classic phenotype (95-98%) associated with a homozygous GAA triplet repeat expansion (in the first intron) on both alleles has an age of onset before 25 years, wheelchair dependence within a decade, and death typically due to cardiac compromise by the fourth decade. Repeat expansion size was inversely correlated with the age at onset, duration to wheelchair, and development of cardiomyopathy [10]. Variability in clinical presentations included either late or very late presentations, retained tendon reflexes, or Acadian type (original French people living in North America, intermediate repeats, milder course, and lower incidence of cardiomyopathy) and was usually associated with lower GAA repeat expansion sizes or genetic modifiers.

Compound heterozygous (2-5%) individuals possess a GAA trinucleotide repeat expansion on one allele and a point mutation on the other allele. Diseases causing alterations include frameshift, missense, splice site, in/dels, and nonsense mutations. The two largest case series of Friedrich's ataxia patients with point mutations have been described by Cossee et al. [11] (25 patients) and Gellera et al. [12] (12 patients). Recently Galea et al. [13] compared clinical information from 131 individuals with homozygous expansions and 111 compound heterozygotes. Structural modeling and stability analyses were used to predict protein stability and protein interaction disruption of the various missense mutations. Within the 111 compound heterozygotes (81 were from previous literature review) 50 were predicted to be null alleles representing 38 different types of mutations. These consisted mostly of splice site or in/del mutations that resulted in truncating mutations. Very few were nonsense point mutations as they are rare among the point mutations that have been detected to date. It has been observed that null mutations have earlier onset and higher incidence of diabetes compared to homozygous GAA expansions. On the other hand, there is a higher rate of cardiomyopathy in homozygous GAA expansion than any type of compound heterozygous mutation.

Here we report the case of a child with Friedrich's ataxia found to harbor a W155X nonsense mutation that has to our knowledge, only been described once before [14]. We discuss the clinical phenotype while drawing comparisons with point mutations in general and the previously published cases of nonsense point mutations.

2. Case Description

A 7.5-year-old boy presented with progressive gait disturbance and falls. History included a full-term birth with no pregnancy or delivery complications. Developmental milestones including sitting up without support, walking, and speech were all within the normal range. Family history was remarkable for tremors in grandfather. He was first seen by the pediatric neurologist for unsteady gait and toe walking at the age of 3.5 years with the gait unsteadiness commencing around the age of 2.5 years with frequent falls. Tremors in the hands were noted sometime previous to the clinic visit. Examination was notable for a well-developed child with a normal funduscopic exam, no cardiac murmur, and normal mental status including speech, normal cranial nerves, and strength. He had 1+ deep tendon reflexes (DTRs) in both upper and lower extremities with down going toes. Gait was wide based and unsteady. He had a tremor in both hands.

By the age of 6.5 years he had progressed to more falls and worsening handwriting. Examination revealed pes cavus, mild scoliosis, and absence of cardiac murmur. Neurological exam was notable for trace to absent DTRs, loss of position sense, positive Romberg, downgoing toes, slowed rapid alternating movements, tremor on finger to nose exam, and wide based unsteady gait.

By the age of 7 years he had more frequent falls and worsening handwriting. Examination showed progression with respect to ataxia in upper and lower limbs with wider based gait. DTRs were absent and a positive Babinski was noted.

At last exam around the age of 7.5 years he was falling more, and exam showed evidence of increased tone in lower extremities with foot drop and steppage gait in addition to decreased proprioception in the lower extremities and inconsistent responses in the upper extremities.

Magnetic resonance imaging of the brain was normal. Laboratory testing including quantitative immunoglobulins, alpha fetoprotein, thyroid profile, serum lactate, vitamin E levels, creatine kinase, serum amino acids, and serum acylcarnitine profile were all normal. Echocardiogram showed global hypertrophy of both ventricles. Ophthalmological examination did not show any evidence of optic atrophy.

Mutation analysis showed one allele with a GAA trinucleotide repeat expansion of approximately 1000. Since the index of suspicion was high, frataxin sequencing was done which demonstrated another allele harboring a c.464G>A nucleotide change. The nucleotide change predicted an amino acid substitution of tryptophan to a premature stop codon at residue 155 (W155X).

3. Discussion

The classic Friedreich's ataxia phenotype (95-98%) is due to a homozygous GAA triplet repeat expansion in intron 1 of the FXN gene (Figure 1(a)), which results in low frataxin protein levels, whereas compound heterozygous (2-5%) individuals possess GAA trinucleotide repeat expansion on one allele and point mutation on the other allele, as seen in our patient (Figure 1(b)).

Including our patient there are four other reported nonsense mutations. Campuzano et al. [9] published the case of a French family with 2 affected siblings with a T to G transversion in exon 3 that changed a leucine to a stop codon (L106X). De Castro et al. [14] reported a Cuban patient from Florida, USA, with a G to A nucleotide change in exon 4 that resulted in substitution of tryptophan to a stop codon, similar to our patient (W155X). Gellera et al. [12] reported an Italian patient with a C to G transversion leading to a substitution of tyrosine to a stop codon (Y118X) in exon 3 (Figure 1(c)).

Clinical features of the known nonsense Friedrich's ataxia patients are listed in Table 1. All patients were males. Age at onset of symptoms was before 15. All patients presented with gait ataxia, upper motor neuron signs, dysarthria, decreased vibration, and scoliosis. Upper and lower limb areflexia and cardiomyopathy were present in all except sibling 2 from the French family. Diabetes was not found in any patients. Hearing loss was not present in most of the patients and presence or absence of hearing was not mentioned in the siblings from France.

From the collective works of Cossee et al. [11] and Gellera et al. [12], some patterns have emerged with respect

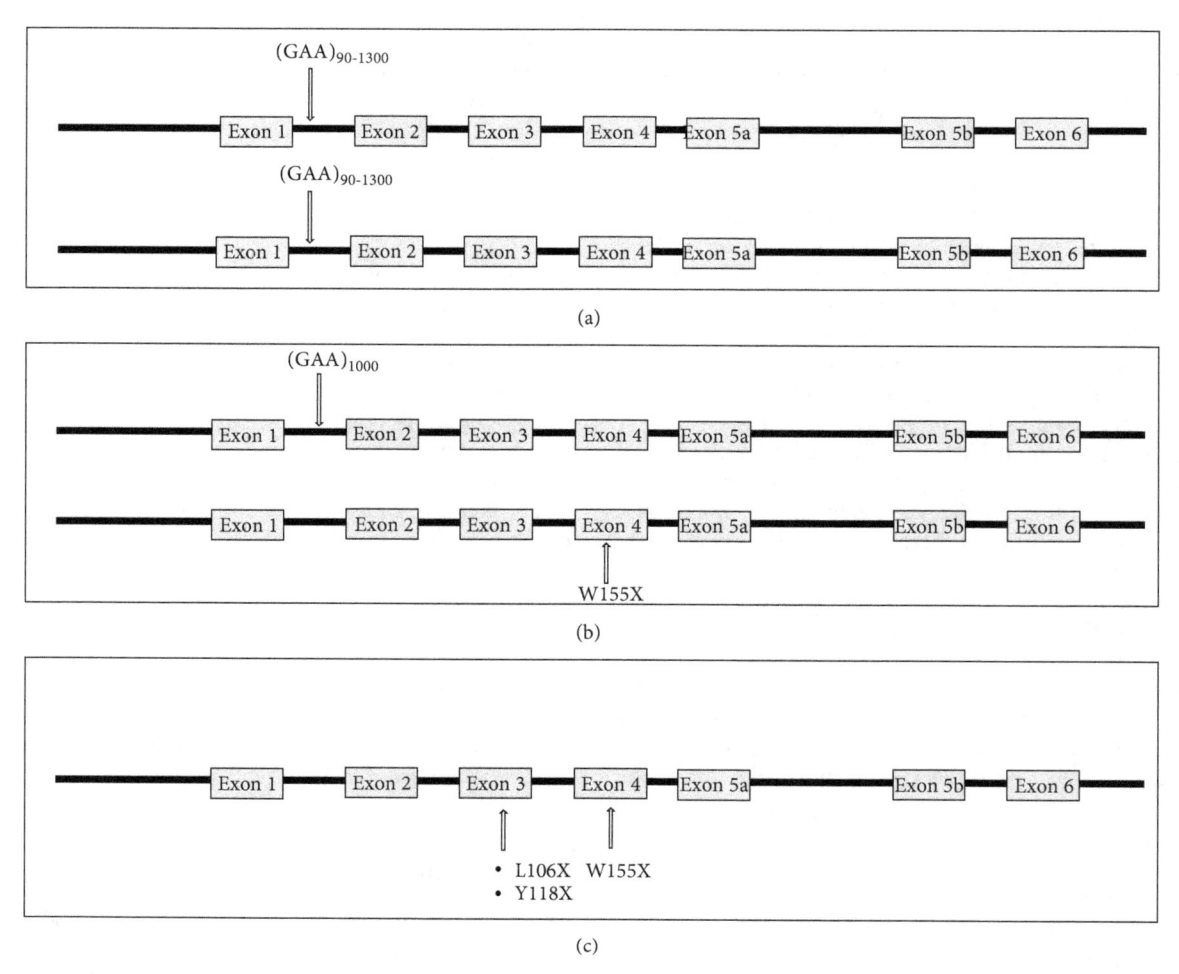

FIGURE 1: (a) Homozygous GAA triplet repeat expansion. (b) Compound heterozygosity with a point mutation in the second allele resulting in a stop codon, as in our patient. (c) Other known compound heterozygous cases resulting in a nonsense mutation from review of literature.

to disease onset and clinical features when homozygous trinucleotide repeat expansion is compared to those with compound heterozygosity. As discussed in those papers, the onset of symptoms is significantly earlier in the compound heterozygous patients (before 25 years of age). The offered explanation is that the repeat expansion in the homozygous patients is significantly smaller and becomes the determinant of the age of onset. This seems to suggest that the residual expression of frataxin protein determines the clinical phenotype. Therefore, in compound heterozygotes the frataxin protein is very low in quantity with a larger repeat expansion on one allele and no protein is expressed with the point mutation on the other allele. Other clinical features that have been noted from the work of Cossee and Gellera et al. is the lower incidence of dysarthria and higher incidence of optic atrophy (especially where expansions were greater than 700 repeats).

Interestingly enough, all the patients with the known nonsense mutations were male. The nonsense mutation hot spots seem to center in exons 3 and 4 of the frataxin gene. Some features were consistent with what is known about compound heterozygotes with an early onset, upper motor signs, gait ataxia, decreased vibratory sensation, and cardiomyopathy. Age at onset was directly proportional to the number of trinucleotide repeat expansion sizes in the nonsense mutations too. Our patient demonstrated the earliest onset which correlated with approximately 1000 repeats, higher than the other patients. Our patient's ancestry on the paternal side was Cuban which was similar to the W155X nonsense mutation described by De Castro et al. [14].

The sample size for phenotypic generalization of children presenting with nonsense mutations is small and our patient is only 8 years of age. As such clinical pattern recognition with respect to absence of diabetes, hearing loss and optic atrophy in our patient cannot be thought of as unique. Furthermore, genetic and clinical heterogeneity has emerged within compound heterozygous mutations. Although lower levels of frataxin are seen in compound heterozygotes compared to homozygous GAA repeat expansions, levels of frataxin can be significantly different in tissues among different mutations, leading to variabilities in clinical phenotype [15]. There is evidence that certain mutations such as G130V or I154F, although compound heterozygote, have milder clinical phenotypes [16].

Table 1: Clinical features of Friedrich's ataxia patients with nonsense mutations.

Mutation	L106X (Sibling 1)	L106X (Sibling 2)	W155X	Y118X	W155X Our patient
Geographical origin	France	France	USA (Cuban origin)	Italy	USA (Father Cuban)
GAA repeat size	733	700	850	640	1000
Gender	Male	Male	Male	Male	Male
Age at onset (years)	9	13	4	14	2.5
Age at last exam (years)	35	32	Unknown	27	8
Gait ataxia	+	+	+	+	+
Nystagmus	+	+	-	+	-
Deep Tendon Reflexes	-	+, upper limbs	-	-	-
Babinski sign	+, unilateral	+	+	+	+
Vibration sense	↓	↓	↓	↓	↓
Foot deformity	+	+	+	-	+
Cardiomyopathy	+	-	+	+	+
Scoliosis	+	+	+	+	+
Optic disks	Pallor	Pallor	No atrophy	No atrophy	No atrophy
Dysarthria	+	+	+	+	+
Diabetes	-	-	-	-	-
Hearing loss	Not reported	Not reported	-	-	-

In conclusion, if the index of suspicion is high for Friedrich's ataxia then frataxin sequencing should be performed if there is a repeat expansion detected only on one allele. Secondly, for the most part, compound heterozygous patients have an earlier age of onset that directly correlates with the trinucleotide expansion size. Finally, whether there is a unique phenotype to the nonsense mutations requires further study before counseling families regarding natural history of disease.

References

[1] A. H. Koeppen, "Friedreich's ataxia: Pathology, pathogenesis, and molecular genetics," *Journal of the Neurological Sciences*, vol. 303, no. 1-2, pp. 1–12, 2011.

[2] F. Taroni and S. DiDonato, "Pathways to motor incoordination: The inherited ataxias," *Nature Reviews Neuroscience*, vol. 5, no. 8, pp. 641–655, 2004.

[3] P. Salazar, R. Indorkar, M. Dietrich, and A. Farzaneh-Far, "Cardiomyopathy in Friedreich's ataxia," *European Heart Journal*, vol. 39, no. 7, p. 631, 2018.

[4] A. Pappa, M. G. Häusler, A. Veigel et al., "Diabetes mellitus in Friedreich Ataxia: A case series of 19 patients from the German-Austrian diabetes mellitus registry," *Diabetes Research and Clinical Practice*, vol. 141, pp. 229–236, 2018.

[5] A. E. Harding, "Friedreich's ataxia: a clinical and genetic study of 90 families with an analysis of early diagnostic criteria and intrafamilial clustering of clinical features," *Brain*, vol. 104, no. 3, pp. 589–620, 1981.

[6] M. B. Delatycki and L. A. Corben, "Clinical features of Friedreich ataxia," *Journal of Child Neurology*, vol. 27, no. 9, pp. 1133–1137, 2012.

[7] S. Chamberlain, J. Shaw, A. Rowland et al., "Mapping of mutation causing Friedreich's ataxia to human chromosome 9," *Nature*, vol. 334, no. 6179, pp. 248–250, 1988.

[8] L. Montermini, F. Rodius, L. Pianese et al., "The Friedreich ataxia critical region spans a 150-kb interval on chromosome 9q13," *American Journal of Human Genetics*, vol. 57, no. 5, pp. 1061–1067, 1995.

[9] V. Campuzano, L. Montermini, M. D. Moltò et al., "Friedreich's ataxia: autosomal recessive disease caused by an intronic GAA triplet repeat expansion," *Science*, vol. 271, no. 5254, pp. 1423–1427, 1996.

[10] A. Filla, G. De Michele, F. Cavalcanti et al., "The relationship between trinucleotide (GAA) repeat length and clinical features in Friedreich ataxia," *American Journal of Human Genetics*, vol. 59, no. 3, pp. 554–560, 1996.

[11] M. Cossée, A. Dürr, M. Schmitt et al., "Friedreich's ataxia: Point mutations and clinical presentation of compound heterozygotes," *Annals of Neurology*, vol. 45, no. 2, pp. 200–206, 1999.

[12] C. Gellera, B. Castellotti, C. Mariotti et al., "Frataxin gene point mutations in Italian Friedreich ataxia patients," *neurogenetics*, vol. 8, no. 4, pp. 289–299, 2007.

[13] C. A. Galea, A. Huq, P. J. Lockhart et al., "Compound heterozygous FXN mutations and clinical outcome in friedreich ataxia," *Annals of Neurology*, vol. 79, no. 3, pp. 485–495, 2016.

[14] M. De Castro, J. García-Planells, E. Monrós et al., "Genotype and phenotype analysis of Friedreich's ataxia compound heterozygous patients," *Human Genetics*, vol. 106, no. 1, pp. 86–92, 2000.

[15] M. Lazaropoulos, Y. Dong, E. Clark et al., "Frataxin levels in peripheral tissue in Friedreich ataxia," *Annals of Clinical and Translational Neurology*, vol. 2, no. 8, pp. 831–842, 2015.

[16] E. Clark, J. S. Butler, C. J. Isaacs, M. Napierala, and D. R. Lynch, "Selected missense mutations impair frataxin processing in Friedreich ataxia," *Annals of Clinical and Translational Neurology*, vol. 4, no. 8, pp. 575–584, 2017.

Never Too Old? Occurrence of Medulloblastoma in the Elderly beyond the 70th Year of Life

Homajoun Maslehaty,[1] Johannes Van de Nes,[2] Sarah Teuber-Hanselmann,[2] Christoph Moenninghoff,[3] Ulrich Sure,[4] and Neriman Oezkan[4]

[1]Department of Neurosurgery, Nordstadt Hospital, Hannover, Germany
[2]Institute of Neuropathology, Faculty of Medicine, University Duisburg-Essen, University Hospital Essen, Germany
[3]Institute of Neuroradiology, Faculty of Medicine, University Duisburg-Essen, University Hospital Essen, Germany
[4]Department of Neurosurgery, University Duisburg-Essen, University Hospital Essen, Germany

Correspondence should be addressed to Homajoun Maslehaty; h.maslehaty@gmx.de

Academic Editor: Mehmet Turgut

The occurrence of medulloblastoma (MB) in the elderly is an absolutely rare event. Concerning this issue we report on two MB patients beyond the 70th year of life. Two patients older than 70 years presented with a mass in the posterior fossa without evidence of a preexisting malignant tumor. After careful radiological work-up the suspected diagnosis was metastasis of an unknown primary tumor. Both patients underwent surgery and histopathological analysis revealed MB in both cases (classical MB and desmoplastic type). The two cases presented here represent also one classical MB and one additional desmoplastic MB. To our knowledge we report for the first time that there are different molecular subtypes of MB in the elderly patients that seem to be consistent with those subtypes mainly occurring in young adults. Unfortunately the patients died within one week after surgery due to respiratory insufficiency and an unclear cause. The presented cases show that MB can occur in the elderly. Although this constellation is absolutely rare, MB should be considered in the differential diagnosis, especially when a primary tumor is not known or detected.

1. Introduction

Medulloblastomas (MB) are small, round, blue cell, neuroectodermal tumors with neuronal differentiation in the cerebellum. These tumors usually occur in childhood. The incidence of MB in young adults is estimated to be less than 1% of all intracranial neoplasms [1, 2]. The mean age at time of diagnosis is estimated with 26 years [3]. The occurrence of MB in the elderly is an absolutely rare event. Concerning this issue we report on two MB patients beyond the 70th year of life.

2. Case Reports

Case 1 concerned a 71-year-old male presenting with gait difficulties and vertigo. Cranial MRI revealed a low and focal contrast-enhancing nodular tumor in the left cerebellar hemisphere and upper vermis (Figure 1). The lesion appeared hypointense relative to gray matter on T1 weighted (T1w) images and moderately hyperintense on T2w images. Tumor margins were best displayed on diffusion weighted images (DWI). The suspected clinical diagnosis was metastasis from an unknown primary tumor. Microsurgical resection of the tumor was performed. Histopathological work-up revealed a highly cellular tumor consisting of small cells with scant cytoplasm and round-oval or pleomorphic, hyperchromatic cells in the cerebellum. A part of the tumor showed a nodular architecture and a desmoplastic component (Gomori staining). Some tumor cells expressed the neuronal differentiation marker synaptophysin. The diagnosis was paucinodular desmoplastic MB (WHO grade IV). Tumor cells showed nuclear YAP1 and cytoplasmic GAB1 staining, while nuclear staining for ß-catenin and staining for p53 was negative. There was no MYC- or MYCN-amplification detectable (Figure 2). The patient's condition was stable in the continuing

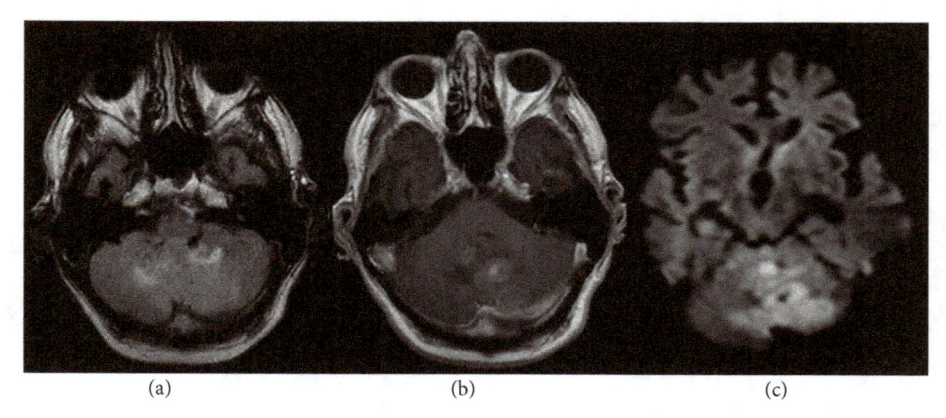

FIGURE 1: Transversal 1.5 Tesla FLAIR images (a) of a left cerebellar and vermal medulloblastoma show poor tumor delineation and inhomogeneous hyperintensity. Medulloblastomas normally appear hypointense relative to gray matter on T1w images with minimal to patchy contrast enhancement (b) and moderate restriction on diffusion weighted images (c).

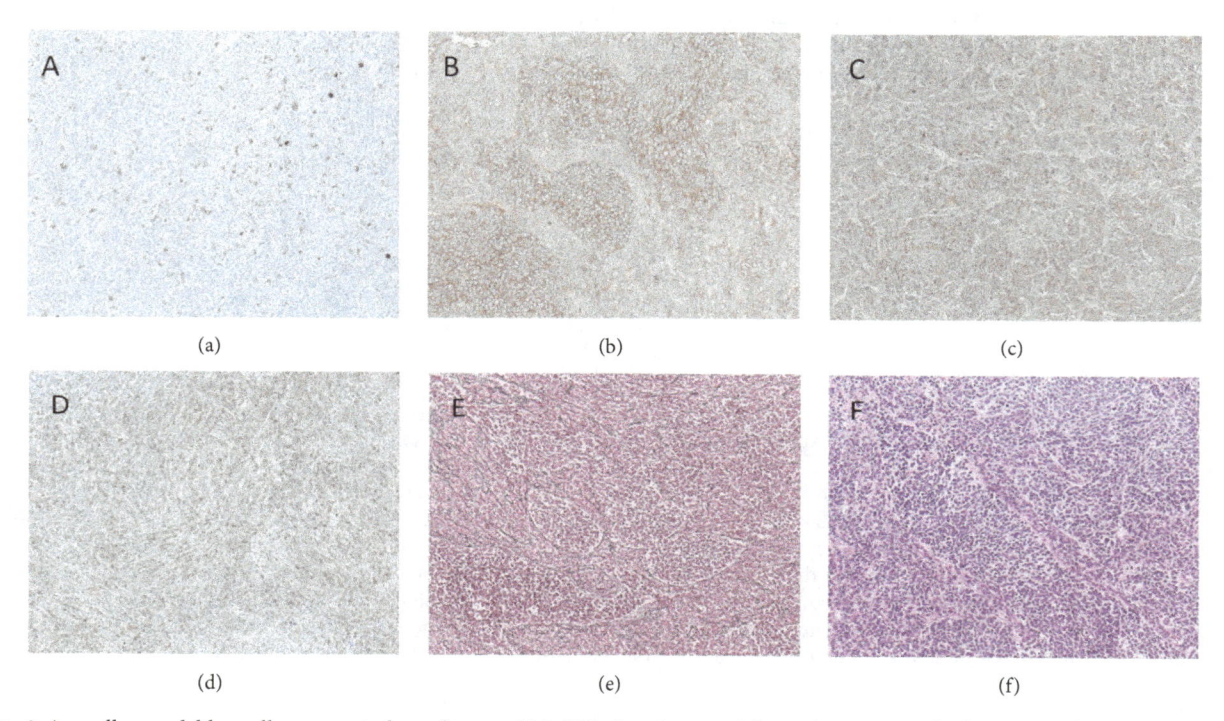

FIGURE 2: A small, round, blue cell, neuroectodermal tumor ((a), HE) showing a nodular architecture and a dense reticulin fiber network ((b), Gomori). Tumor cells showed nuclear expression of YAP1 (c) and cytoplasmic expression of GAB1 (d) while there was no nuclear expression of beta-catenin (e). Ki67-labelling reveals high proliferative activity (f).

course; however a week later he was affected by a severe pneumonia and died due to respiratory insufficiency.

Case 2 was a 72-year-old male who was referred to the hospital because of change of personality and loss of weight. Cranial MRI showed a large low contrast-enhancing mass in the right cerebellar hemisphere consisting of a lateral solid component and a small medial cystic. The tumor caused occlusive hydrocephalus but no surrounding edema (Figure 3). MR revealed diffusion restriction of the solid tumor part and peripheral susceptibility effects, e.g., hemosiderin deposits. Once again, the first suspected diagnosis was metastasis without presence of any neoplasm in the patient history; the second radiological diagnosis was MB. The possibility of a high-grade glioma was discussed but neglected due to its rare occurrence in the cerebellum in this age group. Prior to surgery an external ventricular drainage was inserted. Complete tumor resection was performed. Histopathological examination showed a highly cellular cerebellar tumor consisting of sheets of uniform cells with a high nuclear/cytoplasmic ratio and round to oval hyperchromatic nuclei. Many tumor cells reacted for synaptophysin. There was no evidence of a nodular or desmoplastic component

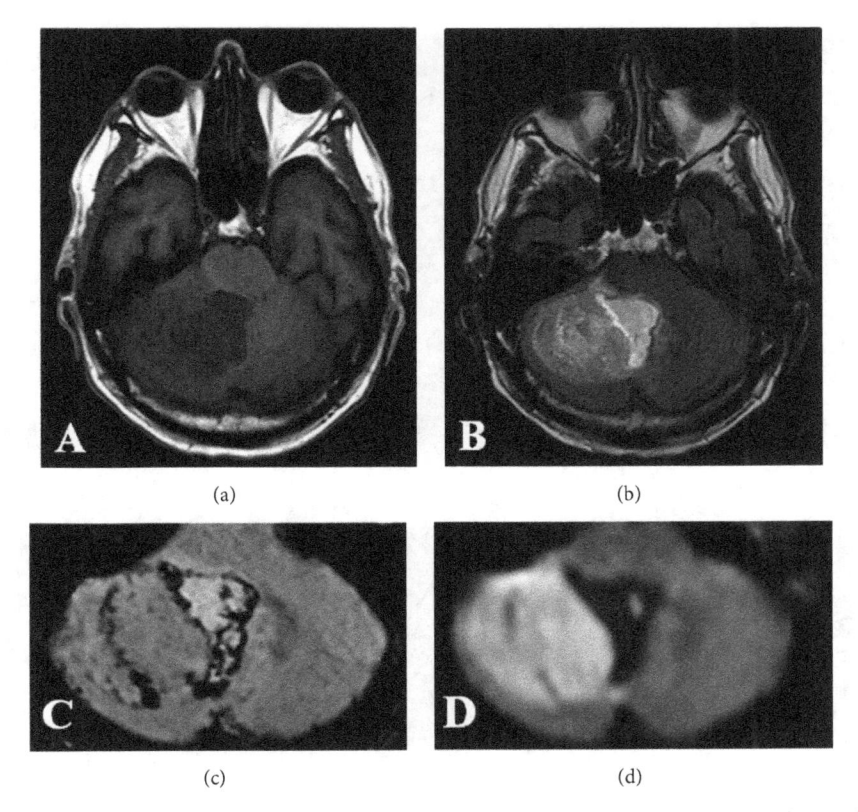

FIGURE 3: Transversal T1w image at 1.5 Tesla (a) shows a large hypointense tumor of the right cerebellar hemisphere with a hyperintense cyst on FLAIR images (b), which fills most of the fourth ventricle and causes obstructive hydrocephalus (not shown). Susceptibility weighted images (c) reveal hemosiderin deposits in the caudal tumor parts. Because of its dense cellularity, this tumor shows moderate restriction on diffusion weighted images (d).

in the Gomori staining. The diagnosis was that of a classical MB (WHO grade IV) (Figure 4). The tumor cells did not show staining for YAP1, GAB1, and p53 or nuclear staining for ß-catenin. Evidence of MYC- or MYCN-amplification was not found. The postoperative course was uneventful and the ventricular drainage was removed without evidence of an enlarged ventricular system. However, the patient was found dead seven days later in his room. The cause of unexpected death could not be clarified, since an autopsy was not allowed.

3. Discussion

Up to now there are four different molecular subtypes of MBs recognized, including activation of WNT-signaling pathway, SHH-signaling pathway, and the Non-WNT-/Non-SHH-subtype, which can be subdivided into group 3 (mostly MYC-amplified) and group 4 (often MYCN-amplified). Most of the desmoplastic MBs are of the SHH-activated subtype, whereas classic MBs are of the WNT- or the Non-WNT-/Non-SHH-subtype.

In contrast to children, in young adults the most common molecular subtypes are the SHH-activated/p53-wildtype and group 4 MB [4, 5]. Only five cases of MB occurring beyond the 70th year of life have been reported [6, 7]. All the reported cases were diagnosed as classical MB (WHO grade IV).

The two cases presented here represent also one classical MB and one additional desmoplastic MB. To our knowledge we report for the first time that there are different molecular subtypes of MB in the elderly patients that seem to be consistent with those subtypes mainly occurring in young adults.

Unfortunately the presented cases had a very unsatisfactory postoperative course, so that we cannot report any response of the patients to the planned radiotherapy in case 1 and combined radiochemotherapy in case 2.

Regarding the radiologic findings, we could not detect any differences to MB in younger ages. A moderate contrast-enhancing mass in T1-weighted sequences in the posterior fossa with surrounding brain edema and anatomical contact to the vermis and the fourth ventricle were typical findings. Histologic examination did not show any differences compared to the findings of MB occurring in younger patients.

The presented cases show that MB can occur in the elderly. Although this constellation is absolutely rare, MB should be considered in the differential diagnosis, especially when a primary tumor is not known or detected.

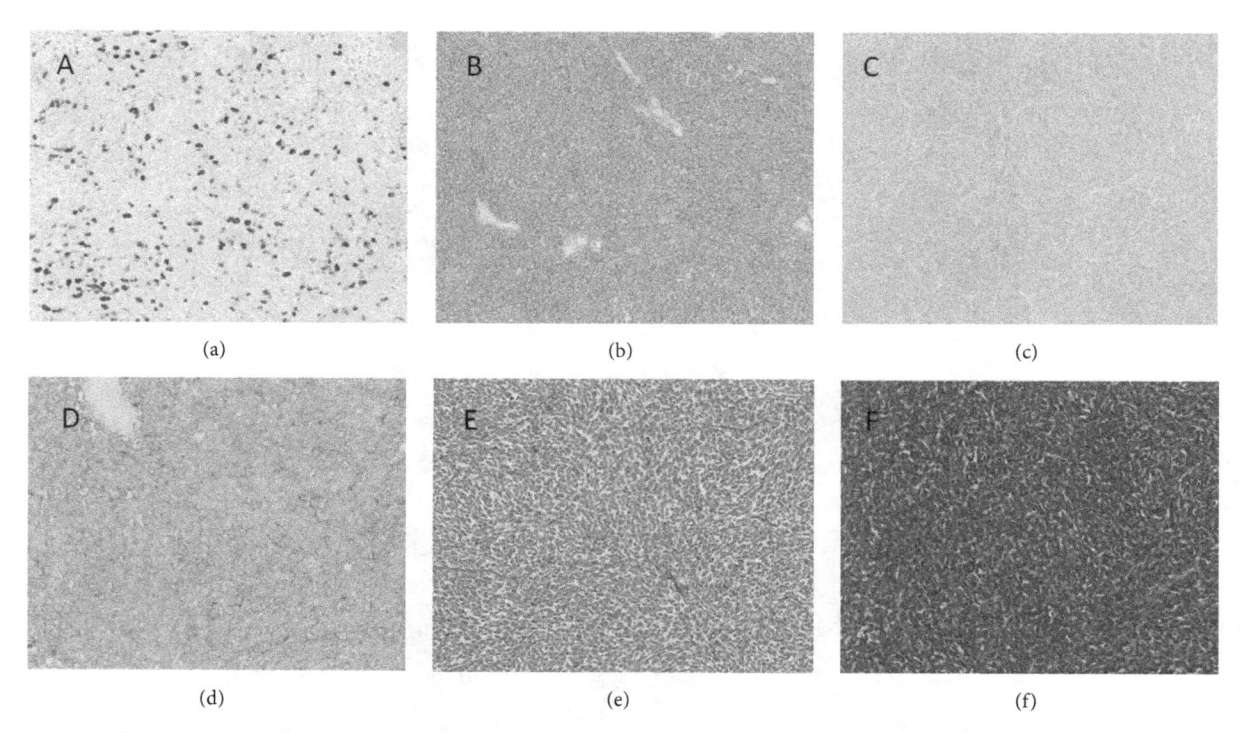

FIGURE 4: A small, round, blue cell, neuroectodermal tumor ((a), HE) without nodular architecture and without reticulin fiber network ((b), Gomori). Tumor cells showed expression of synaptophysin (c) but no expression of YAP1 and GAB1 (d). There was no nuclear expression of beta-catenin (e). Ki67-labelling reveals high proliferative activity (f).

References

[1] U. Abacioglu, O. Uzel, M. Sengoz, S. Turkan, and A. Ober, "Medulloblastoma in adults: Treatment results and prognostic factors," *International Journal of Radiation Oncology • Biology • Physics*, vol. 54, no. 3, pp. 855–860, 2002.

[2] N. Zhang, T. Ouyang, H. Kang, W. Long, B. Thomas, and S. Zhu, "Adult medulloblastoma: clinical characters, prognostic factors, outcomes and patterns of relapse," *Journal of Neuro-Oncology*, vol. 124, no. 2, pp. 255–264, 2015.

[3] C. Vigneron, D. Antoni, A. Coca et al., "Adult medulloblastoma: Retrospective series of 21 patients," *Cancer Radiothérapie*, vol. 20, no. 1, pp. 14–17, 2016.

[4] F. Zhao, H. Ohgaki, L. Xu et al., "Molecular subgroups of adult medulloblastoma: A long-term single-institution study," *Neuro-Oncology*, vol. 18, no. 7, pp. 982–990, 2016.

[5] F. J. Rodriguez, C. Eberhart, B. P. O'Neill et al., "Histopathologic grading of adult medulloblastomas," *Cancer*, vol. 109, no. 12, pp. 2557–2565, 2007.

[6] A. R. Huppmann, J. M. Orenstein, and R. V. Jones, "Cerebellar medulloblastoma in the elderly," *Annals of Diagnostic Pathology*, vol. 13, no. 1, pp. 55–59, 2009.

[7] B. Liang, E. Feng, Q. Wang et al., "Medulloblastoma in an elderly patient: A case report and literature review," *Molecular and Clinical Oncology*, vol. 5, no. 3, pp. 312–314, 2016.

Effect of Spinal Cord Stimulation on Gait in a Patient with Thalamic Pain

Arito Yozu,[1] Masahiko Sumitani,[2] Masahiro Shin,[3] Kazuhiko Ishi,[3] Michihiro Osumi,[4] Junji Katsuhira,[5] Ryosuke Chiba,[6] and Nobuhiko Haga[1]

[1]*Department of Rehabilitation Medicine, The University of Tokyo Hospital, 7-3-1 Hongo, Bunkyo-ku, Tokyo 113-8655, Japan*
[2]*Department of Pain and Palliative Medicine, The University of Tokyo Hospital, 7-3-1 Hongo, Bunkyo-ku, Tokyo 113-8655, Japan*
[3]*Department of Neurosurgery, The University of Tokyo Hospital, 7-3-1 Hongo, Bunkyo-ku, Tokyo 113-8655, Japan*
[4]*Neurorehabilitation Research Center, Kio University, 4-2-2 Umaminaka, Koryo-cho, Kitakatsuragi-gun, Nara 635-0832, Japan*
[5]*Department of Prosthetics and Orthotics and Assistive Technology, Faculty of Medical Technology, Niigata University of Health and Welfare, 1398 Shimami-cho, Kita-ku, Niigata, Niigata 950-3198, Japan*
[6]*Research Center for Brain Function and Medical Engineering, Asahikawa Medical University, 1-1-1 Higashi-2-jyou, Midorigaoka, Asahikawa, Hokkaido 078-8510, Japan*

Correspondence should be addressed to Arito Yozu; yodu-jscn@umin.net

Academic Editor: Paola Sandroni

Thalamic pain is a central neuropathic pain disorder which occurs after stroke. Its severe chronic pain is often intractable to pharmacotherapies and affects the patients' activities of daily living (ADL) and quality of life (QOL). Recently, spinal cord stimulation (SCS) has been reported to be effective in relieving the pain of thalamic pain; however, the effect of SCS on gait performance in patients is unknown. Therefore, we evaluated the gait performance before and after SCS in a case with thalamic pain. A 73-year-old male with thalamic pain participated in this study. We evaluated the gait of the patient two times: before SCS insertion and after 6 days of SCS. At the second evaluation, we measured the gait in three conditions: stimulation off, comfortable stimulation, and strong stimulation. SCS succeeded in improving the pain from 7 to 2 on an 11-point numerical rating scale. Step frequency and the velocity of gait tended to increase between pre- and poststimulation periods. There were no apparent differences in gait among the three stimulation conditions (off, comfortable, and strong) at the poststimulation period. SCS may be effective on gait in patients with thalamic pain.

1. Introduction

Thalamic pain is a central neuropathic pain disorder, which occurs after thalamic stroke. Of all the stroke survivors, 2.7%–8% patients suffer from thalamic pain [1, 2]. They generally experience severe chronic pain in the hemibody opposite to the thalamic lesion, and thalamic pain is often intractable to various pharmacotherapies. Consequently, thalamic pain generally affects the activities of daily living (ADL) and quality of life (QOL) in patients after stroke [3].

Spinal cord stimulation (SCS) is used to treat intractable pain disorders, including both central and peripheral neuropathic pain. For peripheral neuropathic pain, SCS has proven to be effective in relieving pain [4–8]. For thalamic pain (central neuropathic pain), the analgesic effect of SCS used to be uncertain; however, two recent studies showed its effectiveness in patients with central neuropathic pain [9, 10]. Lopez et al. reported that pain relief was satisfactory in 6 of 8 patients [10]. Aly et al. reported that half of the 30 patients experienced good or fair pain relief during the SCS trial [9].

Considering the clinical usefulness of SCS in patients with thalamic pain, we should focus not only on pain relief but also on its effect on gait because gait performance is the critical element of ADL and has a heavy impact on QOL [11–15]. Rijken et al. examined the effect of SCS on gait in peripheral neuropathic pain and found no significant change in step frequency, velocity, and step length [16]. However, there is no study that examined the effect of SCS on gait in central neuropathic pain. Therefore, how gait performance would change by SCS in central neuropathic pain is unknown. We may expect an increase in gait performance due to the pain relief. In this study, we first evaluated the gait performance before and after SCS in a single patient with thalamic pain.

2. Subject and Methods

2.1. Patient. A 73-year-old male with thalamic pain in his right hemibody for 2 years participated in this study. After left thalamic hemorrhage, he suffered from right hemiparesis and poststroke thalamic pain, mainly in his right upper and lower extremities. Thalamic pain was resistant to some pharmacotherapies, including pregabalin, antidepressants, and opioid, and he subsequently received SCS treatment. The patient provided his written informed consent prior to the study. All the procedures were performed in accordance with the Declaration of Helsinki, and they were approved by the institutional ethics committee.

2.2. SCS Procedure. The operation for SCS lead insertion was performed under local anesthesia with the guidance of fluoroscopy. Two eight-electrode leads (Octrode; St. Jude Medical, Inc., St. Paul, Minnesota, USA) were implanted at the 5th cervical (C5) and 8th thoracic (Th8) vertebrae-level epidural space. The upper lead treated pain in the upper extremity and the lower in the lower extremity. The leads were connected to a pulse generator (Genesis Patient Programmer; St. Jude Medical, Inc., St. Paul, Minnesota, USA).

Stimulation was initiated 1 day after the operation. A daily stimulation protocol was set at the discretion of the patient. Basically, the patient switched on the SCS generator during daytime and switched it off when he was asleep. When it was switched on, the amplitude was set between 0.8 and 8.0 mA, a rate of 4 Hz, and pulse width with 210–300 μsec. The stimulation protocol was selected by himself to induce the distribution of "comfortable" sense to his upper and lower extremities.

2.3. Pain Assessment. We used an 11-point numerical rating scale (NRS) for pain assessment [17–20]. The NRS is a segmented numerical version of the visual analog scale. The most commonly used is the 11-item NRS, in which the patient selects a whole number (0–10) that best reflects the intensity of his pain [17–20]. Here, 0 represents "no pain" and 10 represents "pain as bad as you can imagine."

2.4. Gait Assessment. We evaluated the gait of the patient two times: the day before SCS insertion and after 6 days of SCS period (Figure 1). His gait was measured by the motion analysis system (VICON MX; VICON Motion Systems Ltd., Oxford, UK). Reflective markers were placed on the body according to the modified Helen Hayes marker set [21]. Spatiotemporal parameters (step frequency, velocity, and stride length) and kinematics (range of motion (ROM) in extension/flexion of the hip, knee, and ankle during the gait) were calculated.

At the first evaluation, we could collect nine gait cycles from three trials. This was our best effort before the patient became too tired to continue. At the second evaluation,

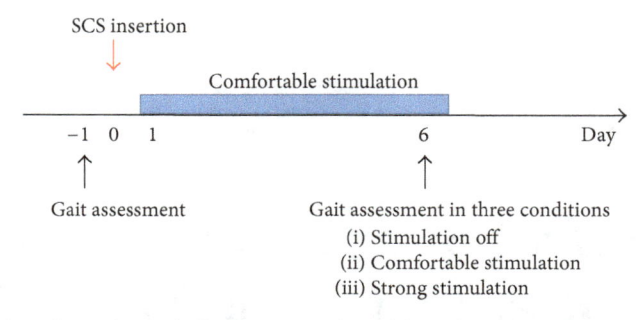

Figure 1: The study design. We evaluated the gait two times: the day before spinal cord stimulation (SCS) insertion and after 6 days of SCS period. At the second evaluation, we measured three conditions: SCS off, SCS comfortable, and SCS strong.

we measured the gait in three conditions: stimulation off, stimulating the SCS lead for the lower extremity under a "comfortable" setting, and stimulating under a "strong (but not noxious)" setting. We measured the gait of each condition immediately after switching to each condition during the second evaluation. The comfortable setting showed the amplitude of 3 mA for the lower SCS lead, and the strong setting showed 5 mA. Using 5 mA amplitude stimulation, he experienced a slight muscle twitch in his right foot. To extract the effect of SCS in the lower extremity, we did not stimulate the upper SCS lead for the upper extremity in any of these three conditions. In these three conditions of the second evaluation, we could collect 12 gait cycles from four trials for each condition. In total, it took 16 minutes to measure the three conditions.

2.5. Statistical Analysis. In total, we measured the gait in four conditions: (1) pre-SCS insertion, (2) stimulation off after 6 days of the SCS period, (3) "comfortable" stimulation after 6 days of the SCS period, and (4) "strong" stimulation after 6 days of the SCS period. We compared the spatiotemporal parameters and kinematics of these conditions using one-way analysis of variance (ANOVA). We set the significant level strictly at $p < 0.01$ to avoid false positives because of a single-case study. Multiple comparisons were made with the use of the Bonferroni method. Statistical analyses were performed using the Statistical Package for the Social Sciences (SPSS) (ver. 22, IBM Corp., NY, USA).

3. Results

3.1. Pain. The pain existed in the patient's whole right lower limb (from the toes to the hip and inguinal region) and in his right hand. The pain was 7 on the NRS before SCS and improved to 2 after 6 days of SCS. Because of the residual effect of SCS, the pain did not deteriorate even under the SCS-off condition in the post-SCS measurement.

3.2. Spatial and Temporal Parameters. The measurements of step frequency, velocity, and stride length in four conditions are shown in Figure 2. The step frequency significantly increased at the three postperiod conditions compared with

TABLE 1: Range of motion in extension/flexion during gait.

	Pre-SCS		SCS off		SCS comfortable		SCS strong	
	Mean	SD	Mean	SD	Mean	SD	Mean	SD
Left hip	31.8	2.1	37.5	2.6*	35.8	1.7*	36.4	2.8*
Right hip	31.0	6.3	33.4	3.4	31.4	2.4	30.9	3.5
Left knee	46.7	3.6	48.2	2.5	47.8	1.9	48.2	2.0
Right knee	41.8	11.4	37.7	5.8	34.4	2.9	35.3	7.3
Left ankle	25.0	4.8	29.9	4.8	30.9	2.6	29.6	4.0
Right ankle	11.4	2.8	13.4	2.1	13.0	1.5	13.4	4.2

*$p < 0.01$; significant difference between pre-SCS and SCS off, between pre-SCS and SCS comfortable, and between pre-SCS and SCS strong.
SCS, spinal cord stimulation.
SD, standard deviation.

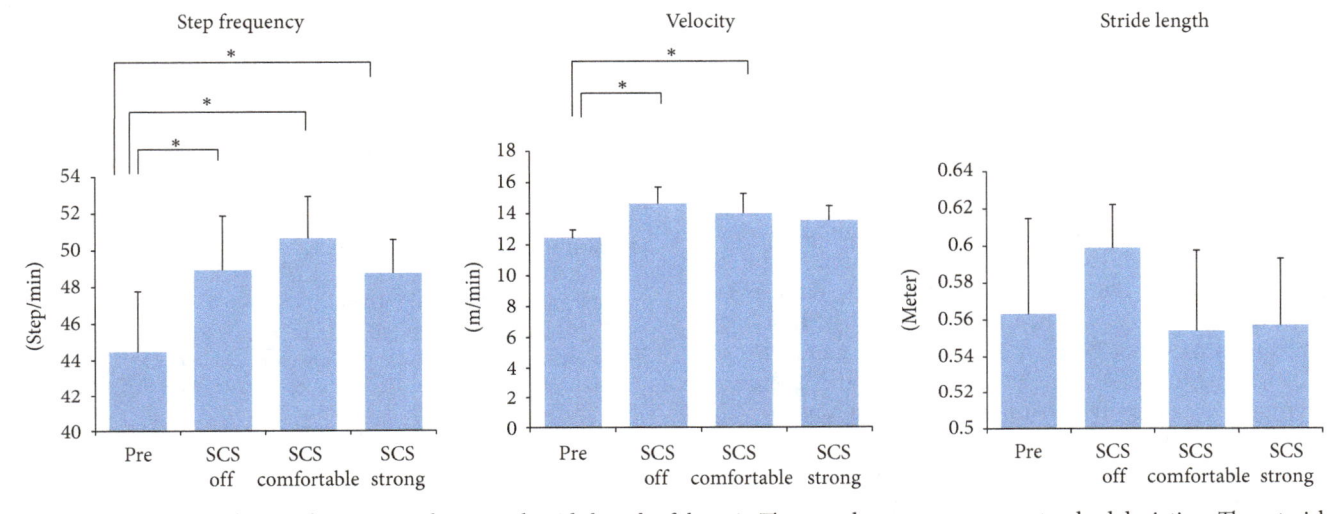

FIGURE 2: Mean values for step frequency, velocity, and stride length of the gait. The error bars represent one standard deviation. The asterisks indicate significant difference ($p < 0.01$).

that at the preperiod. There were no significant differences among the three poststimulation period conditions with respect to the step frequency.

The velocity of gait increased significantly between preperiod and SCS off at the postperiod and between preperiod and comfortable SCS at the postperiod. There were no significant differences among the three postperiod conditions with respect to the velocity.

Further, there were no differences in the stride length among the four conditions.

3.3. Kinematics. ROM in extension/flexion during the gait in the lower extremities is shown in Table 1. The motion of the left hip increased significantly between the prestimulation period and the other three poststimulation period conditions. However, the other remaining joints did not show any apparent change after 6 days of the SCS period.

4. Discussion

This study is the first to report the effect of SCS on gait in a patient with thalamic pain. SCS succeeded in improving the pain from 7 to 2 on an 11-point NRS. Step frequency and the velocity of gait tended to increase between pre- and poststimulation periods. There were no apparent differences in gait among the three stimulation conditions (off, comfortable, and strong) at the poststimulation period.

4.1. Pre- versus Poststimulation Period. The velocity of the gait tended to increase at the poststimulation period. Because velocity is the multiplication of length by frequency and because the stride length did not differ apparently between the conditions, the increase in velocity is due to the increase in step frequency.

The result of our study was different from that of Rijken et al. [16], which examined the effect of SCS in peripheral neuropathic pain and found no significant change in step frequency or velocity. Such a difference may exist on the original motor performances of the participants and also on methodological issues. The participants of the previous study had moderate gait impairment (e.g., the velocity was approximately 50 m/min), whereas our participant had more severe gait impairment (e.g., the velocity was approximately 14 m/min), and the impact of SCS did not appear in the previous study. Furthermore, the previous study used a treadmill to measure the gait performance. Generally, in treadmill walking, participants must adapt to the belt; therefore, measurements obtained by a treadmill are not necessarily similar to their natural gait performance. On the other hand, our study examined level gait, which would reflect more natural motor performance.

One most possible mechanism for the increase of the frequency is that the pain relief permitted the patient to move more freely. An intimate relationship between pain and motor dysfunction is known. For example, a study on patients with intermittent claudication demonstrated that the pain was related to the impairment of step frequency and walking speed [22]. This pattern is similar to our study's pattern.

The gait performance was improved even in the SCS-off condition compared with the pre-SCS condition. SCS has a residual effect on pain relief, and the patient did not complain of pain deterioration even when the SCS was turned off at post-SCS measurement. Compared with the pre-SCS condition, the patient had less pain in the SCS-off condition. We think this is why the gait improved in the SCS-off condition compared with the pre-SCS measurement.

Despite pain being present in the right hemibody, which was relieved by SCS, the joint motion increased in the left hip and not in the right. This is not surprising because the right hip is also the side of hemiparesis, and the effect of the pain relief might not be seen. On the other hand, the left hip is a proximal joint and adjacent to the right. Therefore, SCS may release the left hip from its restriction caused by the surrounding pain.

Another possibility for gait restoration is the effect of SCS apart from pain relief. There are studies on Parkinson's disease, spinal cord injury, and ataxia, where gait was improved by SCS [23–27]. The mechanism for this effect is unclear. One proposed is that locomotion is increased by the disruption of antikinetic oscillatory synchronization in the corticobasal ganglia circuits through the activation of lemniscal and brainstem pathways [24].

4.2. Poststimulation Period. There were no apparent differences among three stimulating conditions at the poststimulation period. SCS stimulates the dorsal column of the spine, including the medial lemniscal tract, which is the pathway of proprioception. Thus, SCS may interfere with proprioception and might affect the gait [28]. However, our data showed no apparent change even in strong stimulation. We tested level gait in our study, whereas dual-task gait or eye-closed-balance test may extract the effect on proprioception more sensitively. This will be our future work.

4.3. Limitations. This study examined only a single subject. Furthermore, we only studied one point after the insertion of SCS. The patient might adapt to SCS, and gait performance may change in the long term. A group study with a long-term follow-up is needed to evaluate the definite effect of SCS on gait in patients with thalamic pain. Nonetheless, this was the first study to highlight the gait performance in central neuropathic pain after SCS.

Competing Interests

The authors declare that there are no competing interests regarding the publication of this paper.

Acknowledgments

This research was supported partly by the Japan Society for the Promotion of Science KAKENHI (nos. 25870170, 15K01361, 15H01671, 26120006, and 26120008).

References

[1] G. Andersen, K. Vestergaard, M. Ingeman-Nielsen, and T. S. Jensen, "Incidence of central post-stroke pain," *Pain*, vol. 61, no. 2, pp. 187–193, 1995.

[2] M. J. O'Donnell, H.-C. Diener, R. L. Sacco, A. A. Panju, R. Vinisko, and S. Yusuf, "Chronic pain syndromes after ischemic stroke: PRoFESS trial," *Stroke*, vol. 44, no. 5, pp. 1238–1243, 2013.

[3] M. Widar and G. Ahlström, "Disability after a stroke and the influence of long-term pain on everyday life," *Scandinavian Journal of Caring Sciences*, vol. 16, no. 3, pp. 302–310, 2002.

[4] Health Quality Ontario, "Spinal cord stimulation for neuropathic pain: an evidence-based analysis," *Ontario Health Technology Assessment Series*, vol. 5, no. 4, pp. 1–78, 2005.

[5] K. Kumar, G. Hunter, and D. Demeria, "Spinal cord stimulation in treatment of chronic benign pain: challenges in treatment planning and present status, a 22-year experience," *Neurosurgery*, vol. 58, no. 3, pp. 481–496, 2006.

[6] A. Mailis-Gagnon, A. D. Furlan, J. A. Sandoval, and R. Taylor, "Spinal cord stimulation for chronic pain," *Cochrane Database of Systematic Reviews*, no. 3, Article ID CD003783, 2004.

[7] L. Manchikanti, S. Datta, S. Gupta et al., "A critical review of the American pain society clinical practice guidelines for interventional techniques: part 2. Therapeutic interventions," *Pain Physician*, vol. 13, no. 4, pp. E215–E264, 2010.

[8] R. S. Taylor, M. J. Desai, P. Rigoard, and R. J. Taylor, "Predictors of pain relief following spinal cord stimulation in chronic back and leg pain and failed back surgery syndrome: a systematic review and meta-regression analysis," *Pain Practice*, vol. 14, no. 6, pp. 489–505, 2014.

[9] M. M. Aly, Y. Saitoh, K. Hosomi, S. Oshino, H. Kishima, and T. Yoshimine, "Spinal cord stimulation for central poststroke pain," *Neurosurgery*, vol. 67, no. 1, pp. ons206–ons212, 2010.

[10] J. A. Lopez, L. M. Torres, F. Gala, and I. Iglesias, "Spinal cord stimulation and thalamic pain: long-term results of eight cases," *Neuromodulation*, vol. 12, no. 3, pp. 240–243, 2009.

[11] E. Andrenelli, E. Ippoliti, M. Coccia et al., "Features and predictors of activity limitations and participation restriction 2 years after intensive rehabilitation following first-ever stroke," *European Journal of Physical and Rehabilitation Medicine*, vol. 51, no. 5, pp. 575–585, 2015.

[12] C. Barrett and P. Taylor, "The effects of the odstock drop foot stimulator on perceived quality of life for people with stroke and multiple sclerosis," *Neuromodulation*, vol. 13, no. 1, pp. 58–64, 2010.

[13] K. H. Cho, J. Y. Lee, K. J. Lee, and E. K. Kang, "Factors related to gait function in post-stroke patients," *Journal of Physical Therapy Science*, vol. 26, no. 12, pp. 1941–1944, 2014.

[14] R. F. Macko, F. Benvenuti, S. Stanhope et al., "Adaptive physical activity improves mobility function and quality of life in

chronic hemiparesis," *Journal of Rehabilitation Research and Development*, vol. 45, no. 2, pp. 323–328, 2008.

[15] M. H. Ursin, H. Ihle-Hansen, B. Fure, A. Tveit, and A. Bergland, "Effects of premorbid physical activity on stroke severity and post-stroke functioning," *Journal of Rehabilitation Medicine*, vol. 47, no. 7, pp. 612–617, 2015.

[16] N. H. Rijken, L. H. Vonhögen, J. Duysens, and N. L. Keijsers, "The effect of spinal cord stimulation (SCS) on static balance and gait," *Neuromodulation*, vol. 16, no. 3, pp. 244–250, 2013.

[17] J. T. Farrar, J. P. Young Jr., L. LaMoreaux, J. L. Werth, and R. M. Poole, "Clinical importance of changes in chronic pain intensity measured on an 11-point numerical pain rating scale," *Pain*, vol. 94, no. 2, pp. 149–158, 2001.

[18] G. A. Hawker, S. Mian, T. Kendzerska, and M. French, "Measures of adult pain: Visual Analog Scale for Pain (VAS Pain), Numeric Rating Scale for Pain (NRS Pain), McGill Pain Questionnaire (MPQ), Short-Form McGill Pain Questionnaire (SF-MPQ), Chronic Pain Grade Scale (CPGS), Short Form-36 Bodily Pain Scale (SF-36 BPS), and Measure of Intermittent and Constant Osteoarthritis Pain (ICOAP)," *Arthritis Care and Research*, vol. 63, no. 11, pp. S240–S252, 2011.

[19] M. P. Jensen and C. A. McFarland, "Increasing the reliability and validity of pain intensity measurement in chronic pain patients," *Pain*, vol. 55, no. 2, pp. 195–203, 1993.

[20] C. S. Rodriguez, "Pain measurement in the elderly: a review," *Pain Management Nursing*, vol. 2, no. 2, pp. 38–46, 2001.

[21] T. D. Collins, S. N. Ghoussayni, D. J. Ewins, and J. A. Kent, "A six degrees-of-freedom marker set for gait analysis: repeatability and comparison with a modified Helen Hayes set," *Gait and Posture*, vol. 30, no. 2, pp. 173–180, 2009.

[22] K. A. Mockford, N. Vanicek, A. Jordan, I. C. Chetter, and P. A. Coughlin, "Kinematic adaptations to ischemic pain in claudicants during continuous walking," *Gait and Posture*, vol. 32, no. 3, pp. 395–399, 2010.

[23] T. Agari and I. Date, "Spinal cord stimulation for the treatment of abnormal posture and gait disorder in patients with Parkinson's disease," *Neurologia Medico-Chirurgica*, vol. 52, no. 7, pp. 470–474, 2012.

[24] R. Fuentes, P. Petersson, and M. A. L. Nicolelis, "Restoration of locomotive function in Parkinson's disease by spinal cord stimulation: mechanistic approach," *European Journal of Neuroscience*, vol. 32, no. 7, pp. 1100–1108, 2010.

[25] R. Fuentes, P. Petersson, W. B. Siesser, M. G. Caron, and M. A. L. Nicolelis, "Spinal cord stimulation restores locomotion in animal models of Parkinson's disease," *Science*, vol. 323, no. 5921, pp. 1578–1582, 2009.

[26] U. S. Hofstoetter, M. Krenn, S. M. Danner et al., "Augmentation of voluntary locomotor activity by transcutaneous spinal cord stimulation in motor-incomplete spinal cord-injured individuals," *Artificial Organs*, vol. 39, no. 10, pp. E176–E186, 2015.

[27] C. Sidiropoulos, K. Masani, T. Mestre et al., "Spinal cord stimulation for gait impairment in spinocerebellar ataxia 7," *Journal of Neurology*, vol. 261, no. 3, pp. 570–574, 2014.

[28] R. Chiba, K. Takakusaki, J. Ota, A. Yozu, and N. Haga, "Human upright posture control models based on multisensory inputs; in fast and slow dynamics," *Neuroscience Research*, vol. 104, pp. 96–104, 2016.

Profound Autonomic Instability Complicated by Multiple Episodes of Cardiac Asystole and Refractory Bradycardia in a Patient with Anti-NMDA Encephalitis

Stephanie R. Mehr,[1] Roy C. Neeley,[2] Melissa Wiley,[1] and Avinash B. Kumar[2]

[1]Department of Anesthesiology, Vanderbilt University, Nashville, TN 37212, USA
[2]Department of Anesthesiology, Division of Critical Care, Vanderbilt University, Nashville, TN 37212, USA

Correspondence should be addressed to Avinash B. Kumar; avinash.b.kumar@vanderbilt.edu

Academic Editor: Chin-Chang Huang

Anti-N-methyl-D-aspartate receptor encephalitis (anti-NMDARE) is autoimmune encephalitis primarily affecting young adults and children. First described about a decade ago, it frequently manifests as a syndrome that includes progressive behavioral changes, psychosis, central hypoventilation, seizures, and autonomic instability. Although cardiac arrhythmias often accompany anti-NMDARE, the need for long-term electrophysiological support is rare. We describe the case of NMDARE whose ICU course was complicated by progressively worsening episodes of tachyarrhythmia-bradyarrhythmia and episodes of asystole from which she was successfully resuscitated. Her life-threatening episodes of autonomic instability were successfully controlled only after the placement of a permanent pacemaker during her ICU stay. She made a clinical recovery and was discharged to a skilled nursing facility after a protracted hospital course.

1. Introduction

Anti-N-methyl-D-aspartate receptor encephalitis (anti-NMDARE) is a severe form of autoimmune encephalitis resulting from autoantibodies directed against GluN1 subunits of the NMDA receptor in the central nervous system. Dalmau and colleagues described this condition, which primarily affects young adults and children, for the first time as recently as 2007 [1, 2]. Patients frequently present with variable neuropsychiatric symptoms ranging from psychosis to seizures to catatonia, adding to the complexity of an early diagnosis. We obtained written consent from the patient's family to present a complex case of anti-NMDARE with catatonia, seizures, acute respiratory failure, and profound autonomic instability requiring aggressive interventions including multiple rounds of CPR and cardiac pacing in the ICU. We seek to focus on the ICU course of illness in this complex patient with a protracted hospital course.

2. Case Report

Our patient was a 31-year-old African American female with a 2-3-week history of acute behavioral changes, personality breakdown, sexual inappropriateness, and religious grandiosity. Her past medical history was significant for asthma, genital HSV, and polycystic ovarian syndrome. She was admitted to the psychiatry service for evaluation of her acute behavioral changes and cognitive decline. During her admission, she developed new onset grand-mal seizures and was transferred to the neurologic intensive care unit. She continued to have frequent seizures and began to develop worsening catatonia. The neurological workup included multimodal imaging and CSF studies that were positive for GluN1 antibodies, supporting a diagnosis of anti-NMDARE. Subsequent workup including CT scans of the chest, abdomen, and pelvis, ultrasound of the pelvis, and a PET scan was negative for a tumor etiology. Our patient did not have a tumor etiology.

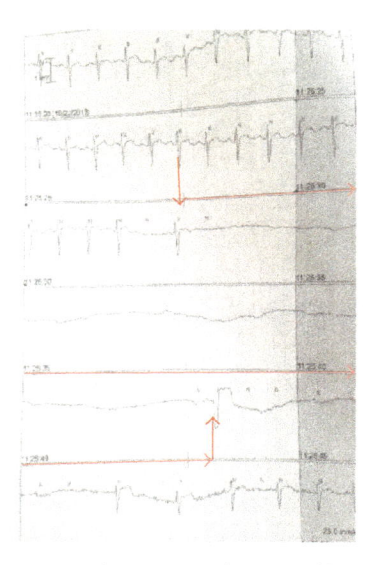

FIGURE 1: EKG strips with arrows outlining sudden progression of sinus tachycardia to asystole for more than 15 seconds before an escape beat and return of sinus rhythm (spontaneously).

FIGURE 2: EKG strips with arrows outlining progression of severe bradycardia to transient asystole with return of sinus rhythm (spontaneously).

As the frequency of seizures increased, her mental status deteriorated and she was intubated for airway protection on hospital day 18. She had escalating episodes of autonomic instability, manifested by episodes ranging from narrow complex tachycardia with heart rates in the 140–160 bpm to severe bradycardia induced by vasovagal maneuvers such as coughing, suctioning of the endotracheal tube, and defecation. These episodes were initially self-limited but over subsequent days necessitated active pharmacologic intervention including combination of multiple rounds of glycopyrrolate and/or atropine and low doses of epinephrine during the episodes.

The initial treatment of the bradycardic episodes was targeted at reduction of vagal stimuli and triggers for bradycardia. This included suppression of coughing episodes with intravenous fentanyl and premedication with inhaled lidocaine before endotracheal suctioning. Intermittent propofol and ketamine sedation were also attempted to decrease vasovagal triggers but no clinical efficacy was appreciated. An early tracheostomy (ICU day 5) was done to help alleviate the airway irritation, decrease IV sedation, and facilitate mobilization.

The patient continued to have two further episodes of severe bradycardia that progressed to cardiac asystole necessitating cardiopulmonary resuscitation. The period of asystole was recognized early and immediate initiation of CPR and chest compressions were carried out for two minutes with return of circulation. The EKG recordings showing progression to severe bradycardia are shown in Figures 1 and 2. She was transcutaneously paced during one episode to manage severe bradyarrhythmias as doses of glycopyrrolate and atropine (aliquots of 0.2 mg IV doses) were ineffective. Cardiac workup, including electrocardiogram, cardiac enzymes, and echocardiogram, was all within normal limits. Episodes of bradycardia and SVT occurred daily, until twenty days after the first episode of bradycardia, when a permanent pacemaker was placed. A snapshot of the episodes of autonomic instability is outlined in Figure 3.

The patient received multiple therapies including high dose methylprednisolone and IVIg, immunotherapy with rituximab, intrathecal methotrexate, and an extended course of electroconvulsive therapy (ECT) for her profound catatonia. A visual snapshot of treatments offered is outlined in Figure 4.

The patient was discharged initially to a skilled nursing facility and then home. She made a good clinical recovery with the ability to take care of herself and family in due time.

Posthospital discharge interrogation of the pacemaker revealed 32 episodes of SVT (the longest lasting six and a half minutes) but no further severe bradycardia episodes beyond four days after pacemaker insertion.

3. Discussion

Our case illustrates the variable presentation and multisystem complexities that are involved in the care of this relatively new entity: anti-NMDA receptor encephalitis. From an epidemiological perspective, anti-NMDARE may be one of the more common causes of autoimmune encephalitis. The reported frequency of tumor or paraneoplastic association is also evolving as the literature accumulates about anti-NMDARE [3]. A recent large multicenter observational study of 577 patients found the association with a tumor etiology (teratomas) in less than 40% of cases [3]. Tumor etiology was ruled out in our patient.

We focus on the cardiovascular and autonomic instability in our case presentation. Bradycardia related to seizure activity and autonomic instability in anti-NMDARE has been previously reported [3, 4]. Central autonomic control of heart rate is surprisingly complex. Simplistically the resting

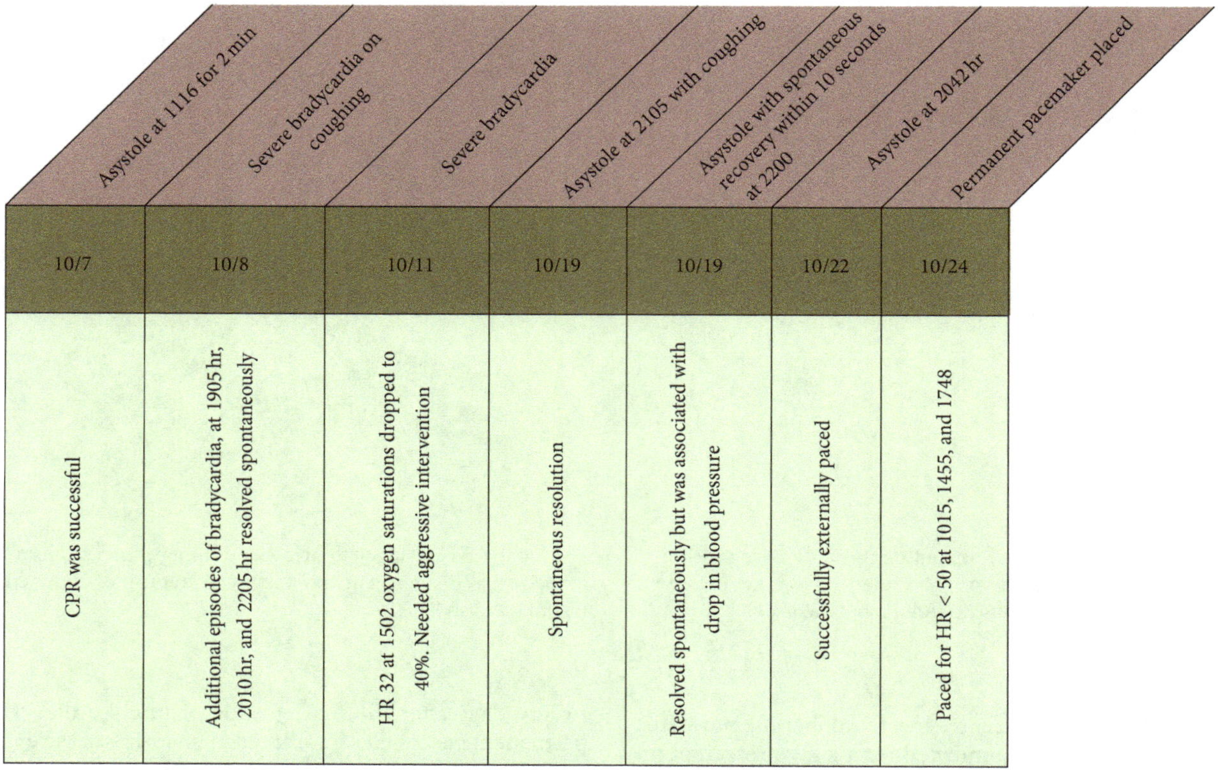

	10/7	10/8	10/11	10/19	10/19	10/22	10/24
Event	Asystole at 1116 for 2 min	Severe bradycardia on coughing	Severe bradycardia	Asystole at 2105 with coughing	Asystole with spontaneous recovery within 10 seconds at 2200	Asystole at 2042 hr	Permanent pacemaker placed
Intervention	CPR was successful	Additional episodes of bradycardia, at 1905 hr, 2010 hr, and 2205 hr resolved spontaneously	HR 32 at 1502 oxygen saturations dropped to 40%. Needed aggressive intervention	Spontaneous resolution	Resolved spontaneously but was associated with drop in blood pressure	Successfully externally paced	Paced for HR < 50 at 1015, 1455, and 1748

Figure 3: Timeline of autonomic instability and interventions in the ICU.

heart rate is a function of the cardiogenic pacemaker and a balance between the bradycardiogenic parasympathetic system and the positive chronotropic sympathetic system. Mapping studies in animals have shown that several regions of the telencephalon, including the insula, anterior cingulate cortices, and amygdala, are involved in modulation of cardiac sympathetic and parasympathetic outflow. These connections eventually influence the preganglionic sympathetic and parasympathetic neurons of the heart [1]. Seizure induced activation can result in a synchronization of cardiac autonomic discharges with epileptogenic activity called the "lockstep" phenomenon and induces a lethal bradyarrhythmia or even asystole [4]. However in our case, not all bradycardia episodes were precipitated by vagal or epileptogenic stimuli. As the frequency of episodes escalated, several episodes of bradycardia did not have a clear precipitating factor and moreover these episodes were progressively more resistant to pharmacological interventions.

Class I indications for temporary pacemakers in the ICU include asystole, symptomatic bradycardia with hypotension and/or not responsive to atropine, and bifascicular blocks. Other common indications for temporary pacing include drug toxicities (digoxin toxicity, beta-blocker) and hyperkalemic bradycardia [5]. Frequently cardiologists will refrain from placing a pacemaker if the underlying mechanism of tachyarrhythmia-bradyarrhythmia is deemed episodic and/or related to the hyperacute phase of an illness. There is variability in the practice of implanting permanent pacemakers in noncardiac diseases especially if the indication is perceived to be reversible or time limited [6]. In case of anti-NMDARE, the autonomic instability can last for several weeks to months after the disease onset [1].

Anti-NMDARE patients frequently present to psychiatry services as the first point of contact. The psychiatric symptoms range from psychosis, auditory and visual hallucinations, aggression, anxiety, obsessive-compulsive behaviors, and depression to frank catatonia [7, 8]. The diagnosis is established by a positive serum or CSF sample screening for antibodies to the NMDA receptor subunit. Admission brain MRI scans have been reported as normal in as high as 70% of cases and EEG may show nonspecific slowing or slow continuous rhythmic activity during the later catatonic phase of illness [9]. There are small case series that describe a pattern of rhythmic delta activity (1–3 Hz) with superimposed bursts of rhythmic (20–30 Hz) beta activity that has been labeled "extreme delta brush" [10]. Multiple EEGs in our patient at the time of ICU admission were reviewed as delta waves with intermixed beta activity suggestive of an extreme delta brush pattern. This pattern was noticeably absent prior to the patient's transfer out of the ICU.

The key to an early diagnosis is often having a high index of suspicion in this younger patient cohort with new onset of neuropsychiatric symptoms combined with autonomic instability with or without seizures [3]. Prognosis of patients

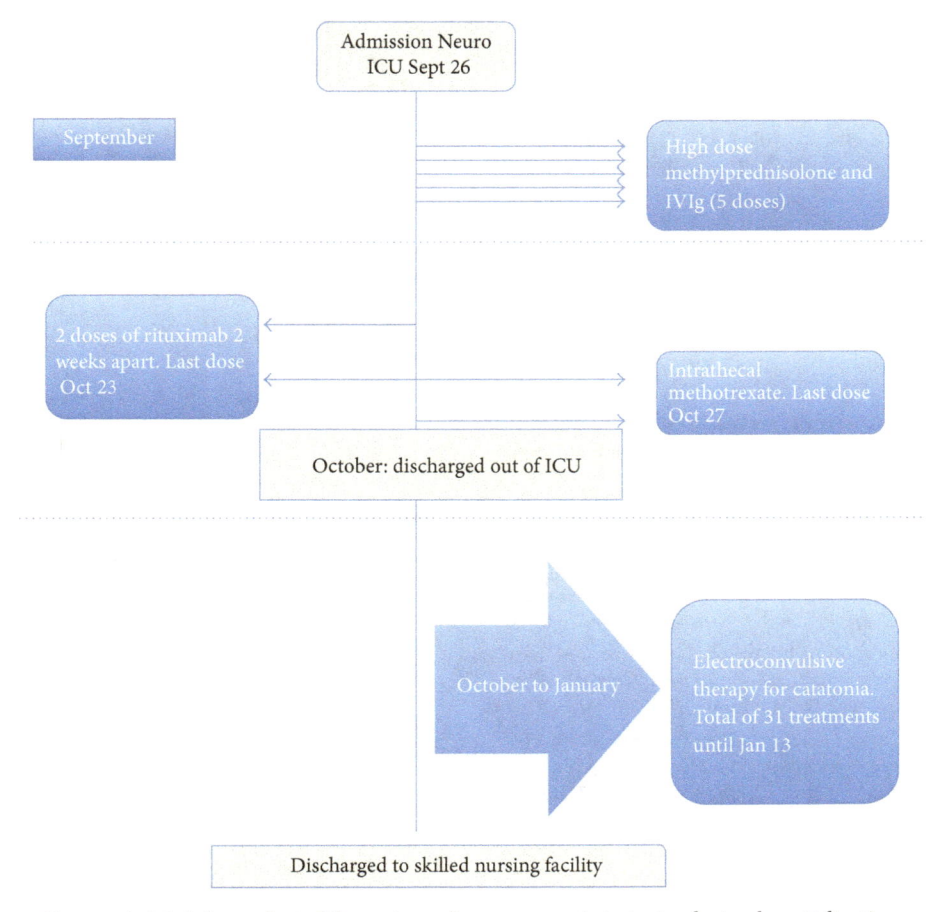

Figure 4: A brief snapshot of therapies and management strategies during hospitalization.

depends on early diagnosis, appropriate immunomodulatory therapy, and, in paraneoplastic cases, complete tumor removal. First-line immunotherapy is typically corticosteroids, intravenous immunoglobulins, or plasma exchange. Second-line therapy in resistant cases may necessitate using rituximab or cyclophosphamide and supportive care. Our patient underwent two courses of rituximab and intrathecal methotrexate as well.

The debilitating outcomes of anti-NMDARE are primarily from the persistent long-term cognitive deficits. It is worth noting that impairments in executive functions and memory can persist for an extended period of time even after clinical recovery and hospital discharge. Role of the NMDA receptors in the hippocampus is central to the postulated mechanism of cognitive and memory deficits. Connectivity to other areas such as the frontal cortices may play a role in the cognitive deficits as well [11].

Electroconvulsive therapy has been successfully tried in patients with severe psychiatric symptoms such as catatonia. Our patient underwent immunotherapy, immunosuppression, and long course of ECT prior to discharge. A schematic of the time course and treatments is outlined in Figure 3. Our patient had a recalcitrant course complicated by cardiorespiratory, psychiatric, and neurocognitive issues in spite of multimodal medical therapy until discharge from the hospital to a skilled nursing facility.

4. Conclusion

Early recognition, aggressive cardiorespiratory support in the ICU, and multistep pharmacological and supportive care by our multidisciplinary teams lead to a good outcome in our specific patient. Guidelines for early electrophysiological support in the setting of hemodynamic instability in anti-NMDARE are needed in the future.

Competing Interests

The authors declare that they have no competing interests.

Acknowledgments

This study is supported by departmental funding only.

References

[1] M. J. Titulaer, L. McCracken, I. Gabilondo et al., "Treatment and prognostic factors for long-term outcome in patients with anti-NMDA receptor encephalitis: an observational cohort study," *The Lancet Neurology*, vol. 12, no. 2, pp. 157–165, 2013.

[2] J. Dalmau, A. J. Gleichman, E. G. Hughes et al., "Anti-NMDA-receptor encephalitis: case series and analysis of the effects of antibodies," *The Lancet Neurology*, vol. 7, no. 12, pp. 1091–1098, 2008.

[3] L. H. Sansing, E. Tüzün, M. W. Ko, J. Baccon, D. R. Lynch, and J. Dalmau, "A patient with encephalitis associated with NMDA receptor antibodies," *Nature Clinical Practice Neurology*, vol. 3, no. 5, pp. 291–296, 2007.

[4] J. W. Britton and E. Benarroch, "Seizures and syncope: anatomic basis and diagnostic considerations," *Clinical Autonomic Research*, vol. 16, no. 1, pp. 18–28, 2006.

[5] K. Jansen and L. Lagae, "Cardiac changes in epilepsy," *Seizure*, vol. 19, no. 8, pp. 455–460, 2010.

[6] A. E. Epstein, J. P. Dimarco, K. A. Ellenbogen et al., "ACC/AHA/HRS 2008 guidelines for device-based therapy of cardiac rhythm abnormalities," *Heart Rhythm*, vol. 5, pp. e1–e62, 2008.

[7] B. L. Sullivan, K. Bartels, and N. Hamilton, "Insertion and management of temporary pacemakers," *Seminars in Cardiothoracic and Vascular Anesthesia*, vol. 20, no. 1, pp. 52–62, 2016.

[8] B. Ziaeian and K. Shamsa, "Dazed, confused, and asystolic: possible signs of anti–N-methyl-D-aspartate receptor encephalitis," *Texas Heart Institute Journal*, vol. 42, no. 2, pp. 175–177, 2015.

[9] E. Lancaster, E. Martinez-Hernandez, and J. Dalmau, "Encephalitis and antibodies to synaptic and neuronal cell surface proteins," *Neurology*, vol. 77, no. 2, pp. 179–189, 2011.

[10] S. E. Schmitt, K. Pargeon, E. S. Frechette, L. J. Hirsch, J. Dalmau, and D. Friedman, "Extreme delta brush; a unique EEG pattern in adults with anti-NMDA receptor encephalitis," *Neurology*, vol. 79, no. 11, pp. 1094–1100, 2012.

[11] C. Finke, U. A. Kopp, H. Prüss, J. Dalmau, K.-P. Wandinger, and C. J. Ploner, "Cognitive deficits following anti-NMDA receptor encephalitis," *Journal of Neurology, Neurosurgery and Psychiatry*, vol. 83, no. 2, pp. 195–198, 2012.

Acute Stroke due to Electrocution: Uncommon or Unrecognized?

Laxmi Kokatnur[1,2] and Mohan Rudrappa[1,2]

[1]Louisiana State University Health Sciences Center Shreveport, 1501 Kings Hwy, Shreveport, LA 71104, USA
[2]Overton Brooks VA Medical Center, 510 E Stoner Ave, Shreveport, LA 71101, USA

Correspondence should be addressed to Laxmi Kokatnur; drlaxmisk@gmail.com

Academic Editor: Andreas K. Demetriades

The growing dependence on electricity in our daily lives has increased the incidence of electrocution injuries. Although several neurological injuries have been described previously, acute stroke due to electrocution is rare. Our patient, a previously healthy man, was electrocuted after he grabbed a "live" high-voltage wire. Although he was hemodynamically stable, he remained confused with language defects. MRI of the brain showed acute stroke in the bilateral anterior cerebral artery territory and watershed regions of the left middle cerebral artery territory. MR angiogram incidentally showed A1 segment aplasia of the right anterior cerebral artery. Electrocution is known to cause vasospasm leading to end-organ damage similar to that seen in stroke. In our patient, vasospasm of the left anterior circulation likely led to watershed infarcts in the left parietal lobe and bilateral frontal lobes. Due to aplasia of the A1 segment on the right side, perfusion to both frontal lobes was solely from the left anterior cerebral artery.

1. Introduction

Electricity played a crucial role in building modern civilization, and humans have paid the price for it. On an average, 411 people will be electrocuted every year [1]. Despite improvements in overall safety measures, this number is likely to increase as we depend more on electricity in every aspect of our lives. The severity of injury depends on the type and strength of current and ranges from a barely perceptible tingling sensation to instant death. Even though several neurological injuries have been described before, acute stroke due to electrocution is only reported in a handful of cases. This underreporting might be due to uncommon occurrence or under recognition. We present a case of acute stroke due to electrocution along with a review of the literature to increase awareness of this rare condition among medical professionals. The early diagnosis and treatment of this condition will have therapeutic implications.

2. Case Presentation

A 38-year-old white male was found down in the field after he reportedly grabbed a "live" electrical wire. On the way to the local hospital, he regained consciousness but remained confused thereafter. He had sustained second-degree burns at the entry wound in the right palm and had a small exit wound in the right foot. Ecchymosis was also noted on right side of the body over the knee, thigh, and shoulder. A pan CT scan of the body did not reveal any major abnormality, including fractures. He remained hemodynamically stable but was pleasantly confused with a nonfocal neurological examination. A CT scan of the brain showed multiple hypodensities in the left parietal region and frontal region bilaterally. All serology labs were normal except total creatinine kinase levels, which peaked at 1100 U/L. Hence, he was transferred to the burn unit in our hospital for further management of burns with rhabdomyolysis. On examination, he was a pleasant gentleman with complete amnesia of the inciting event. He was alert but disoriented to all spheres. Most of the responses were limited to either head nodding or a few words associated with tangentiality and paraphasia. Repetition was impaired, but comprehension was preserved for simple commands. The cranial nerves and motor and sensory systems were clinically normal except limitation of the right arm's movement due to pain. MRI of the brain using 1.5 Tesla MRI machine showed multiple areas of diffusion restriction

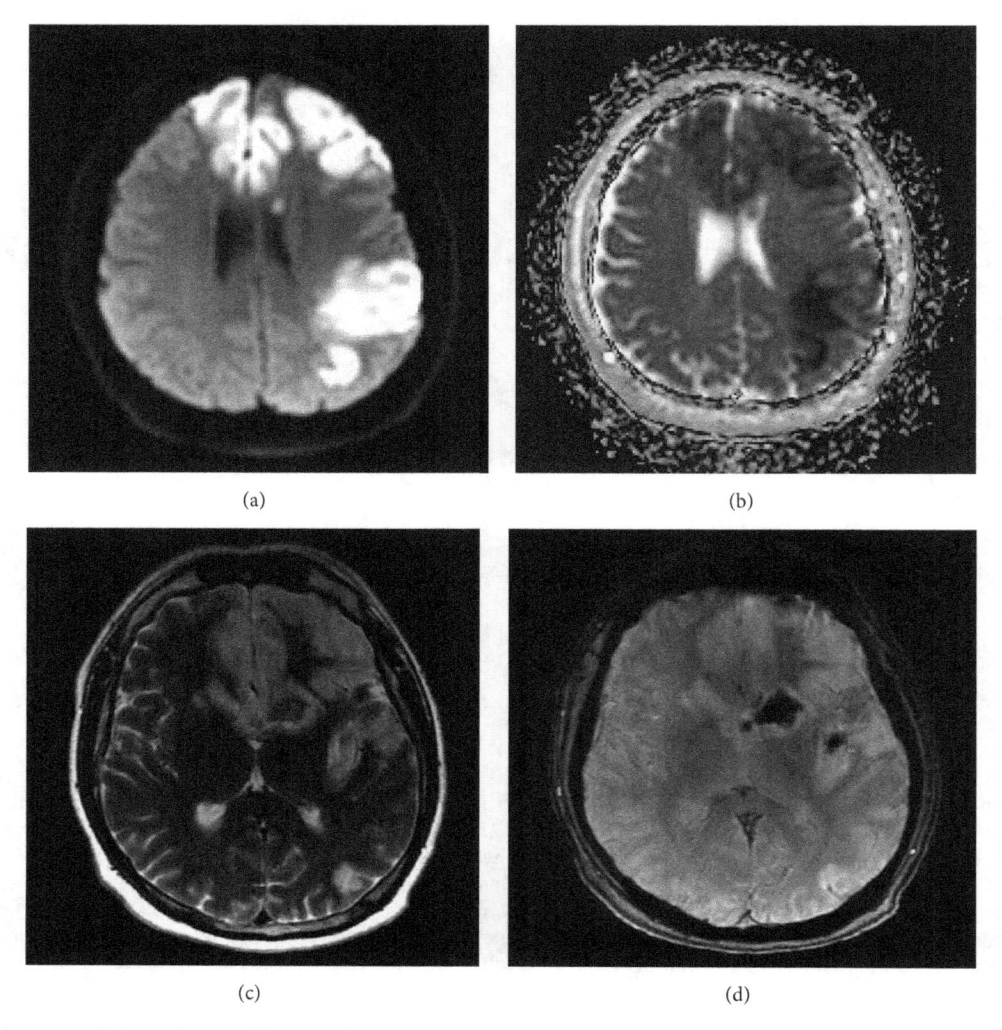

FIGURE 1: Selected images of MRI of brain. ((a) and (b)) (DWI/ADC) image showing restriction diffusion in bilateral medial frontal lobes and watershed areas in frontal and temporal lobes. (c) T2-weighted image showing hyperintensities in basal ganglia (recurrent artery of Heubner). (d) SWI sequence showing hemorrhagic changes in left basal ganglia and insula.

in the bilateral medial frontal lobe and bilateral basal ganglia along with watershed areas in the left frontal and temporal regions (Figure 1). Susceptibility-weighted images showed hemorrhage in the left basal ganglia and insula (Figure 1). T2-weighted images showed hyperintensity in the corresponding regions. MR angiogram did not reveal any filling defect or obvious vasospasm but showed aplastic A1 segment of the right anterior cerebral artery (Figure 2). Based on these findings, acute stroke was diagnosed, likely due to vasospasm of the left anterior cerebral circulation due to electrocution. As the patient had presented 3 days after the injury and had shown clinical improvement, it was hypothesized that vasospasm of cerebral vessels might have been resolved when MR angiogram was performed. No hypotension in the field was reported by the first responders and no hypotension was documented during the initial intensive care unit stay at the outside hospital and telemetry monitoring at our center. Also, there was no evidence of end-organ injury due to hypotension induced hypoperfusion arguing against hypotension induced watershed cerebral infarction. Due to aplasia of the right A1 segment, both frontal lobes were supplied by the anterior cerebral artery and vasospasm of the left anterior cerebral circulation might have led to both frontal lobe infarcts along with watershed infarcts of the left middle cerebral artery territory.

An extensive work-up did not reveal any other risk factors for stroke. Transthoracic echocardiogram showed normal structural and functional heart without any intracardiac thrombus; vegetation and bubble study did not show any right to left shunt. Telemetry cardiac monitoring also failed to detect any cardiac arrhythmia. MRA neck did not show any evidence of carotid or vertebral artery disease. The patient's family denied that the patient had any preexisting medical or surgical conditions, including a substance abuse problem. He was an anthropology graduate working as a stunt man for movies and reported being healthy before this event. Despite extensive interviews, the circumstances of the electrocution could not be elucidated, except that he was barefoot at the

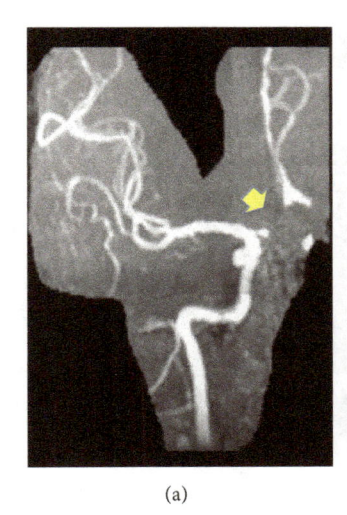

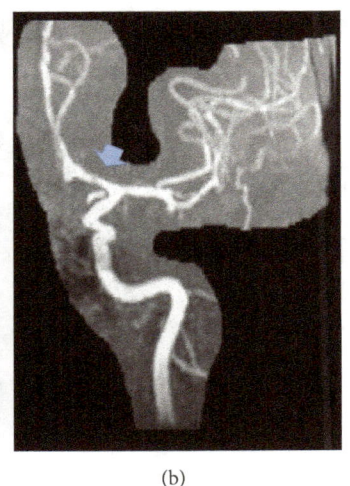

FIGURE 2: Selected images of MR angiogram. (a) Aplastic A1 segment of right ACA (yellow arrow). (b) Normal A1 segment of left ACA (blue arrow) supplying both frontal lobes.

time of the accident and it was a high-voltage electrical wire. People visiting a local church found him confused on the ground and called for emergency medical services. With supportive treatment, the patient's overall condition improved with some residual language defects. The mild rhabdomyolysis improved after hydration. The entry and exit electric burn wounds responded to local wound care. He was transferred to the neurorehabilitation center for further management and is reported to be recovering well.

3. Discussion

Electricity is the flow of electrons through a conductor and is the main source of energy in the 21st century. Voltage is the force responsible for the flow and is measured in volts. Current is the strength of the flow and is measured in amperes. Direct current (DC) flows in only one direction, but alternating current (AC) changes its direction based on the set frequency. Electricity is transported from the production site as AC at a high voltage of 230–700 kV and is gradually reduced to 220–120 V using transformers before it reaches domestic customers. The severity of electrocution injuries depends on the strength of the current and duration of contact. While 1 milliamp (mA) barely causes a tingling sensation, 20 mA can paralyze respiratory muscles. Electrocution with more than 2 amps of current causes significant internal organ and cardiac damage, leading to sudden death [1]. Most electrocution injuries occur in domestic settings with low-voltage current. They rarely require medical attention and are underreported. Injuries from high-voltage electrocution (more than 600 volts) account for 3%–5% of admissions to burn units and 7% of all work-related fatalities [1, 2].

After electrocution, the tissues sustain injuries based on their resistance to the flow of current. The nervous system, blood vessels, and mucous membrane are more prone to injuries as they offer less resistance. Bones, fat, and tendons offer more resistance, but they generate more heat and suffer

TABLE 1: Neurological injuries caused by electrocution.

Type of nervous system	Immediate	Delayed
Central nervous system	Confusion Loss of consciousness Amnesia Acute stroke Seizure Headache Focal brain necrosis Transection of spinal cord Rupture of aneurysm	Transverse myelitis Amyotrophic lateral sclerosis Ascending paralysis Personality changes Delayed brain atrophy
Peripheral nervous system	Nerve palsy	Neuropathies
Autonomic nervous system	Raynaud phenomenon Horner's syndrome Keraunoparalysis	Complex regional pain syndrome

thermal injury. AC causes tetanic contraction of muscles and the victim is thrown away, breaking the circuit. In contrast, DC of the same strength causes continuous contraction of muscles, making the victim hold on to the source of the current, leading to further electrocution [12, 13]. The nervous system, by virtue of its electrochemical properties, offers the least resistance to the flow of current and hence it is commonly involved in electrocution injuries. Most patients show transient confusion due to alteration of the electrical potential in the brain, which resolves with time. If the brainstem is directly involved, even a low-strength current can cause death due to the involvement of cardiorespiratory centers. Even though most recover from the initial injury, several delayed-onset symptoms of electrocution have also been described [12]. The spectrum of neurological injuries due to electrocution is noted in Table 1.

Table 2: Published case reports of acute stroke due to electrocution.

Author, year	Age Sex	Voltage	Entry site/exit site	CT head findings	MRI brain findings	Angiogram*	Follow-up**	Other key findings
Singh Jain et al., 2015 [3]	40 Male	High 11000 V	Right arm/axilla	Bilateral, cerebellar, and left occipital hypodensity	Bilateral, cerebellar, and left occipital stroke	Normal	Symptoms improved	18% burns
Bell et al., 2014 [4]	32 Male	High 50000 V Taser gun	NP/NP	Left MCA territory infarct	Left MCA territory ischemic stroke	Distal M1 and proximal M2 left middle cerebral artery filling defect	NP	
Kim et al., 2014 [5]	52 Male	Low 220 V	Right hand/left hand		Left MCA territory ischemic stroke	Focal stenosis of left MCA, left proximal ACA, and proximal basilar artery	Symptoms resolved	Radial nerve neuropathy
Jain et al., 2014 [6]	55 Male	High 66000 V	NP/NP	NP	Left cerebellum ischemia stroke with mass effect	Diffuse narrowing/vasospasm of left vertebral artery	Symptoms improved. Vasospasm resolved at 6 months	
Johl et al., 2012 [7]	43 Male	Low 440 V	Scalp/left foot	NP	Bilateral medullary pyramids and pons	NP	Symptoms improved. MRI changes resolved	Spinal card infarction
Chen et al., 2012 [8]	62 Female	Low 110 V	Left hand/NP	NP	Left paramedian pons ischemic stroke	Narrowing of proximal basilar artery, bilateral distal vertebral artery, and MCA likely due to thrombosis	Symptoms resolved. Stenosis progressed	Protein C deficiency
Verma et al., 2014 [9]	30 Male	Low 240 V	NP/NP	Right MCA infarct with mass effect	NP	NP	Symptoms improved. Mass effect resolved	Acute myocardial infarction
Huan-Jui et al., 2010 [10]	50 Male	Low 110 V	Both hands/NP	Normal	Right frontotemporal area, basal ganglia, and corona radiate stroke	Segmental narrowing of siphon of right internal carotid artery and M1 segment of middle cerebral artery	Symptoms did not improve. Vasospasm resolved	TPA was given. Vasospasm improved with intra-arterial nimodipine
Kamyar and Trob, 2009 [11]	28 Male	Low 220 V	Both hands/left foot	Normal	Mesial occipital bilateral infarction	NP	Symptoms improved	Cardiac arrest for 10 min. Cardiogenic-ischemic encephalopathy

NP: not reported. * refers to either CT MR or digital subtraction angiogram. ** indicates that most cases report short follow-up period.

Acute stroke due to electrocution is uncommon and has been described in only nine cases in the English literature to the best of our knowledge. The salient features of these cases are summarized in Table 2. As the available evidence is from case reports, there is paucity of knowledge regarding the pathophysiology, clinical features, treatment, and outcomes of stroke due to electrocution. Most cases are reported in young males involving low-voltage current. Interestingly, acute stroke can occur even when the central nervous system is not in the direct path of the current, as seen in our patient.

Blood vessels, due to their high water content, can transmit electric current easily to distant sites and cause metastatic injuries. In animal models, direct electrical stimulation of cerebral vessels can cause vasospasm and this effect has been seen at distant sites [14]. In a study looking at vascular injuries due to electrocution in humans, vasospasm was seen in 8 of 12 patients on angiogram [15]. Electrostatic energy in blood vessels can initiate vascular mediopathy and/or intravascular coagulation even when the surrounding tissues appear to be normal [8]. In fact, electricity is used for thrombus generation in animal models when studying carotid artery clots [16]. Acute stroke is also described in electric injury due to lightning [17].

All reported cases were treated as per standard guidelines for the management of acute stroke. Thrombolysis was administered in one patient with no benefit. Later, intra-arterial nimodipine showed a favorable response [10]. Most cases showed clinical improvement, some with complete radiological resolution. The interesting but unfortunate finding of A1 segment aplasia contributed to significant bilateral frontal lobe injury in our patient. A1 segment aplasia is an uncommon developmental defect seen in approximately 2% of cases of stroke on angiograms [18]. Bilateral frontal lobe stroke due to A1 segment aplasia has been reported in only three case reports [19].

4. Conclusion

Neurological injuries are common after electrocution injuries. Physicians should be wary of neurological injuries including acute stroke, even when the nervous system does not fall in the path of the current. Timely neuroimaging is helpful and if vasospasm is noted on an angiogram, intra-arterial nimodipine can be considered. The prognosis is excellent with supportive treatment.

Competing Interests

The authors, Dr. Laxmi Kokatnur and Dr. Mohan Rudrappa, declare that there are no competing interests regarding the publication of this paper.

References

[1] S. Kisner and V. Casini, "Epidemiology of electrocution fatalities," Worker Death by Electrocution, A Summary of Niosh Surveillance and Investigative Findings, Department of Health and Human Resource, Washington, DC, USA, no. 98-131, pp. 9–19, May 1998, http://www.cdc.gov/niosh/docs/98-131/pdfs/98-131.pdf.

[2] A. A. Mohammadi, M. Amini, D. Mehrabani, Z. Kiani, and A. Seddigh, "A survey on 30 months electrical burns in Shiraz University of Medical Sciences Burn Hospital," Burns, vol. 34, no. 1, pp. 111–113, 2008.

[3] R. Singh Jain, S. Kumar, D. T. Suresh, and R. Agarwal, "Acute vertebrobasilar ischemic stroke due to electric injury," The American Journal of Emergency Medicine, vol. 33, no. 7, pp. 992–992.e6, 2015.

[4] N. Bell, M. Moon, and P. Dross, "Cerebrovascular accident (CVA) in association with a Taser-induced electrical injury," Emergency Radiology, vol. 21, no. 2, pp. 211–213, 2014.

[5] H. M. Kim, Y. Ko, J. S. Kim, S. H. Lim, and B. Y. Hong, "Neurological complication after low-voltage electric injury: a case report," Annals of Rehabilitation Medicine, vol. 38, no. 2, pp. 277–281, 2014.

[6] R. S. Jain, P. K. Gupta, R. Handa, K. Nagpal, S. Prakash, and R. Agrawal, "Vertebrobasilar territory ischemic stroke after electrical injury: delayed sequelae," Journal of Stroke and Cerebrovascular Diseases, vol. 23, no. 6, pp. 1721–1723, 2014.

[7] H. K. Johl, A. Olshansky, S. R. Beydoun, and R. A. Rison, "Cervicothoracic spinal cord and pontomedullary injury secondary to high-voltage electrocution: a case report," Journal of Medical Case Reports, vol. 6, article 296, 2012.

[8] W.-H. Chen, C. Chui, C.-C. Lui, and H.-L. Yin, "Ischemic stroke after low-voltage electric injury in a diabetic and coagulopathic woman," Journal of Stroke and Cerebrovascular Diseases, vol. 21, no. 8, pp. 913.e1–913.e4, 2012.

[9] G. C. Verma, G. Jain, A. Wahid et al., "Acute Ischaemic stroke and acute myocardial infarction occurring together in domestic low-voltage (220–240V) electrical injury: a rare complication," Journal of Association of Physicians of India, vol. 62, no. 7, pp. 620–623, 2014.

[10] Y. Huan-Jui, L. Chih-Yang, L. Huei-Yu, and C. Po-Chih, "Acute ischemic stroke in low-voltage electrical injury: a case report," Surgical Neurology International, vol. 1, no. 1, p. 83, 2010.

[11] R. Kamyar and J. D. Trobe, "Bilateral mesial occipital lobe infarction after cardiogenic hypotension induced by electrical shock," Journal of Neuro-Ophthalmology, vol. 29, no. 2, pp. 107–110, 2009.

[12] A. C. Koumbourlis, "Electrical injuries," Critical Care Medicine, vol. 30, no. 11, pp. S424–S430, 2002.

[13] J. A. Martinez, T. Nguyen, and K. J. Buechter, "Electrical Injuries," Southern Medical Journal, vol. 93, no. 7-12, pp. 1165–1168, 2000.

[14] F. A. Echlin, "Vasospasm and focal cerebral ischemia an experimental study," Archives of Neurology & Psychiatry, vol. 47, no. 1, pp. 77–96, 1942.

[15] J. L. Hunt, W. F. McManus, W. P. Haney et al., "Vascular lesions in acute electric injuries," Journal of Trauma—Injury, Infection & Critical Care, vol. 14, no. 6, pp. 461–473, 1974.

[16] A. Kusada, N. Isogai, and B. C. Cooley, "Electric injury model of murine arterial thrombosis," Thrombosis Research, vol. 121, no. 1, pp. 103–106, 2007.

[17] M. Cherington, P. R. Yarnell, and S. F. London, "Neurologic complications of lightning injuries," Western Journal of Medicine, vol. 162, no. 5, pp. 413–417, 1995.

[18] G. Makowicz, R. Poniatowska, and M. Lusawa, "Variants of cerebral arteries—anterior circulation," Polish Journal of Radiology, vol. 78, no. 3, pp. 42–47, 2013.

[19] M. Krishnan, S. Kumar, S. Ali, and R. S. Iyer, "Sudden bilateral anterior cerebral infarction: unusual stroke associated with unusual vascular anomalies," Postgraduate Medical Journal, vol. 89, no. 1048, pp. 120–121, 2013.

A Patient with Eight Intracranial Aneurysms: Endovascular Treatment in Two Sessions

Erol Akgul,[1] Hasan Bilen Onan,[1] Huseyin Tugsan Balli,[1] and Nuri Eralp Cetinalp[2]

[1]Radiology Department of Medical Faculty, Cukurova University, Adana, Turkey
[2]Neurosurgery Department of Medical Faculty, Cukurova University, Adana, Turkey

Correspondence should be addressed to Erol Akgul; akgulerol@gmail.com

Academic Editor: Hidetoshi Ikeda

The frequency of multiple intracranial aneurysms seen in patients with or without subarachnoid hemorrhage is high. The advancement of the endovascular technique and devices has ensured that endovascular treatment of intracranial aneurysms is the first choice in most cases, especially in unruptured ones. Different combinations of treatment modalities and techniques can be used in the management of multiple aneurysms. But in selected patients without subarachnoid hemorrhage, treatment of all aneurysms in one or more sessions with endovascular techniques is less traumatic than that with surgery. In the literature, the maximum number of aneurysms in one patient treated endovascularly and/or surgically is seven. In this case report, we present, with a review of the literature, a patient with eight intracranial aneurysms, all of which were treated in two sessions with various endovascular techniques. A 40-year-old female patient was admitted due to headache. Angiography showed eight aneurysms in the posterior circulation and, bilaterally, in the anterior circulation. All aneurysms were treated endovascularly in two sessions. In the treatment of the aneurysms, different endovascular techniques were used including flow diverters stents, stent-assisted coiling, Y-stent-assisted coiling, and coiling alone.

1. Introduction

The frequency of multiple intracranial aneurysms seen in patients with or without subarachnoid hemorrhage (SAH) is high. In many published articles, the rate of multiple intracranial aneurysms has been reported as being between 7% and 45% [1–6]. The advancement of endovascular techniques and devices has ensured that endovascular treatment of intracranial aneurysms is the first choice in most cases, especially for unruptured aneurysms. Surgical treatment of multiple intracranial aneurysms requires multiple craniotomies in most cases. There are some articles reporting the treatment of multiple intracranial aneurysms using 1-stage clipping or coiling, or a combination of both techniques [5–10]. The decision of the best treatment modality should be made utilizing a multidisciplinary approach [7, 8, 11]. In the literature, the maximum number of aneurysms in one patient treated endovascularly and/or surgically is seven [5, 11].

In this case report, we present, with a review of the literature, a patient with eight intracranial aneurysms, all of which were treated in two sessions with various endovascular techniques.

2. Case Presentation

A 40-year-old female patient was admitted due to headache beginning one month previously and steadily worsening. A nonenhanced CT was performed due to high suspicion of SAH. The CT showed no SAH but round hyperdensities adjacent to the sphenoid corpus on the left, in front of the mesencephalon, and in the Sylvian fissure on the left implied internal carotid artery (ICA) cavernous segment, basilar tip, and middle cerebral artery (MCA) aneurysms, respectively (Figures 1(a) and 1(b)). Angiography was performed. Eight aneurysms were seen in the posterior circulation and, bilaterally, in the anterior circulation (Figure 1). Table 1 shows the details of the aneurysm locations, characteristics, treatment technique, and stents.

The fusiform aneurysm of the left ICA cavernous segment was partially thrombosed, and there was a severe stenosis at

(a)

(b)

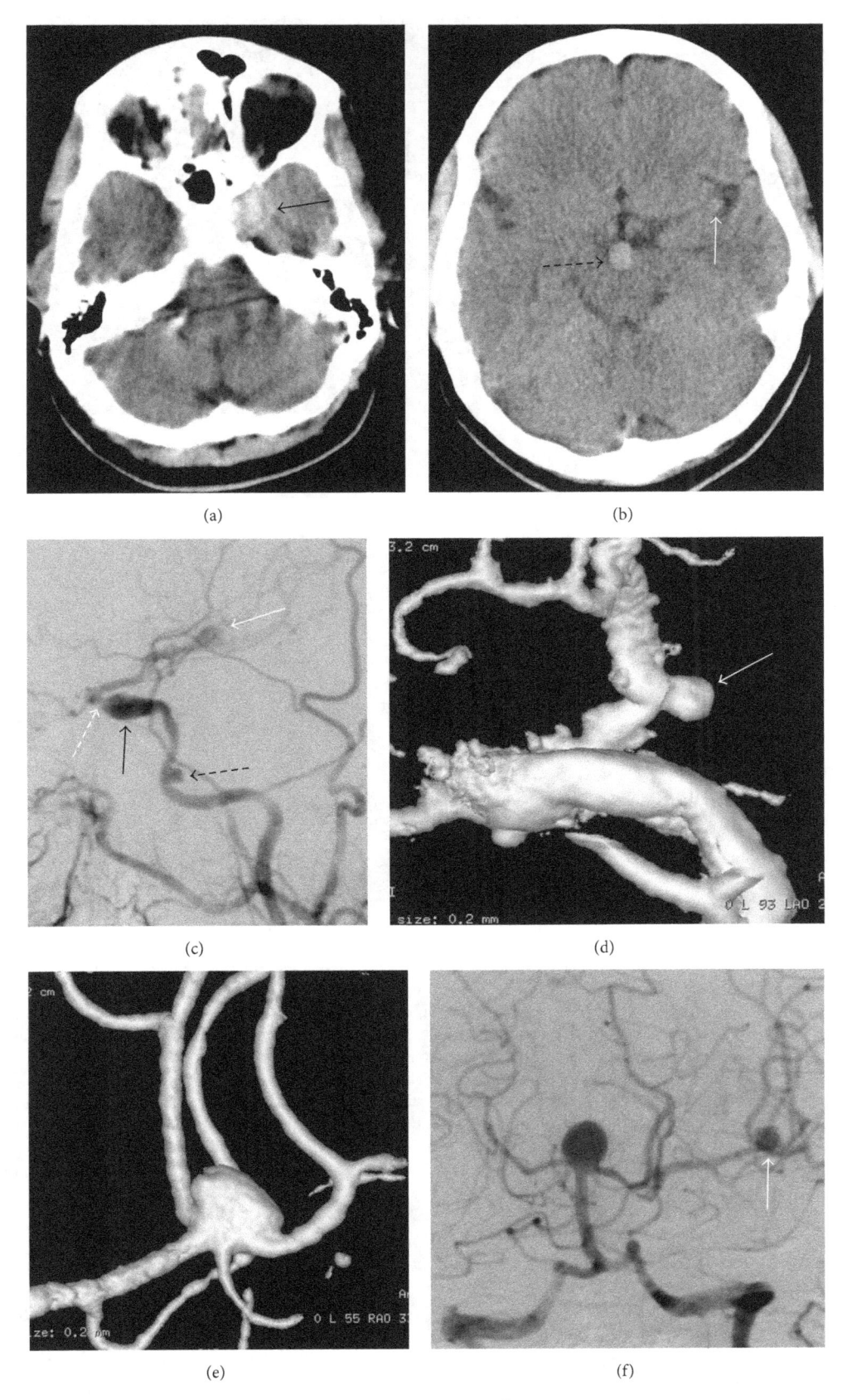

(c)

(d)

(e)

(f)

Figure 1: Continued.

(g)

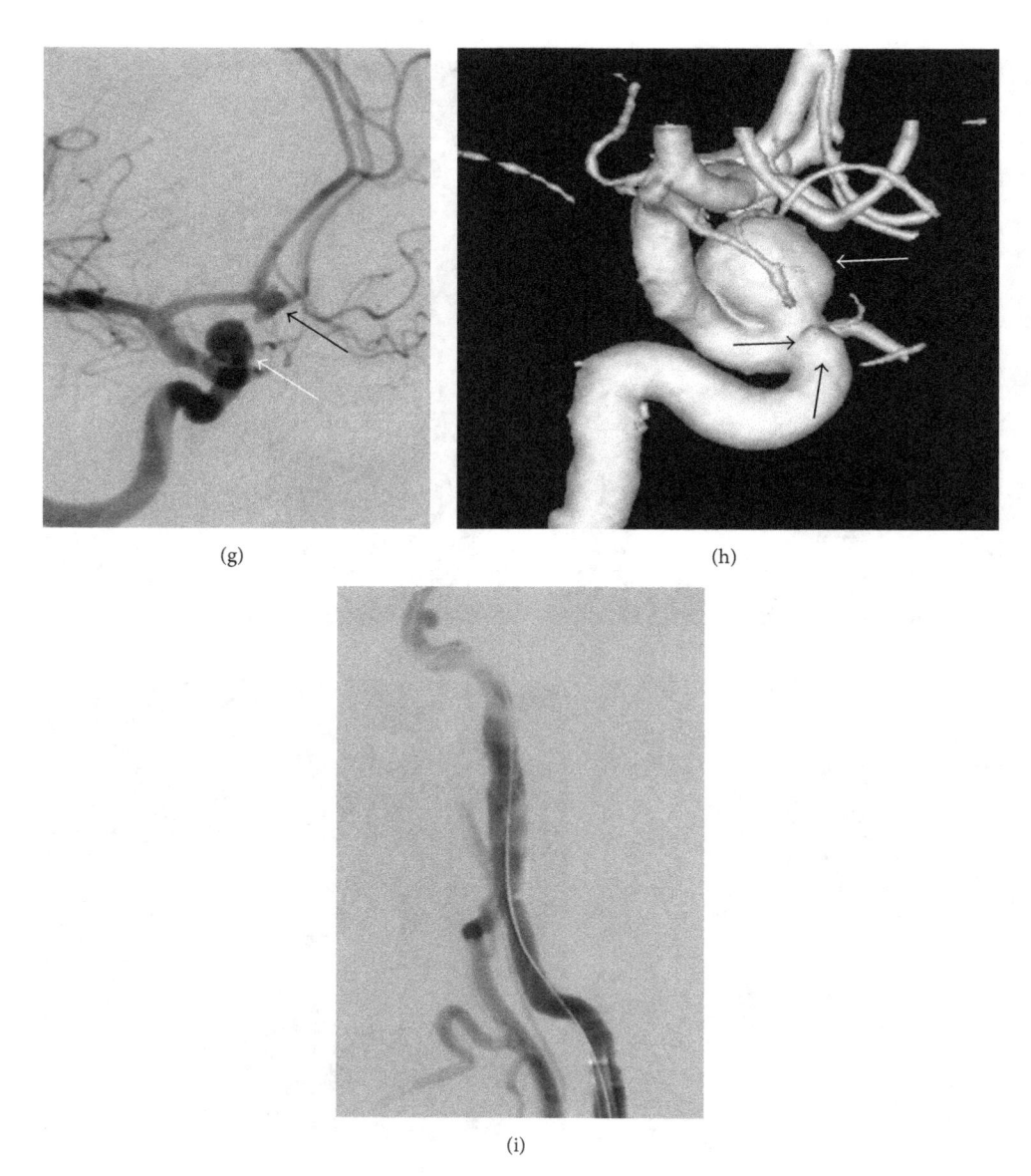

(h)

(i)

Figure 1: Nonenhanced axial CT slices ((a) and (b)) show three round hyperdensities: one adjacent to the sphenoid corpus on the left, another in front of the mesencephalon, and the third in the Sylvian fissure on the left, implying aneurysms of the internal carotid artery (ICA) cavernous segment (arrow, (a)), basilar tip (dashed arrow, (b)), and middle cerebral artery (white arrow, (b)), respectively. The DSA of the left carotid artery (c) reveals a small wide-necked aneurysm of the ICA lacerum segment (black dashed arrow, (c)), a fusiform aneurysm of the ICA cavernous segment (black arrow, (c)), and a middle cerebral artery bifurcation aneurysm (white arrows, (c) and (f)). A severe stenosis (white dashed arrow, (c)) adjacent to the fusiform aneurysm was also seen, resulting in reduced distal flow (c). 3D images ((d) and (e)) show the small saccular narrow-necked aneurysm of the anterior choroidal artery (white arrow, (d)) and the small saccular wide-necked aneurysm of the middle cerebral artery (e). A saccular wide-necked basilar tip aneurysm (f), a fusiform aneurysm of the anterior communicating artery (black arrow, (g)), and a saccular narrow-necked aneurysm (white arrows, (g) and (h)) and a blister-like (black arrows, (h)) aneurysm of the right ICA ophthalmic segment are seen in the DSA ((f) and (g)) and 3D (h) images. The ICA cervical segment dissection (i) possibly occurred during embolization of the aneurysms.

the distal part of the aneurysm (Figure 1(c)). The distal flow beyond the stenosis was reduced significantly. Most of the left MCA blood flow came from the posterior communicating artery (PComA) due to the stenosis (Figure 1(f)).

All aneurysms were decided to be treated endovascularly in two sessions. In the morning, about 8 hours before the procedure, 500 mg of acetylsalicylic acid (Aspirin; Bayer Healthcare, Germany) and two tablets of clopidogrel (Plavix; Bristol-Myers Squibb/Sanofi Pharmaceuticals, NY, USA) were loaded.

After administering general anesthesia, the left common carotid artery (CCA) was catheterized with a long 6F introducer (NeuronMax 6F, Penumbra Inc., Alameda, CA, USA) and the ICA with a 5F distal access guiding catheter (Navien,

Table 1: Aneurysm locations, characteristics, and treatment techniques.

Aneu. no.	Location	Type	Size/neck (mm)	Treatment	Stents	Treat. session
1	Lacerum segment of left ICA	Saccular	3 × 4/4	FD	Surpass 4 × 30	1st
2	Cavernous segment of left ICA	Fusiform	11 × 6	FD	Surpass 4 × 20	1st
3	Left AChorA	Saccular	3 × 3/2	Coil		1st
4	Bifurcation of left middle cerebral artery	Saccular	6 × 4/4	Stent and coil	LeoBaby 2.5 × 25	1st
6	AComA	Fusiform	4 × 5.5	Stent and coil	LeoBaby 2.5 × 25	1st
5	Basilar tip	Saccular	10 × 10/6	Y stenting and coil	Neuroform EZ 3 × 30 and Enterprise 4.5 × 22	2nd
7	Ophthalmic segment of right ICA	Saccular	8 × 8/2.5	FD and coil	Surpass 4 × 20	2nd
8	Ophthalmic segment of right ICA	Blood blister	2.5 × 2.5	FD	Surpass 4 × 20	2nd

AComA: anterior communicating artery, Aneu: aneurysm, AChorA: anterior choroidal artery, FD: flow diverter, ICA: internal carotid artery, and treat: treatment.

Covidien AG, Paris, France). After insertion of the latter, 5000 IU heparin was administered IV, targeting two or three times the baseline value, and the serum-activated coagulation time (ACT) was checked. During the procedure, 1000 IU or more of heparin was administered per hour to keep the ACT level stable. After the procedure, 750–1000 IU/h heparin was infused for 24 hours.

Before the treatment of the cavernous segment fusiform aneurysm, the stenosis adjacent to aneurysm was dilated with two Gateway balloons with diameters of 1.5 × 15 and 2.5 × 15 mm (Stryker Neuroendovascular, Kalamazoo, MI, USA). Then, two Surpass flow diverter (FD) (Stryker) stents were implanted to cover the fusiform cavernous and saccular lacerum segment aneurysms. To provide proper apposition of the Surpass stents, a Scepter C balloon (Microvention Terumo, Tustin, CA, USA) with a diameter of 4 × 15 mm was used.

The small anterior choroidal artery aneurysm was embolized with bare coils only, using an Excelsior SL-10 microcatheter (Stryker) and a 0.012 hydrophilic microguide wire with a double-angled tip (Terumo Medical Corporation, Tokyo, Japan). The bifurcation aneurysm of the left MCA was totally closed with stent-assisted (LeoBaby, Balt, Montmorency, France) coiling with a jailed microcatheter, Excelsior SL-10. The left ICA cervical segment dissection, which may have occurred during catheterization, was seen in final angiograms of the left side. The dissection was treated with a carotid Wallstent (7 × 30) (Stryker). Then, the right CCA and ICA were catheterized with the same long introducer and distal access guiding catheter. The fusiform aneurysm of the anterior communicating artery was completely filled with coils, using an Excelsior SL-10 microcatheter. Then, a LeoBaby stent was deployed to prevent recanalization. It was decided that the other aneurysms would be treated in a separate session.

One day later, the patient had no complaint except headache and DWI showed no ischemic lesion. Ten days later, the patient was readmitted to the angiosuite for treatment, under general anesthesia, of the other aneurysms. First, a right ICA DSA performed before starting the treatment showed insufficient apposition of the distal part of the second proximal Surpass stent inside the proximal part of the first Surpass. An attempt to ensure sufficient apposition of the second stent using two Gateway balloons (3 × 15 and 3.5 × 15 mm) was unsuccessful. The stents were left as they were; no further attempts at proper apposition were made.

The patient's basilar tip aneurysm was treated with Y-stent-assisted coiling (Table 1), after enabling access to the left vertebral artery using a 6F NeuronMax with a 6F FargoMax (Balt) distal access guiding catheter. A Neuroform EZ stent (Stryker) was deployed as the first stent from the left posterior cerebral artery to the basilar artery. Following catheterization of the aneurysm with an Excelsior SL-10 microcatheter, an Enterprise stent (Codman Neuro, Raynham, MA, USA) was deployed through a Prowler Select Plus microcatheter (Codman Neuro) and the aneurysm was completely coiled via the jailed Excelsior SL-10.

The ophthalmic segment aneurysm of the right ICA was completely coiled; then, a Surpass stent was implanted to prevent recanalization and to cover the blister aneurysm proximal to the aneurysm of the ophthalmic segment. The proximal part of the Surpass was not apposed to the vessel wall due to its acute curvature. To appose the proximal part of the Surpass stent, a Transform occlusion balloon catheter (5 × 15 mm) (Stryker) was used, but the shape of the proximal part of the Surpass did not change. Then, an Enterprise stent (4 × 22) was deployed inside the Surpass and proper apposition was provided.

The patient was awake and had no neurologic symptoms. DWI was again performed and no ischemic lesion was detected. The patient's only complaint at discharge was of a mild headache. 100 mg of Aspirin was ordered to continue indefinitely and one tablet of Plavix for 6 months.

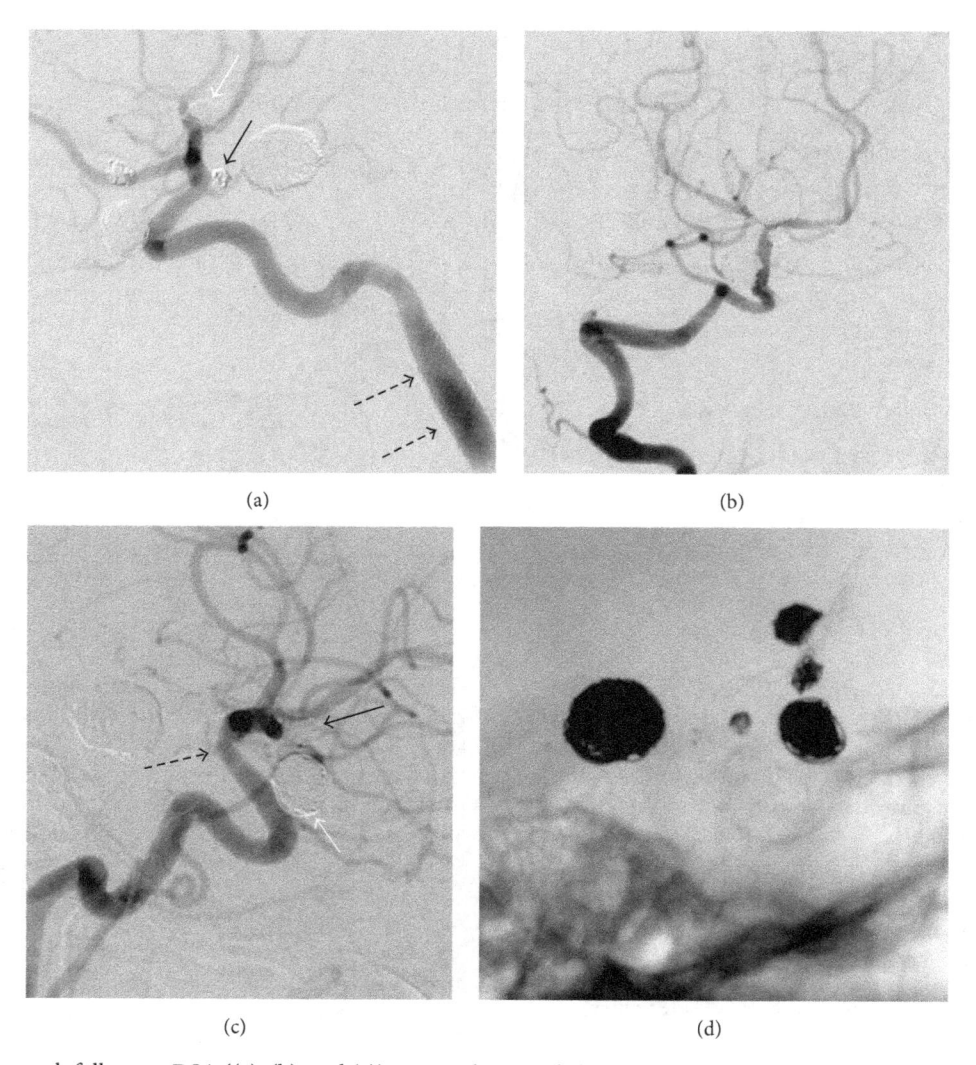

FIGURE 2: The 9th-month follow-up DSA ((a), (b), and (c)) images show total closure of the aneurysms of the left ICA lacerum segment (a) and the cavernous segment (a), the left anterior choroidal artery (black arrow, (a)), the middle cerebral artery (white arrow, (a)), the basilar tip (b), the anterior communicating artery (black arrow, (c)), and the right ICA ophthalmic segment (white arrow, (c)). The intimal hyperplasia inside the stents seen in the 3rd-month follow-up angiograms (not shown here) was totally relieved. The coils and stents used for the treatment of the aneurysms are seen in the fluoroscopic image (d). A slight fusiform dilation and no in-stent stenosis are seen in the left ICA cervical segment dissection, which was treated with a carotid Wallstent (black dashed arrows, (a)). The 3rd-month DSA (not shown here) showed a slight narrowing, due to the fish mouth or foreshortening effect, inside the distal part of the Surpass stent used for the right ophthalmic segment aneurysms. The 9th-month follow-up DSA (c) showed no change (black dashed arrow, (c)) and no intimal hyperplasia.

The 3rd-month follow-up angiograms showed an excellent reconstruction of the cavernous segment aneurysm, as well as disappearance of the petrous segment aneurysm of the left ICA. The anterior choroidal artery (AChorA) aneurysm was still filling but there was no regrowth. The left MCA, anterior communicating artery (AComA), basilar tip, right ICA ophthalmic segment, and right blister aneurysms were fully closed, but there was mild hyperplasia inside the stents used for the MCA, AComA, and basilar tip aneurysms. A slight narrowing was seen inside the distal part of the Surpass stent, due to foreshortening of the Surpass distal part, used for right ICA ophthalmic segment aneurysms. There was no intimal hyperplasia or in-stent stenosis in the left ICA cervical segment dissection treated with Wallstent.

The hyperplasia inside the stents was totally relieved and all aneurysms were closed in the 9th-month follow-up angiograms (Figure 2).

3. Discussion

When surgery is selected for treatment of multiple intracranial aneurysms, multiple craniotomies are usually required [12]. A single-stage procedure is indicated by multiple intracranial aneurysms on the same side of the anterior circulation. But if the aneurysms are located bilaterally in the anterior circulation or if they are in both the anterior and the posterior circulations, a two-stage procedure is suitable [10]. Hydrocephalus and edema of the brain make access to multiple aneurysms more difficult in the first few days following SAH [1]. Many studies showed clipping of multiple aneurysms results in poorer outcomes than in a single aneurysm [4, 12–14]. This can be explained by the increased manipulation of brain tissue and vasculature during multiple-aneurysm surgery [13, 14]. On the other hand, coiling for multiple aneurysms involves no manipulation of cerebral arteries or of brain tissue. As such, when multiple aneurysms are located either on both sides or in both the posterior and anterior circulations, a single-stage treatment with coiling may be more practical than the one with clipping [6]. In Shen et al.'s [9] study of 84 aneurysms in 36 patients, they chose to leave 19 of the aneurysms untreated. Of the remaining 65, two were treated surgically by clipping and the rest using various endovascular techniques. Their conclusion was that endovascular treatment was a more suitable method than surgery for multiple intracranial aneurysms.

Solander et al. [1] performed endovascular treatment by using Guglielmi detachable coils on 93 aneurysms in 38 consecutive patients and reported the overall clinical outcome was excellent in 34 patients (89%), good in one (3%), fair in one (3%), and fatal in two (5%). Xavier et al. [8] treated the 13 aneurysms of six patients using 1-stage coiling. No periprocedural complications were reported in their study. Jeon et al. [6] reported 1-stage coiling of multiple aneurysms seemed to be safe and effective, with low morbidity and mortality in their study including 167 patients having more than two aneurysms each.

In the literature, searched via PubMed, there is no reported case or study concerning a patient with more than seven simultaneous aneurysms, treated in 1 or more stages either endovascularly, surgically, or by both techniques [1, 5, 7, 8, 10, 15]. In Jeon et al.'s [6] cohort including 167 patients with 359 aneurysms, while two patients had six aneurysms, only one patient had seven aneurysms. They attempted to treat all patients with 1-stage coiling. Oh and Lim [5] treated, with coil embolization in single sessions, 28 patients with multiple intracranial aneurysms. In this group, while only one patient had six aneurysms, the others had less than 6. Ahmed et al. [11] reported a patient with seven aneurysms, one of which ruptured. They treated the patient in two surgical sessions, followed by one endovascular session including only coiling and stent-assisted coiling. In Xavier et al.'s [8] report including six patients, the numbers of aneurysms in each patient were between two and five.

Our patient had eight aneurysms, more than any single patient reported in the literature. The patient also had a severe stenosis adjacent to the left ICA fusiform aneurysm. We treated the aneurysms and the stenosis in two sessions due to their large number. The patient had no SAH, so we used all kinds and combinations of endovascular treatment techniques. We started treating the aneurysms from the left side due to the presence of severe stenosis there. An AComA aneurysm seen during the right side carotid angiography was treated because of its bizarre appearance, with nipples implying imminent rupture. While one fusiform, one saccular, and one blood blister aneurysm were treated only with Surpass flow diverters, two saccular aneurysms were treated with stent-assisted coiling. One wide-necked saccular aneurysm, basilar tip, was treated with Y-stent-assisted coiling, one narrow-necked saccular AChorA aneurysm with coiling alone, and one saccular ICA ophthalmic aneurysm with coiling and flow diverter (Table 1 and Figure 2). The treatment of the patient was accomplished with no complication other than the left ICA cervical segment dissection, which was subsequently treated with carotid Wallstent.

4. Conclusion

The rate of multiple intracranial aneurysms is very high and ranges from 7% to 45%. Different combinations of treatment modalities and techniques can be used in the management of multiple aneurysms. But in patients without SAH, treatment of all aneurysms with endovascular techniques in one or more sessions is less traumatic than surgical treatment.

Competing Interests

The authors declare that there is no conflict of interests regarding the publication of this article.

Acknowledgments

The authors thank Lawrence Alan Chambers for his help in linguistic corrections of the manuscript.

References

[1] S. Solander, A. Ulhoa, F. Viñuela et al., "Endovascular treatment of multiple intracranial aneurysms by using Guglielmi detachable coils," Journal of Neurosurgery, vol. 90, no. 5, pp. 857–864, 1999.

[2] H. E. Ellamushi, J. P. Grieve, H. R. Jäger, and N. D. Kitchen, "Risk factors for the formation of multiple intracranial aneurysms," Journal of Neurosurgery, vol. 94, no. 5, pp. 728–732, 2001.

[3] M. Kaminogo, M. Yonekura, and S. Shibata, "Incidence and outcome of multiple intracranial aneurysms in a defined population," Stroke, vol. 34, no. 1, pp. 16–21, 2003.

[4] T. Inagawa, "Incidence and risk factors for multiple intracranial saccular aneurysms in patients with subarachnoid hemorrhage in Izumo City, Japan," Acta Neurochirurgica, vol. 151, no. 12, pp. 1623–1630, 2009.

[5] K. Oh and Y. C. Lim, "Single-session coil embolization of multiple intracranial aneurysms," Journal of Cerebrovascular and Endovascular Neurosurgery, vol. 15, no. 3, pp. 184–190, 2013.

[6] P. Jeon, B. M. Kim, D. J. Kim, D. I. Kim, and S. H. Suh, "Treatment of multiple intracranial aneurysms with 1-stage coiling," American Journal of Neuroradiology, vol. 35, no. 6, pp. 1170–1173, 2014.

[7] J. Chung and Y. S. Shin, "Multiple intracranial aneurysms treated by multiple treatment modalities," Neurosurgery, vol. 69, no. 4, pp. E1030–E1032, 2011.

[8] A. R. Xavier, M. Rayes, P. Pandey, A. Tiwari, A. Kansara, and M. Guthikonda, "The safety and efficacy of coiling multiple aneurysms in the same session," Journal of NeuroInterventional Surgery, vol. 4, no. 1, pp. 27–30, 2012.

[9] X. Shen, T. Xu, X. Ding, W. Wang, Z. Liu, and H. Qin, "Multiple intracranial aneurysms: endovascular treatment and

complications," *Interventional Neuroradiology*, vol. 20, no. 4, pp. 442–447, 2014.

[10] S. Guo and Y. Xing, "Surgical treatment of multiple intracranial aneurysms," *Turkish Neurosurgery*, vol. 24, no. 2, pp. 208–213, 2014.

[11] O. Ahmed, P. Kalakoti, M. Hefner, H. Cuellar, and B. Guthikonda, "Seven intracranial aneurysms in one patient: treatment and review of literature," *Journal of Cerebrovascular and Endovascular Neurosurgery*, vol. 17, no. 2, pp. 113–119, 2015.

[12] J. Vajda, "Multiple intracranial aneurysms: a high risk condition," *Acta Neurochirurgica*, vol. 118, no. 1-2, pp. 59–75, 1992.

[13] K. Mizoi, J. Suzuki, and T. Yoshimoto, "Surgical treatment of multiple aneurysms: review of experience with 372 cases," *Acta Neurochirurgica*, vol. 96, no. 1-2, pp. 8–14, 1989.

[14] J. Rinne, J. Hernesniemi, M. Niskanen, M. Vapalahti, D. G. Piepgras, and S. J. Peerless, "Management outcome for multiple intracranial aneurysms," *Neurosurgery*, vol. 36, no. 1, pp. 31–38, 1995.

[15] Y. Xu, S.-D. Chen, B. Lei, W.-H. Zhang, and W.-Y. Wang, "One-stage operation for rare multiple mirror intracranial aneurysms: a case report and literature review," *Turkish Neurosurgery*, vol. 24, no. 4, pp. 598–601, 2014.

Limb Pain as Unusual Presentation of a Parietal Intraparenchymal Bleeding Associated with Crack Cocaine Use: A Case Report

Alan Lucerna,[1] James Espinosa,[1] Taimur Zaman,[2] Risha Hertz,[3] and Douglas Stranges[1]

[1]*Department of Emergency Medicine, Rowan University SOM/Jefferson Health, Stratford, NJ, USA*
[2]*Department of Neurology, Jefferson Health, Stratford, NJ, USA*
[3]*Penn Medicine, Gibbsboro, NJ, USA*

Correspondence should be addressed to Alan Lucerna; lucernaa@gmail.com

Academic Editor: Peter Berlit

Limb pain as a presenting feature of an ischemic or hemorrhagic stroke is extremely rare. Here we present a case of a 65-year-old male with complaints of left arm pain and allodynia (specifically light touch to any part of the left arm produced significant discomfort) who was found to have a right parietal lobe intraparenchymal bleed after smoking crack cocaine. Acute central pain is mainly associated with parietal, thalamic, and brainstem lesions. It has been proposed that acute limb pain from a parietal lobe stroke is due to the disconnection of the parietal cortex from the thalamus secondary to the interruption of the pathways between the hemisphere and thalamus/basal ganglia.

1. Introduction

Acute limb pain as a stroke presentation is extremely rare. Central causes of pain are well accepted and understood, explained by physiologic and neuroanatomical principles [1, 2]. Central pain syndrome is a neurological condition secondary to damage or dysfunction of the central nervous system (CNS), which is comprised of the brain, brainstem, and spinal cord. In addition to stroke, central pain syndrome has also been associated with multiple sclerosis, tumors, epilepsy, brain or spinal cord trauma, and Parkinson's disease [3].

2. Case Report

A 65-year-old right hand dominant, African American male presented to the ED via emergency medical service. He had just finished smoking crack cocaine when he developed left arm pain that he described as "cramping". He reported that the pain was so intense that he became weak causing him to fall onto the ground. The pain made him feel like "jumping out of the window." He denied any head injury and he had no loss of consciousness (LOC). The patient had no chest, shortness of breath, or dyspnea on exertion. He denied any neck, back, or abdominal pain.

The patient's past medical history included diabetes, hypertension, hepatitis C, sick sinus syndrome, paroxysmal atrial fibrillation, hyperlipidemia, deep vein thrombosis, chronic kidney disease, hilar mediastinal adenopathy, diastolic heart failure, valvular heart disease, and cardiac arrhythmia of nonsustained ventricular tachycardia with a permanent pacemaker. The patient admitted to intermittent cocaine abuse. His medications include atorvastatin, furosemide, isosorbide mononitrate, acetaminophen with codeine, apixaban, hydralazine, metformin, albuterol sulfate, amlodipine, and tamsulosin.

Vital signs were essentially within normal limits with the exception of a blood pressure of 142/83 mmHg.

The patient had a strong left radial pulse and brisk capillary refill of the left hand with no tenderness or deformity. The patient was noted to have left arm weakness and what looked like choreiform or clumsy left arm movements. His left leg was also noted to be weak. There was no numbness.

Interestingly, light touch to any part of the left arm produced significant discomfort to the point where he did not want anything touching the left arm. He was noted to have decreased rapid alternating movements on the left upper extremity as well as mild difficulty with fine motor control. His left arm and left leg motor strength was 4/5. His cranial nerves II to XII were grossly intact. There were no visual fields cuts noted. Extraocular motility was intact. The grimace was symmetric. There was no evidence of double simultaneous extinction.

There were no pulsatile abdominal masses on exam and the bilateral radial pulses were equal. The patient was unable to tell the exact time of onset of his symptoms. The patient's left arm pain improved with morphine 4 mg intravenously.

The electrocardiogram (ECG) showed sinus tachycardia with first degree atria-ventricular block, as well as ST and T wave abnormality suggestive of lateral ischemia [Figure 1]. This is however unchanged compared to his ECG from two years previously [Figure 2]. His cardiac enzyme was negative.

A computed tomography (CT) scan of the head without contrast showed an acute 2.2 cm intraparenchymal hemorrhage with vasogenic edema in the posterior right parietal lobe [see Figure 3]. X-rays of the upper extremity were unremarkable. The chest X-ray showed normal cardiac silhouette and pulmonary vasculature.

Laboratory data showed a creatinine of 1.34 mg/dL. The urine drug screen showed cocaine.

The patient was placed on a continuous nicardipine infusion to maintain a systolic blood pressure of 140 mm Hg as per neurosurgical consultation. He was transferred to a neurointensive care unit. His left arm pain resolved after 24 hours. The carotid ultrasound showed no hemodynamically significant carotid stenosis and antegrade flow was present in the bilateral vertebral arteries. A CT angiography of the head and neck did not show any aneurysms. His serial cardiac enzymes remained negative throughout his hospitalization. A cardiac catheterization was not performed as the patient had it done one year previously showing angiographically normal coronaries. A cardiology consult was obtained and the patient was found to have no evidence of acute coronary syndrome (ACS) or ischemia. He was subsequently discharged to a rehabilitation facility.

3. Discussion

Cocaine is a known cause of intracerebral hemorrhage (ICH). Cocaine can cause a rapid rise in blood pressures and can promote aneurysmal ruptures [4]. In addition, intracranial vasospasms from cocaine can lead to ischemia and hemorrhagic strokes [5]. Cocaine induced cerebral vasculitis has also been reported [6]. The most likely cause of the hemorrhage in our patient was a blood pressure spike related to cocaine use in someone who was also being treated with apixaban. His work-up did not reveal any brain aneurysms.

However, no matter the cause, reports of intracranial hemorrhage manifesting as acute limb pain are rare. Our patient complained of intense "cramping pain" of the left arm and the pain was worsened by nonnoxious stimuli like light touch. This is consistent with allodynic pain. Allodynia is a painful sensation caused by innocuous stimuli [7].

Acute central pain is thought to be secondary to interruptions of the spino-thalamo-parietal projections leading to spontaneous pain. Acute central pain is mainly associated with parietal, thalamic, or brainstem lesions [8]. Rossetti et al. reported that "*Pathophysiologically, a disinhibition of the phylogenetically old pain pathway that passes through the intralaminar thalamic nuclei and projects to the anterior cingulate cortex and an imbalance of the putative modulatory action of the lemniscal system on the pain pathways have been postulated.*" It has also been proposed that the hyperactivity of the differentiated parietal neurons as a result of their disconnection leads to spontaneous painful sensations [8]. Rossetti also pointed out that spontaneous pain following a hemispheric stroke had mainly right parietal lobe lesions and typically last 2 days. Our patient also had right parietal lobe bleed and his pain resolved after 24 hours.

The role of the parietal lobe in terms of pain perception is compelling. Epileptic events are usually associated with motor findings; however, lesions involving the parietal cortex can present as focal sensory seizures, which often present a diagnostic dilemma as the symptoms may be tingling, numbness, or dysesthesias [1].

Acute limb pain from stroke should be differentiated from central post stroke pain (CPSP). CPSP is well reported and is suspected to affect more than 8% of all patients after a stroke [9]. Dejerine-Roussy Syndrome was originally described by Dejerine and Roussy in 1906 [10]. It is also known as thalamic syndrome or poststroke syndrome and is secondary to an infarction in the thalamus. The resulting injury has been speculated to involve lesions of the spinothalamic pathways with disinhibition and excitation of NMDA receptors in the thalamus [11].

Alvarez-Perez described the symptoms to include "...transient mild hemiparesis, superficial hemianaesthesia (which can be replaced by cutaneous hyperaesthesia and is always accompanied by persistent disturbances of deep sensation), allodynia, mild hemiataxia, astereognosia, severe and paroxysmal pain on the hemiparetic side, and choreoathetoid movements in the limbs on the paralyzed side. The sensory disorder involves both superficial (touch, pain and temperature) and deep (position, vibration) modalities and is associated with a sensation of pain on the affected side which may start a few months after the first clinical manifestations. The pain is continuous, with paroxysmal exacerbations, and it is not suppressed by conventional analgesic treatment" [10].

In the 1950s, thalamic pain was replaced with central post stroke pain (CPSP) as thalamic syndrome was thought to be a misnomer. Thalamic syndrome cannot be considered synonymous with all central pain as thalamic damage does not exclusively precipitate the same constellation of symptoms [9]. CPSP however occurs weeks or months after a thalamic or parietal lesion [8]. Ranges of the reported onset vary from one month to 34 months after [9].

Acute hemiconcern can be mistaken as acute limb pain. It is a motor and visual behavior that can occur during the acute phase of the stroke. In 1995, Bogousslavsky et al. observed

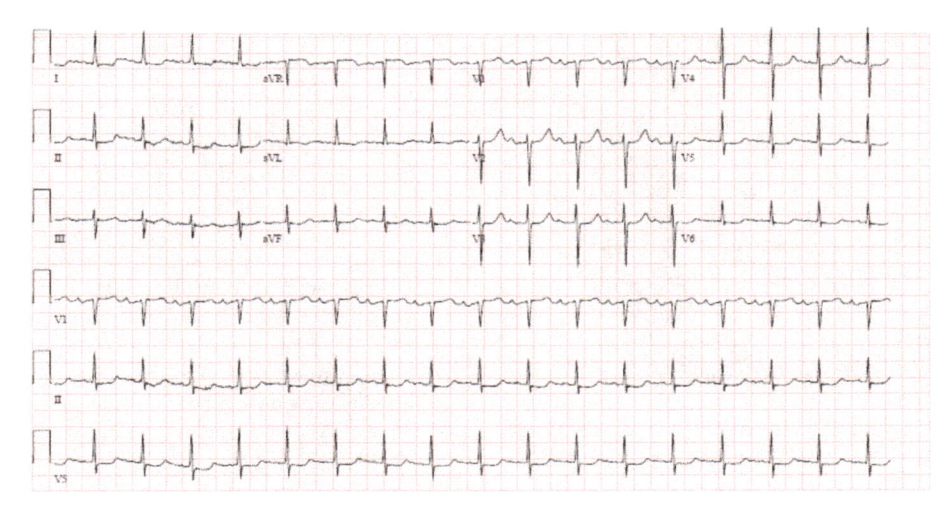

FIGURE 1: Electrocardiogram (ECG) showing sinus tachycardia with first degree atria-ventricular block, as well as ST and T wave abnormality suggestive of lateral ischemia.

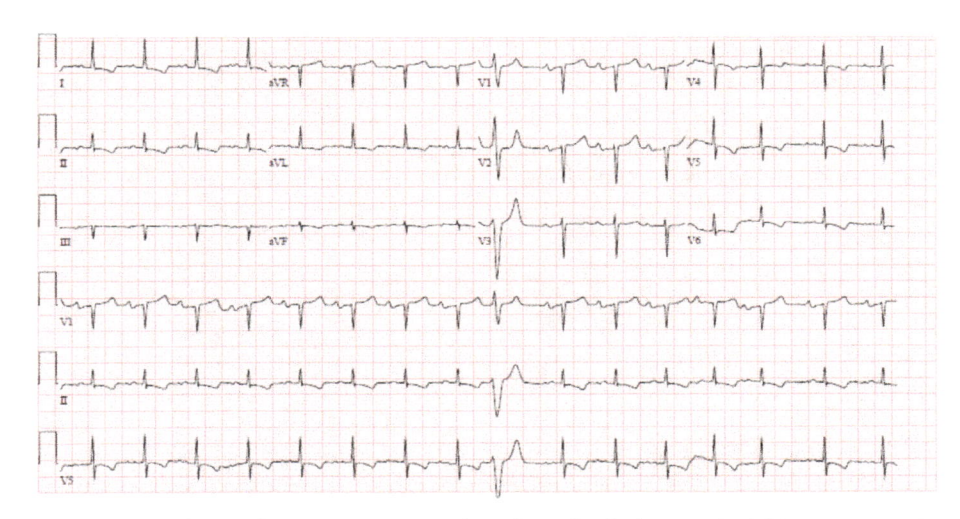

FIGURE 2: Patient's ECG from 2 years previously with similar findings to the ECG on presentation.

patients with strokes involving the territory of the right anterior parietal artery concentrating on the left side of their bodies, relentlessly rubbing, touching, pinching, pressing, lifting, and manipulating parts of the left arm, trunk, and leg with their contralateral hand or foot. These patients had severe loss of elementary sensation on the left (touch, pain, temperature, vibration, and position). This behavior lasted a few days [12]. Acute hemiconcern is easily distinguished from acute limb pain as it is not associated painful symptom [8].

Cocaine has been known to cause coronary vasoconstriction leading to ACS that can manifest as left chest pain or left arm pain or both. While ACS was considered in our patient due to the acute nature of his symptoms, the location of pain, and his multiple risk factors, the pain description was more consistent with allodynia and his clinical exam was consistent with a stroke. His ECG was unchanged from his baseline and the serial troponins during his hospitalization remained negative.

Interestingly, strokes with sensory symptoms have in the past been reported to mimic myocardial ischemia. Gorson et al. have reported patients with prominent unilateral chest wall discomfort associated with sensory symptoms, including burning dysesthesias, alterations in temperature perception, numbness, or tingling, who were first evaluated as cardiac ischemia only to be found later on to have sensory strokes presenting with acute central pain mimicking the discomfort associated with ACS [13]. Since cerebrovascular accidents (CVA) and ACS have the same risk factors, concurrent workups should be initiated in the emergency department.

4. Conclusion

Acute limb pain as a stroke presentation is extremely rare and should be considered in patients presenting with neurological findings such as weakness. Lesions involving the parietal lobe, the thalamus, and the brainstem can result in acute limb

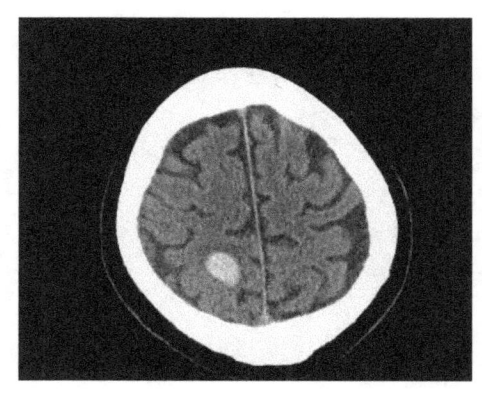

FIGURE 3: CT scan of the brain without contrast showing an acute 2.2 cm intraparenchymal hemorrhage with vasogenic edema in the posterior right parietal lobe.

pain. Other syndromes should be distinguished from acute limb pain from a stroke and include central post stroke pain, which takes time to manifest, and acute hemiconcern, that while acute, it is not associated with pain syndromes. Lastly, strokes with sensory symptoms can mimic ACS. A careful neurological exam is therefore important in patients thought to have a cardiac emergency. Additionally, a concurrent cardiac and neurological work-up should also be considered.

References

[1] J. Michael, Aminoff., and K. Arthur, *Harrisons Neurology in Clinical Medicine*, 15, 3 edition.

[2] A. Malavera, F. A. Silva, F. Fregni, S. Carrillo, and R. G. Garcia, "Repetitive Transcranial Magnetic Stimulation for Phantom Limb Pain in Land Mine Victims: A Double-Blinded, Randomized, Sham-Controlled Trial," *The Journal of Pain*, vol. 17, no. 8, pp. 911–918, 2016.

[3] https://www.ninds.nih.gov/disorders/all-disorders/central-pain-syndrome-information-page.

[4] S. Martin-Schild, K. C. Albright, H. Hallevi et al., "Intracerebral hemorrhage in cocaine users," *Stroke*, vol. 41, no. 4, pp. 680–684, 2010.

[5] P. García-Bermejo, C. Rodríguez-Arias, E. Crespo, S. Pérez-Fernández, J. F. Arenillas, and M. Martínez-Galdámez, "Severe cerebral vasospasm in chronic cocaine users during neurointerventional procedures: A report of two cases," *Interventional Neuroradiology*, vol. 21, no. 1, pp. 19–22, 2015.

[6] E. Pieterse and J. van der Vlag, "Cracking the pathogenesis of cocaine-induced vasculitis," *Rheumatology*, vol. 56, no. 4, pp. 503–505, 2017.

[7] S. Lolignier, N. Eijkelkamp, and J. N. Wood, "Mechanical allodynia," *Pflügers Archiv - European Journal of Physiology*, vol. 467, no. 1, pp. 133–139, 2014.

[8] A. O. Rossetti, J. A. Ghika, F. Vingerhoets, J. Novy, and J. Bogousslavsky, "Neurogenic pain and abnormal movements contralateral to an anterior parietal artery stroke," *JAMA Neurology*, vol. 60, no. 7, pp. 1004–1006, 2003.

[9] J. L. Henry, C. Lalloo, and K. Yashpal, "Central poststroke pain: An abstruse outcome," *Pain Research & Management*, vol. 13, no. 1, pp. 41–49, 2008.

[10] F. J. Alvarez-Perez, "Déjerine-Roussy-Like Syndrome in a Patient with an Ischemic Lesion of the Right Dorsal Protuberance: A Different Cause of Central Neuropathic Pain," *SM Journal of Case Reports*, vol. 2, no. 2, 2016.

[11] M. N. Siddiqui, F. Furgang, S. M. Siddiqui, and J. Sue Ranasinghe, "Dejerine roussy syndrome: The role of methadone in the treatment of a central pain syndrome," *The Internet Journal of Pain, Symptom Control and Palliative Care*, vol. 2, no. 1, pp. XV–XVI, 2001.

[12] J. Bogousslavsky, E. Kumral, F. Regli, G. Assal, and J. Ghika, "Acute hemiconcern: A right anterior parietotemporal syndrome," *Journal of Neurology, Neurosurgery & Psychiatry*, vol. 58, no. 4, pp. 428–432, 1995.

[13] K. C. Gorson, M. S. Pessin, L. D. DeWitt, and L. R. Caplan, "Stroke with sensory symptoms mimicking myocardial ischemia," *Neurology*, vol. 46, no. 2, pp. 548–551, 1996.

Rheumatoid Meningitis Occurring during Etanercept Treatment

Koji Tsuzaki,[1] Takashi Nakamura,[1,2] Hiroyuki Okumura,[1,3] Naoko Tachibana,[1] and Toshiaki Hamano[1]

[1]Department of Neurology, Kansai Electric Power Hospital, Osaka, Japan
[2]Department of Neurology, National Cerebral and Cardiovascular Center, Osaka, Japan
[3]Okumura Clinic, Shiga, Japan

Correspondence should be addressed to Koji Tsuzaki; tsuzaki.koji@b4.kepco.co.jp

Academic Editor: Chin-Chang Huang

We report a 65-year-old man who had repetitive seizures 6 months after receiving etanercept, methotrexate, and prednisolone for rheumatoid arthritis. Mononuclear cells were mildly increased in the cerebrospinal fluid (CSF). Brain magnetic resonance imaging (MRI) showed high intensity along sulci of the frontal and parietal lobes. Brain biopsy revealed lymphocyte and plasma cell infiltration in the meninges, confirming the diagnosis of rheumatoid meningitis. After steroid pulse therapy, seizures resolved and clinical findings improved. When etanercept was replaced by tocilizumab, rheumatoid meningitis did not recur. Although TNF-α inhibitors can control joint symptoms of rheumatoid arthritis, they may induce rheumatoid meningitis.

1. Introduction

The common neurological complications of rheumatoid arthritis are peripheral neuropathies, such as carpal tunnel syndrome and myelopathy due to atlantoaxial subluxation. It is very rare to find complications involving pathologies inside the cranium. In the central nervous system, rheumatoid arthritis targets the meninges, resulting in rheumatoid meningitis [1]. We report a case of rheumatoid meningitis that occurred during etanercept and methotrexate treatment.

2. Case Report

A 65-year-old man came to our clinic in September 2012 with a complaint of transient loss of consciousness. His medical history included prostatomegaly, hypertension, and idiopathic thrombocytopenic purpura. He had been diagnosed as having rheumatoid arthritis in February 2012, which was well controlled by methotrexate (12 mg/week), etanercept (50 mg/week), and prednisolone (2 mg/day). There was no notable family history. Figure 1 shows clinical course (Figure 1).

He was neurologically intact. There were no abnormal findings on brain computerized tomography (CT) and MRI. Electroencephalography (EEG) showed intermittent bursts of bilateral delta activity and infrequent high-amplitude sharp waves predominantly in the frontal regions. Carbamazepine (200 mg/day) was administered for suspected epilepsy, which was later changed to sodium valproate (200 mg/day) due to the occurrence of rash.

After this episode, he showed three transient episodes such as loss of consciousness, generalized tonic convulsion followed by consciousness disturbance, and dysarthria associated with left leg weakness during the following 6 months. Each episode led to hospital admission, but the patient had no neurological symptoms when he was investigated. Brain MRI showed abnormal signals and contrast enhancement in sulci of the left frontal and parietal lobes, but no definite epileptiform activity was found on EEG. CSF revealed nonspecific mild pleocytosis. At this point, chronic meningitis was diagnosed, but the cause was not confirmed.

He was admitted for the fourth time in June 2013, because of a seizure continuing for several minutes and persistent disturbance of consciousness. The patient was slightly disorientated. Examinations of the cranial nerves and motor and sensory systems and deep tendon reflexes and coordination were normal. Serological examination showed that blood platelet count was decreased (58000/μL), without elevated white blood cell count. On biochemical examination, hepatic

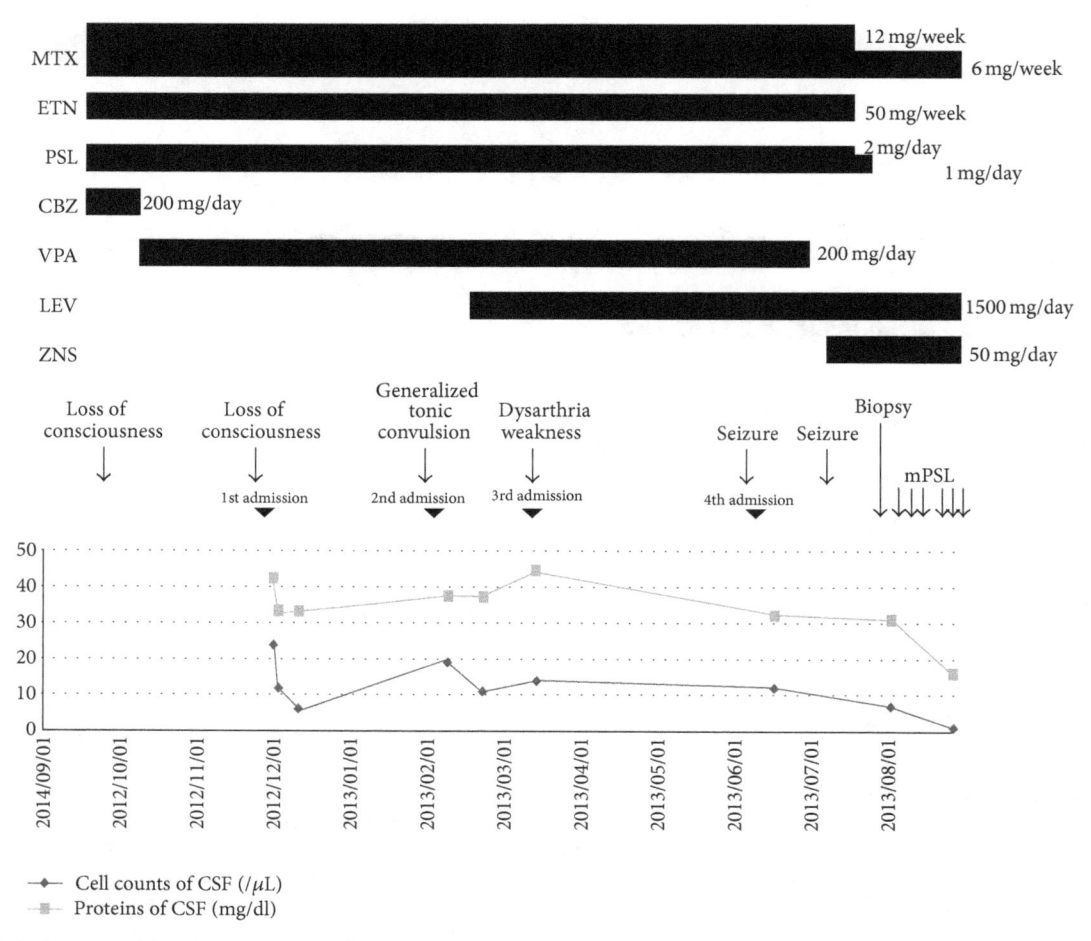

FIGURE 1: Clinical course. After the treatment with intravenous methylprednisolone, cell counts and proteins of CSF decreased, and seizures disappeared. MTX: methotrexate, ETN: etanercept, PSL: prednisolone, CBZ: carbamazepine, VPA: sodium valproate, LEV: levetiracetam, ZNS: zonisamide, and mPSL: methylprednisolone.

enzymes and kidney function were found to be normal, and there were no findings suggesting inflammation. CK was mildly elevated (346 IU/L). Tumor markers were all normal, and sIL2R was mildly elevated at 555 U/mL (reference range: 145–519). Immunological examination showed 12 IU/mL for RF (normal range: 0–10), 80 times for ANA (normal range: 0–40), 297 U/mL for SS-A antibodies (normal range: 0–10), and 18.6 U/mL for SS-B antibodies (normal range: 0–10). PR3-ANCA and MPO-ANCA were normal, and anti-CCP antibodies were 275 U/mL (normal range: 0–4.5). CSF examination showed cell count of 12/μL (mononuclear cells: 12/μL), protein levels of 32 mg/dL, and glucose levels of 55 mg/dL (blood glucose 70 mg/dL). IgG index was 1.7, and cytodiagnosis was negative. CSF culture and PCR for acid-fast bacterium were negative.

Brain MRI showed high intensity areas mainly in the left paracentral sulcus and bilateral superior frontal sulcus in fluid-attenuated inversion recovery and diffusion-weighted imaging scans. Contrast enhancement was observed in the left paracentral sulcus and bilateral superior frontal sulcus. Although the cortex of the left parietal lobe had mild swelling, there were no abnormal findings in the white matter (Figure 2). On EEG, bilateral high-amplitude frontal delta wave bursts of 3–5 Hz occurred in the frontal regions with no epileptiform discharges.

The patient's level of consciousness was improved after hospitalization. Because his rheumatoid arthritis was well controlled and there was thrombocytopenia, methotrexate was reduced to 6 mg/week, and prednisolone and etanercept were discontinued prior to brain biopsy. Zonisamide (50 mg/day) was substituted for sodium valproate, because the patient had another seizure lasting for one hour. New findings on brain CT, MRI, or EEG were not observed at that time.

A brain biopsy from the lesion in the right frontal lobe showed invasion of lymphocytes and plasma cells into the superficial brain layers, resulting in necrosis of the brain surface (Figure 3). The lymphocytes were small; an enzyme antibody technique showed that they were a mixture of CD3- and CD20-positive cells, and light chain restriction was not apparent for plasma cells, indicating that they were unlikely to be tumorous. Flow cytometry also did not show tumor patterns. There were no findings of vasculitis. No fungi or acid-fast bacterium were observed.

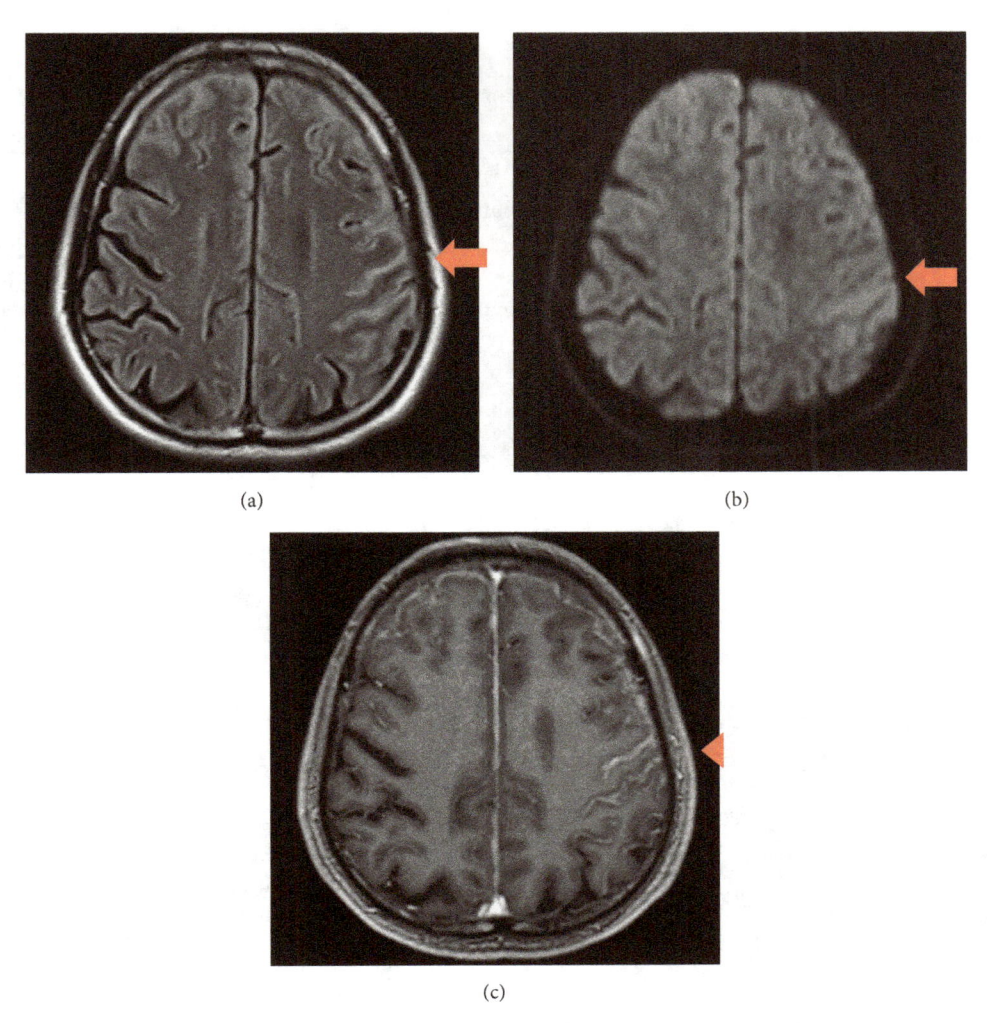

FIGURE 2: Brain MRI findings on the 4th admission. (a) Axial T2 fluid-attenuated inversion recovery (FLAIR) image (1.5 T; TR 10000 ms, TE 108 ms). (b) Diffusion-weighted image (DWI) (1.5 T; TR 5000 ms, TE 75 ms). (c) T1-weighted image (T1WI) enhanced by gadolinium (1.5 T; TR 7.50 ms, TE 2.82 ms). MRI shows extensive thick linear hyperintensity of the leptomeninges in bilateral frontal lobe and the left parietal lobe on T2 FLAIR and DWI (red arrows). T1WI after gadolinium administration shows enhancement of the leptomeninges (red arrowhead).

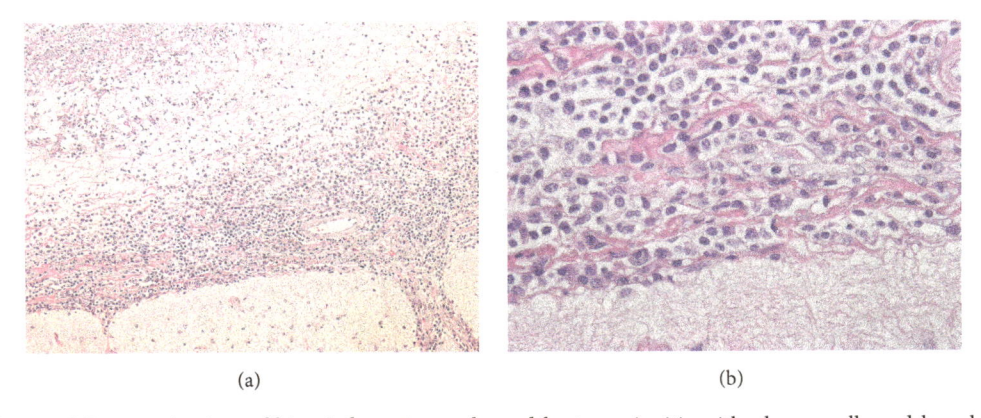

FIGURE 3: Brain biopsy. Microscopic view of biopsied specimen showed leptomeningitis with plasma cells and lymphocytes infiltration. Haematoxylin and eosin stain, magnification of (a) 100x and (b) 400x.

Table 1: Cases of rheumatoid meningitis during treatment with a TNF-α blocker.

Case (age, sex)	Symptoms	TNF-α inhibitor	Duration from administration of TNF-α inhibitor to the onset of rheumatoid meningitis	Treatment
58F [9]	Headache, psychomotor retardation, focal seizures	Adalimumab	7 months	Discontinuation of adalimumab Steroid Rituximab
77M [5]	Headache, expressive dysphasia, involuntary movements of upper extremities, confusion	Adalimumab	2 weeks	Discontinuation of adalimumab Steroid
58F [6]	Headache, emotional lability, left facial numbness, slurred speech, weakness and numbness of the extremities, frequent falls, seizures	Infliximab	3 months	Discontinuation of infliximab Steroid Cyclophosphamide
64M [10]	Aphasia, convulsion, focal seizure of the right side of the body	Infliximab	7 months	Discontinuation of infliximab Steroid
65M (present case)	Seizure	Etanercept	6 months	Discontinuation of etanercept Steroid

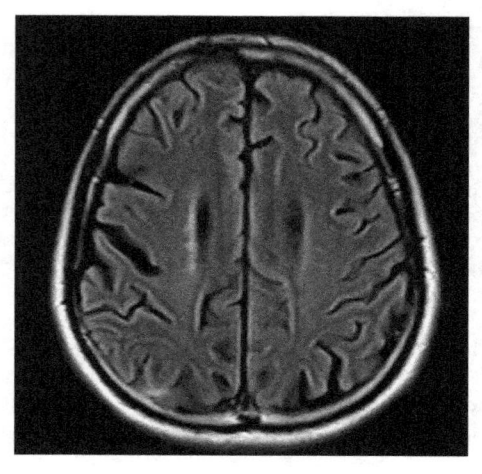

Figure 4: Brain MRI finding 2 years after treatment. T2 FLAIR image (1.5 T; TR 10000 ms, TE 108 ms). MRI performed 2 years after treatment no longer shows linear hyperintensity of the leptomeninges.

Based on the pathological findings, we diagnosed the patient as having rheumatoid meningitis and performed 2 courses of steroid pulse therapy (methylprednisolone 1000 mg/day × 3 days). After the steroid pulse therapy, seizures disappeared and cell counts in the CSF returned to normal. On brain MRI, abnormal signals in the sulci improved (Figure 4), and the slow waves were rarely observed on EEG. In terms of treatment for rheumatoid arthritis, joint symptoms appeared when using methotrexate alone. We added tocilizumab, an IL-6 receptor antagonist, starting in May 2014, and joint symptoms have been well controlled since then. There has also been no recurrence of seizures during the 2 years following the steroid pulse therapy.

3. Discussion

There are no specific biomarkers for rheumatoid meningitis, and brain MRI and biopsy are essential for its diagnosis [2]. On brain MRI, the meninges show contrast enhancement [2, 3]. Pathologically, invasion of lymphocytes in the meninges, vasculitis, and rheumatoid nodules are the typical characteristics [2, 4]. However, it is rare to find all of these characteristics simultaneously [4]. Although there is no consensus for the treatment of rheumatoid meningitis, steroids are often used as the first choice [2, 5]. Our patient also responded well to steroid treatment. When steroid is not effective enough, additional treatment with cyclophosphamide [6], azathioprine [7], cyclosporine [8], and methotrexate [7] may be useful.

To our knowledge, there have been only four case reports of rheumatoid meningitis during treatment with TNF-α inhibitors (Table 1). Huys et al. reported a 58-year-old woman who presented with headache and epilepsy while she was taking methotrexate and adalimumab for rheumatoid arthritis. The meningitis of this patient improved after discontinuation of methotrexate and adalimumab, steroid pulse therapy, and additional administration of rituximab [9]. Ahmed et al. reported a 77-year-old man who had been treated with methotrexate for rheumatoid arthritis. The patient experienced headache, disturbance in consciousness, involuntary movements of the upper and lower limbs, and motor aphasia after adalimumab was added. The symptoms improved after administration of prednisolone, and there was no recurrence after discontinuing adalimumab [5]. Chou et al. reported a 58-year-old woman who presented with headache, slurred speech, numbness of the left side of the face, weakness in the limbs, and seizures. Although her rheumatoid meningitis improved after administration of cyclophosphamide and prednisolone, the symptoms of rheumatoid arthritis deteriorated after discontinuation of cyclophosphamide and reduction of prednisolone. When infliximab was administered, rheumatoid meningitis relapsed. The rheumatoid meningitis improved after discontinuation of infliximab and restarting of cyclophosphamide and prednisolone [6]. Schmid et al. reported a 64-year-old male treated with methotrexate and infliximab. The patient experienced a focal seizure on the right side of the body and aphasia and consciousness disturbance. Symptoms improved after discontinuation of infliximab and steroid pulse therapy [10]. All the patients, including ours, presented with rheumatoid meningitis 2 weeks to 7 months after commencing TNF-α inhibitor treatment, which improved with discontinuation of the treatment and steroid pulse therapy. It is possible that TNF-α inhibitors induce rheumatoid meningitis. It has been pointed out that TNF-α inhibitors can create rheumatoid nodules in a variety of tissues, probably through multiple mechanisms, including modifications of the expression of other cytokines [9, 11]. Another possible explanation is low permeability of etanercept into the brain through the blood-brain barrier [6]. It is possible that etanercept could not suppress the meningitis although it could control the arthritis.

Furthermore, it is widely known that methotrexate can cause aseptic meningitis, particularly in intrathecal administration [12]. In the present patient, methotrexate treatment was reduced prior to biopsy, and there was no recurrence of meningitis after its reduction. Thus, we cannot exclude the possibility that the meningitis was induced by a high dose of methotrexate.

Even when the rheumatoid arthritis is well controlled by TNF-α inhibitors, if seizures and disruption in consciousness occur, biopsy and steroid therapy should be considered immediately, as it is possible that the TNF-α inhibitors can induce rheumatoid meningitis.

Competing Interests

The authors declare that there is no conflict of interests regarding the publication of this paper.

Acknowledgments

The authors thank Dr. Namiko Nishida in the Tazuke Kofukai Medical Research Institute, Kitano Hospital, Department of Neurosurgery, who performed the brain biopsy. They also thank Dr. Yoshiaki Yuba from the Tazuke Kofukai Medical Research Institute, Kitano Hospital, Department of Pathological Diagnosis, for useful advice.

References

[1] T. Kato, K.-I. Hoshi, Y. Sekijima et al., "Rheumatoid meningitis: an autopsy report and review of the literature," *Clinical Rheumatology*, vol. 22, no. 6, pp. 475–480, 2003.

[2] M. Matsushima, H. Yaguchi, M. Niino et al., "MRI and pathological findings of rheumatoid meningitis," *Journal of Clinical Neuroscience*, vol. 17, no. 1, pp. 129–132, 2010.

[3] K. Yamashita, Y. Terasaki, M. Sakaguchi, Y. Nakatsuji, K. Yoshizaki, and H. Mochizuki, "A case of rheumatoid meningitis presented with generalized seizure in whom MRI images were helpful for the diagnosis," *Clinical Neurology*, vol. 55, no. 12, pp. 926–931, 2015.

[4] S. E. Jones, N. A. Belsley, T. C. McLoud, and M. E. Mullins, "Rheumatoid meningitis: radiologic and pathologic correlation," *American Journal of Roentgenology*, vol. 186, no. 4, pp. 1181–1183, 2006.

[5] M. Ahmed, M. Luggen, J. H. Herman et al., "Hypertrophic pachymeningitis in rheumatoid arthritis after adalimumab administration," *Journal of Rheumatology*, vol. 33, no. 11, pp. 2344–2346, 2006.

[6] R. C. Chou, J. W. Henson, D. Tian, E. T. Hedley-Whyte, and A. M. Reginato, "Successful treatment of rheumatoid meningitis with cyclophosphamide but not infliximab," *Annals of the Rheumatic Diseases*, vol. 65, no. 8, pp. 1114–1116, 2006.

[7] D. O. Beck and J. J. Corbett, "Seizures due to central nervous system rheumatoid meningovasculitis," *Neurology*, vol. 33, no. 8, pp. 1058–1061, 1983.

[8] J. Claassen, E. Dwyer, S. Maybaum, and M. S. V. Elkind, "Rheumatoid leptomeningitis after heart transplantation," *Neurology*, vol. 66, no. 6, pp. 948–949, 2006.

[9] A.-C. M. L. Huys, P.-A. Guerne, and J. Horvath, "Rheumatoid meningitis occurring during adalimumab and methotrexate treatment," *Joint Bone Spine*, vol. 79, no. 1, pp. 90–92, 2012.

[10] L. Schmid, M. Müller, T. Treumann et al., "Induction of complete and sustained remission of rheumatoid pachymeningitis by rituximab," *Arthritis and Rheumatism*, vol. 60, no. 6, pp. 1632–1634, 2009.

[11] E. Toussirot, J. M. Berthelot, E. Pertuiset et al., "Pulmonary nodulosis and aseptic granulomatous lung disease occurring in patients with rheumatoid arthritis receiving tumor necrosis factor-α- blocking agent: a case series," *Journal of Rheumatology*, vol. 36, no. 11, pp. 2421–2427, 2009.

[12] C. F. Geiser, Y. Bishop, N. Jaffe et al., "Adverse effects of intrathecal methotrexate in children with acute leukemia in remission," *Blood*, vol. 45, pp. 189–194, 1975.

Advanced Genetic Testing Comes to the Pain Clinic to Make a Diagnosis of Paroxysmal Extreme Pain Disorder

Ashley Cannon,[1,2] Svetlana Kurklinsky,[3] Kimberly J. Guthrie,[1,2] and Douglas L. Riegert-Johnson[1,2]

[1]*The Department of Medical Genetics, Mayo Clinic, Jacksonville, FL 32224, USA*
[2]*Center for Individualized Medicine, Mayo Clinic, Jacksonville, FL 32224, USA*
[3]*Department of Pain Medicine, Mayo Clinic, Jacksonville, FL 32224, USA*

Correspondence should be addressed to Douglas L. Riegert-Johnson; riegertjohnson.douglas@mayo.edu

Academic Editor: Chin-Chang Huang

Objective. To describe the use of an advanced genetic testing technique, whole exome sequencing, to diagnose a patient and their family with a *SCN9A* channelopathy. *Setting*. Academic tertiary care center. *Design*. Case report. *Case Report*. A 61-year-old female with a history of acute facial pain, chronic pain, fibromyalgia, and constipation was found to have a gain of function *SCN9A* mutation by whole exome sequencing. This mutation resulted in an *SCN9A* channelopathy that is most consistent with a diagnosis of paroxysmal extreme pain disorder. In addition to the patient being diagnosed, four siblings have a clinical diagnosis of *SCN9A* channelopathy as they have consistent symptoms and a sister with a known mutation. For treatment, gabapentin was ineffective and carbamazepine was not tolerated. Nontraditional therapies improved symptoms and constipation resolved with pelvic floor retraining with biofeedback. *Conclusion*. Patients with a personal and family history of chronic pain may benefit from a referral to Medical Genetics. Pelvic floor retraining with biofeedback should be considered for patients with a *SCN9A* channelopathy and constipation.

1. Introduction

The *SCN9A* gene encodes the $Na_v1.7$ voltage-gated sodium channel. Mutations in the *SCN9A* gene are the cause of a heterogeneous channelopathy pain syndrome. The $Na_v1.7$ channel is highly expressed in peripheral somatic and visceral sensory neurons, the nociceptive neurons at dorsal root ganglion (DRG), trigeminal ganglion, olfactory sensory neurons, and sympathetic ganglion [1–6]. $Na_v1.7$ amplifies small subthreshold depolarizations [1], regulating excitability of the membrane potential and positioning this sodium channel as a molecular gatekeeper for pain. Heterozygous (monoallelic) gain of function *SCN9A* mutations is associated with multiple phenotypes including small nerve fiber neuropathy (SFN), inherited erythromelalgia (IEM), paroxysmal extreme pain disorder (PEPD) (Table 1), and a novel syndrome of pain dysautonomia [7]. Distinctions between syndromes are made based on presenting symptoms because the same mutation can vary in severity of symptoms and manifest as a different syndrome classification for reasons that are not currently understood. Even in siblings the I228M variant of sodium channel $Na_v1.7$ has been shown to represent itself as both IEM and SFN [8]. The difference in presentation is possibly due to the different patterns of modifier genes, epigenetics, or posttranslational modification, for example, glycosylation [9].

Besides gain of function mutations, biallelic damaging *SCN9A* mutations are associated with congenital insensitivity to pain. A large percentage of small nerve fiber neuropathies have an unknown etiology [10, 11].

Several new technologies, all referred to as next-generation sequencing (NGS), have decreased the cost while increasing the speed of gene sequencing. Using NGS it is now feasible to sequence the coding sequences of all 20,000 genes referred to as the exome. Whole exome sequencing (WES) has been clinically available since 2011 and is now offered by

TABLE 1: Clinical features, triggers, and mutations of sodium channel pain syndromes. Differences between small nerve fiber neuropathy, inherited erythromelalgia, and paroxysmal extreme pain disorder. *The mutations listed are meant to demonstrate phenotypic variability in single mutations; this is not an exhaustive list of mutations.

Pain syndromes	Small nerve fiber neuropathy (SFN)	Inherited erythromelalgia (IEM)	Paroxysmal extreme pain disorder (PEPD)
Clinical features	Cold, burning or electric-like pain, tingling or a pins-and-needles sensation, allodynia and hyperesthesia in feet, and distal extremities [10].	Burning pain, swelling, and skin redness in the distal extremities (feet and, less frequently, the hands). Some individuals have allodynia and hyperalgesia [19, 20].	Skin redness and warmth, severe pain in various parts of the body, typically in the lower part of the body, especially around the rectum, but also can be in head and face, especially the eyes and jaw [16]. Tonic nonepileptic seizures, flushing, watering of eyes or nose, hypersalivation, and weakness (hours to day) related to site of pain [17].
Triggers	None known [10].	Precipitated by mild warmth, standing, exercise, alcohol, and other vasodilating agents, relieved by cooling [16].	Trauma, childbirth, defecation, eating, taking medications, and cold [13].
Duration	Persistent [10].	Occurs multiple times per day and can become constant [4].	Seconds to hours [16].
SCN9A/Na$_v$1.7*	c.554G>A, p.R185H [14] c.684C>G, p.I228M [14] c.1867G>A, p.D623N [14] c.2159T>A, p.I720K [14] c.2215A>G, p.I739V [21] c.2794A>C, p.M932L [14] c.2971G>T, p.V991L [14] c.4596G>A, p.M1532I [14]	c.29A>G, p.Q10R [22, 23] p.L245V [24] c.406A>G, p.I136V [25] c.647T>C, p.F216S [19] c.721T>A, p.S241T [5] c.1185C>A, p.N395K [19] c.2468T>G, p.L823R [26] c.2543T>C, p.I848T [3] c.2573T>A, p.L858H [3] c.2572C>T, p.A863P [27] c.2623C>G, p.Q875E [28] c.4345T>G, p.F1449V [4]	c.2986C>T, p.R996C [13] c.3892G>T, p.V1298F [13] c.3893T>A, p.V1298D [13] c.3895G>T, p.V1299F [13] c.4382T>C, p.I1461T [13] p.F1462V [13] c.4391C>T, p.T1464I [13] G1607K [29] c.4835T>C, p.L1612P [30] c.4880T>A, p.M1627K [13]
SCN10A/Na$_v$1.8*	c.1661T>C, p.L554P [31] c.3910G>A, p.A1304T [31] c.4568G>A, p.C1523Y [31] c.4984G>A, p.G1662S [32] c.5116A>G, p.I1706V [33]		
SCN11A/Na$_v$1.9*	c.1142T>C, p.I381T [34] c.3473T>C, p.L1158P [34]		

several laboratories. Eighty percent of known disease-causing mutations are located in the exome, but the exome represents only 1% of the total genome. Even this 1% of the genome constitutes a vast amount of data, about 30,000,000 base pairs of DNA.

Next-generation sequencing facilitates the identification of individuals with Mendelian disorders that may be underdiagnosed due to variable or relatively nonspecific clinical findings. In this way, such technology will ultimately impact a greater number of medical specialties including Pain Medicine. We describe a case where NGS was used to make a clinically unsuspected diagnosis of PEPD giving the patient a diagnosis and additional treatment options.

PEPD has been described in less than 500 patients [12–15] predominantly in the UK and Netherlands. Clinical features of PEPD are sudden, painful attacks of the anorectal, ocular, and mandibular areas, as well as tonic nonepileptic seizures, flushing, watering of eyes or nose, hypersalivation, and weakness related to the site of pain that can last from hours to days [12, 16–18]. Triggers of the pain can be trauma, childbirth, defecation, cold, and nonphysical triggers such as strong emotions. We describe the use of NGS to make the diagnosis of PEPD and how a mutation reported previously to cause SFN can cause PEPD [14] and give our recommendations for Pain Clinic referrals to Medical Genetics.

2. Case Report

A 61-year-old female of Puerto Rican ancestry was evaluated in Medical Genetics for seemingly separate chronic pain syndromes. She had previously been seen in Family Practice, Gastroenterology, Pain Medicine, Neurology, Physical Medicine and Rehabilitation, Gynecology, and Ophthalmology departments.

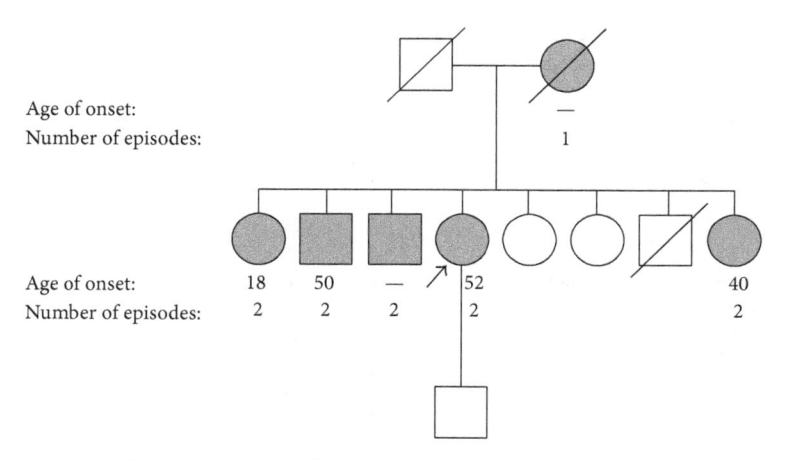

FIGURE 1: *Pedigree.* The patient is indicated by an arrow and all relatives that exhibited at least one episode of extreme facial pain are in grey. The age of onset and number of episodes are indicated beneath each affected individual.

The patient had attacks of facial pain; preliminary diagnosis of Melkersson-Rosenthal syndrome was made. Melkersson-Rosenthal syndrome is a rare nonhereditary disorder characterized by facial weakness, swelling of the face and lips, and furrowing of the tongue. The patient reported similar symptoms in other family members. As familial Melkersson-Rosenthal syndrome had not been reported in the literature, the patient was referred to Medical Genetics for further evaluation. A detailed family history revealed similar facial pain episodes in the patient's mother and four of seven siblings, suggesting a genetic condition of autosomal dominant inheritance (Figure 1). The age of onset of symptoms in the family ranged from 18 to 52 years.

2.1. The Patient Had a Complex Array of Symptoms. The patient had pain involving both sides of the body, both above and below the waistline, including the posterior cervical region. The areas of most severe pain were in the neck, shoulders, both upper extremities, entire back, buttock area, and bilateral lower extremities. Heating pads seem to improve the constant pain and patient preferred a room temperature of 27°C (80°F).

The episodic pain triggers included stressful events (work meetings), defecation, and cold temperatures.

The patient's facial pain symptoms were most consistent with a diagnosis of PEPD. She had two separate episodes of severe facial pain that resulted in hospitalization at the ages of 52 and 61 years. The first episode consisted of severe headache lasting 3 days, right facial swelling, right eye weakness, and forehead paralysis. The second episode consisted of a global thunderclap headache, left orbital eye pain, left facial paralysis with decreased sensation, and right-sided ptosis, in addition to facial swelling and weakness. MR and CT brain imaging were unremarkable.

The facial pain also occurred several times each day and was triggered by cold, smiling, brushing teeth, and chewing, but not by touching the face or food. Paroxysmal type of electrical pain shoots down the right mandible. This may be followed by a pulling sensation in her right cheek and eye. Intensity was typically 5 on a scale of 10, although it may reach 10. The pain was accompanied by dripping lacrimation in the right eye but no facial flushing or sweating (Table 3). The lacrimation was worse when she was eating but she does not describe gustatory sweating (Table 3). Patient's facial pain lasted for several hours. Patient avoids eating cold foods like popsicles and melts ice cream before eating it. Patient also avoids eating in public.

Sinus congestion previously triggered pain, but this mostly resolved after three sinus operations. She denied tear secretion and flushing being triggers for pain (Table 3).

She described often having rectal pain during defecation, consistent with PEPD. This began around the age of 45 and had progressively increased in severity. She described the rectal pain severity to be worse than pain associated with childbirth (10/10); the pain attacks lasted for hours.

She denied having seizures, including the period during childhood; however, patient had several syncope events as an adult.

She reported "fibromyalgia attacks" that occur about twice a month, after stressful events like meetings and cold temperature, which affect the entire body and pain was described as achy and dull; pain lasted for several days. The patient was previously diagnosed with fibromyalgia by Family Medicine at the age of 56 by the American College of Rheumatology 1990 criteria. These findings suggest a complex pain phenotype that consisted of pain attacks akin to PEPD in addition to persistent pain that can be observed in SFN. The patient was also asked about symptoms specific to PEPD.

The patient completed the Neuropathic Pain Scale to evaluate the intensity and characteristics of pain [35]. She described a constant pain that was intense, sharp, deep, and often cold. The intensity was reported as a 5/10 in the coccyx and lower back. She described episodic sharp pain (10/10) in the neck, legs, and back. She reported that the coccyx pain radiates most often to her left leg but sometimes radiates down both legs, lasting for hours. She also described a cold pain (8/10), especially in her feet, even on warm days.

TABLE 2: Small nerve fiber symptom inventory questionnaire: responses of the patient described in this report are marked with x's. The patient has some (0–3) symptoms of small fiber neuropathy.

	Symptoms of small nerve fiber neuropathy	Never	Sometimes	Often	Always
Autonomic	Sweating		x		
	Diarrhea		x		
	Constipation				x
	Urination problems	x			
	Dry eyes				x
	Dry mouth	x			
	Orthostatic complains	x			
	Palpitations	x			
	Hot flashes	x			
Sensory	Sensitive skin	x			
	Burning feet	x			
	Sheet intolerance	x			
	Restless legs	x			

TABLE 3: SCN9A-associated features questionnaire. The responses of the patient described in this case report are shown.

Have you ever had (including early childhood):	Yes/no	If yes, at what age did those features begin?	If yes, how often (sometimes, often, always)
Seizures	No		
Rectal pain	Yes	45-increased in severity	often
Constipation	Yes	3	always
Sensitivity to cold temperatures	Yes	51	always (likes ambient temperature of 27°C)
Redness and swelling of the hands or feet	Yes	36 (during pregnancy)	
Pain during/following tear secretion	No (pain when eyes dry)		
Pain during/following flushing	No		
Pain during/following sinus congestion	Yes	37	sometimes
Pain during/following defecation	Yes	45	always
Pain during/following eating	No		
Pain during/following strong emotions	Yes	53	often

Additionally, the patient completed a small nerve fiber questionnaire (Table 2), which examined the presence and frequency of features associated with SFN such as sweating, diarrhea, constipation, incontinence, dry eyes, dry mouth, dizziness upon standing, palpitations, hot flashes, skin sensitivity, burning feet, sheet intolerance, and restless legs. She reported persistent constipation, dry eyes with occasional diarrhea, and excessive sweating. She denied urination problems, dry mouth, dizziness upon standing, palpitations, hot flashes, sensitive skin, burning feet, sheet intolerance, or restless legs. These findings indicate that the patient exhibits certain features observed in SFN like neuropathic pain, persistent pain, and perhaps some of the autonomic features.

The patient was asked about symptoms of IEM. She did not have severe burning pain in the distal limbs or pain triggered by warmth.

EMG was performed by neurology when patient was 55 and 56 years old for evaluation of Bell's palsy; the first was one was unremarkable, while the second one showed mononeuropathy at the wrist.

2.2. Whole Exome Sequencing (WES) Genomic Testing, Diagnosis, and Treatment. "The patient was referred with a diagnosis of familial Melkersson-Rosenthal syndrome. No gene has been associated with Melkersson-Rosenthal syndrome before. The authors considered several strategies to hunt for the Melkersson-Rosenthal gene. The authors could not identify any strong candidate genes for Sanger sequencing. It was decided to use the WES approach of testing about 20,000 genes with one test."

A sample of the patient's blood was sent to Baylor Medical Genetics Laboratories (Houston, TX) for WES using an Illumina HiSeq platform (San Diego, CA). WES analysis detected a pathogenic heterozygous c.2159T>A (p.I720K) mutation in the *SCN9A* gene. The cost of the WES test was $7000 (USA); the results were available for us after 9 weeks. This patient's testing was paid for by the Mayo Clinic Individualized

Medicine Clinic. We estimate the mean out of pocket expense for WES for patients with commercial insurance at $1000 or less.

Treatment options for *SCN9A* channelopathies are suboptimal. Patients with PEPD have experienced some benefit with carbamazepine [13]. This patient was treated with oxcarbazepine 150 mg twice daily. After 6 weeks of oxcarbazepine treatment she developed Stevens-Johnson syndrome, with skin redness and peeling. Her pain had not improved with oxcarbazepine. Oxcarbazepine was stopped and gabapentin was then begun. The gabapentin regimen was 100 mg three times a day (10 days), 300 mg three times a day (10 days), and finally 600 mg three times per day (10 days). Gabapentin was stopped after the patient reported no improvement and that it was too sedating.

The patient was next offered lacosamide. Lacosamide is an adjunctive treatment for partial onset seizures and diabetic neuropathic pain. Lacosamide enhances slow inactivation of $Na_v 1.7$ and as such may be a valuable choice of treatment. A clinical trial of lacosamide for patients with *SCN9A* mutations has been registered and is recruiting (NCT01911975). The patient declined lacosamide after she was told there was an increased risk of suicidal behavior and ideation (as with all antiepileptic drugs).

The patient reported that nontraditional therapies have been the most effective at treating her pain. Following severe facial pain episodes, her symptoms improved with massage, acupuncture, and cold compresses. Heating pads have improved her constant pain.

The cause of the patient's constipation was diagnosed as pelvic floor dysfunction by anal rectal manometry and MR defecography. The patient described remarkable improvement in constipation after pelvic floor retraining with biofeedback. A physical therapist administered treatment once a week for six weeks (standard regime for our and other centers). Treatment consisted of external therapeutic ultrasound, 5 min of therapeutic exercise, and 30 min of soft tissue mobilization with manual therapy to gluteal muscles, piriformis, coccygeus, ST ligaments, levator ani, and ischiopubic points. At the end of treatment, she was having one bowel movement most days compared to a bowel movement once a month since early childhood.

Return of constipation after pelvic floor retraining with biofeedback occurs in about half of patients at one year [36]. This patient's constipation returned after 4 years and the patient had a second course of pelvic floor retraining with biofeedback. The treatment was again effective and her constipation resolved. We speculate that her pelvic floor dysfunction was a compensatory response to rectal pain during defecation resulting from the *SCN9A* mutation.

3. Discussion

3.1. Patients with SCN9A Mutations Can Present Features of Different Pain Syndromes. Here, we report a patient with an *SCN9A* c.2159T>A mutation that has been reported in one patient before [14]. The patient's clinical presentation is most consistent with PEPD, including severe episodic pain in the facial and anorectal regions that are triggered by stressful events, cold temperatures, and defecation. In addition, she presents with persistent neuropathic pain and autonomic dysfunction, including severe constipation, which is consistent with SFN.

The *SCN9A* c.2159T>A mutation detected in our patient has been reported in a single Dutch patient diagnosed with SFN [14]. This patient experienced severe pain throughout the body with muscle ache before developing the characteristic distal pain of SFN, with burning pain in feet, lower arms, and lower legs, numbness in feet, and hyperhidrosis in feet; the Dutch patient also suffered from hot flashes, skin hyperesthesia, sheet intolerance, restless legs, sweating, diarrhea, micturition, dry eyes and mouth, dizziness, and palpitations [14]. The comparison between the Dutch patient and our patient indicates that even the same *SCN9A* mutation can manifest differently in different patients. Because of the inconsistent relationship between the mutation and the outcome (genotype-phenotype correlation), we and others recommend diagnosis of a specific *SCN9A* channelopathy based on the patient's clinical status.

3.2. SCN9A and Fibromyalgia. The patient suffered from complex pain symptoms, fibromyalgia, and other symptoms of the central sensitization syndrome like depression and anxiety [37, 38]. Stimulation of C-fibers has been implicated in the mechanism of central sensitization syndrome, mainly through the NMDA receptor's role in the spinal transmission of nociceptive signals, and contributes to inflammatory nociceptive sensitization [39, 40]. $Na_v 1.7$ channels have been found on the C-fibers where they could be leading to hyperexcitability and promoting signaling of the NMDA receptors. It would be interesting to see if other patients with fibromyalgia and central sensitization syndrome have mutations in *SCN9A* or proteins that support $Na_v 1.7$ function, like scaffolds of anchoring proteins. Notably, a study of Mexican women demonstrated that an *SCN9A* polymorphism significantly correlated with women diagnosed with fibromyalgia [41]. Because sodium channels located in nociceptors act as molecular gatekeepers for pain stimulation regulating membrane potential, it is possible that fibromyalgia has polygenetic components where sodium channels have an important role.

3.3. Pelvic Floor Biofeedback for PEPD. PEPD is classically associated with rectal pain and constipation. This is the first report of pelvic floor biofeedback for PEPD. Given the excellent response our patient had, we recommend pelvic floor biofeedback be considered for PEPD and *SCN9A* channelopathy patients with rectal pain or constipation. The biofeedback treatment should be tailored to the individual patient.

3.4. WES and the Importance of Making a Diagnosis. WES is a powerful diagnostic technique that can make a diagnosis in 1 of 4 patients in genetics clinics where traditional means of evaluation have failed to make a diagnosis [42]. In our experience, much of the power of WES comes from not being biased by previous clinical judgments and errors. This is illustrated in this case of the diagnosis of Melkersson-Rosenthal syndrome in patient with a clear family history, although Melkersson-Rosenthal syndrome is not known to be hereditary. Additionally, the reported family history of multiple affected family members in two generations increased the likelihood of identifying a single gene disorder by whole exome sequencing.

3.5. The Value of a Diagnosis Cannot Be Overestimated. Although this patient has not had a clear clinical benefit from her diagnosis to date, she has been offered more options (e.g., lacosamide) and may benefit in the future. Individuals attending Medical Genetics clinics often report their primary concern is their children and other family members. The identification of *SCN9A* mutation has benefitted both her son and siblings. The patient's son and siblings can now be tested to determine whether they carry the familial *SCN9A* mutation. Mutation carriers in the family can now have treatment guided by their molecular diagnosis (gabapentin and lacosamide). Also, diagnosed patients can avoid further diagnostic investigations such as EMGs, MRIs, and other tests.

3.6. Recommendations for Referrals from Pain Medicine to Medical Genetics. Individual genetic syndromes are rare, and clinicians must maintain a high degree of suspicion to make a diagnosis. Syndromes associated with chronic pain seen in Medical Genetics clinic include porphyria, hypophosphatasia, Ehlers-Danlos syndrome, and osteogenesis imperfecta. Importantly, many of these syndromes have a disease-specific targeted therapy (e.g., hematin for porphyria).

We recommend that Pain Medicine clinicians consider referring the following patients to Medical Genetics: (a) patients with a pain syndrome and family history of the same syndrome in 2 or more family members, (b) young patients with no explanation for their pain syndrome, (c) individuals of any age with very uncommon presentations, such as the rectal pain of PEPD, and (d) patients with a genetic disorder that may be contributing to their pain (porphyria). These recommendations are based on expert opinion. An online directory of genetic providers isavailable from the National Society of Genetic Counselors (http://www.nsgc.org/).

Competing Interests

The authors declare that they have no competing interests.

Authors' Contributions

Ashley Cannon and Svetlana Kurklinsky contributed equally to this work.

References

[1] S. D. Dib-Hajj, Y. Yang, J. A. Black, and S. G. Waxman, "The Na_v 1.7 sodium channel: from molecule to man," *Nature Reviews Neuroscience*, vol. 14, no. 1, pp. 49–62, 2013.

[2] C. K. Raymond, J. Castle, P. Garrett-Engele et al., "Expression of alternatively spliced sodium channel α-subunit genes. Unique splicing patterns are observed in dorsal root ganglia," *The Journal of Biological Chemistry*, vol. 279, no. 44, pp. 46234–46241, 2004.

[3] Y. Yang, Y. Wang, S. Li et al., "Mutations in SCN9A, encoding a sodium channel alpha subunit, in patients with primary erythermalgia," *Journal of Medical Genetics*, vol. 41, no. 3, pp. 171–174, 2004.

[4] S. D. Dib-Hajj, A. M. Rush, T. R. Cummins et al., "Gain-of-function mutation in Nav1.7 in familial erythromelalgia induces bursting of sensory neurons," *Brain*, vol. 128, no. 8, pp. 1847–1854, 2005.

[5] J. J. Michiels, R. H. M. Te Morsche, J. B. M. J. Jansen, and J. P. H. Drenth, "Autosomal dominant erythermalgia associated with a novel mutation in the voltage-gated sodium channel α subunit Nav1.7," *Archives of Neurology*, vol. 62, no. 10, pp. 1587–1590, 2005.

[6] C. Han, A. M. Rush, S. D. Dib-Hajj et al., "Sporadic onset of erythermalgia: a gain-of-function mutation in Na_v1.7," *Annals of Neurology*, vol. 59, no. 3, pp. 553–558, 2006.

[7] J. G. J. Hoeijmakers, C. Han, I. S. J. Merkies et al., "Small nerve fibres, small hands and small feet: a new syndrome of pain, dysautonomia and acromesomelia in a kindred with a novel Na V1.7 mutation," *Brain*, vol. 135, no. 2, pp. 345–358, 2012.

[8] M. Estacion, C. Han, J.-S. Choi et al., "Intra- and interfamily phenotypic diversity in pain syndromes associated with a gain-of-function variant of Na V1.7," *Molecular Pain*, vol. 7, article 92, 2011.

[9] M. A. Rizzo, J. D. Kocsis, and S. G. Waxman, "Slow sodium conductances of dorsal root ganglion neurons: intraneuronal homogeneity and interneuronal heterogeneity," *Journal of Neurophysiology*, vol. 72, no. 6, pp. 2796–2815, 1994.

[10] A. Hovaguimian and C. H. Gibbons, "Diagnosis and treatment of pain in small-fiber neuropathy," *Current Pain and Headache Reports*, vol. 15, no. 3, pp. 193–200, 2011.

[11] S.-T. Hsieh, "Pathology and functional diagnosis of small-fiber painful neuropathy," *Acta Neurologica Taiwanica*, vol. 19, no. 2, pp. 82–89, 2010.

[12] C. R. Fertleman, C. D. Ferrie, J. Aicardi et al., "Paroxysmal extreme pain disorder (previously familial rectal pain syndrome)," *Neurology*, vol. 69, no. 6, pp. 586–595, 2007.

[13] C. R. Fertleman, M. D. Baker, K. A. Parker et al., "SCN9A mutations in paroxysmal extreme pain disorder: allelic variants underlie distinct channel defects and phenotypes," *Neuron*, vol. 52, no. 5, pp. 767–774, 2006.

[14] C. G. Faber, J. G. J. Hoeijmakers, H.-S. Ahn et al., "Gain of function Na_V1.7 mutations in idiopathic small fiber neuropathy," *Annals of Neurology*, vol. 71, no. 1, pp. 26–39, 2012.

[15] B. A. Brouwer, I. S. J. Merkies, M. M. Gerrits, S. G. Waxman, J. G. J. Hoeijmakers, and C. G. Faber, "Painful neuropathies: the emerging role of sodium channelopathies," *Journal of the Peripheral Nervous System*, vol. 19, no. 2, pp. 53–65, 2014.

[16] R. Dabby, "Pain disorders and erythromelalgia caused by voltage-gated sodium channel mutations," *Current Neurology and Neuroscience Reports*, vol. 12, no. 1, pp. 76–83, 2012.

[17] R. Hayden and M. Grossman, "Rectal, ocular, and submaxillary pain; a familial autonomic disorder related to proctalgia fugax: report of a family," *A.M.A. Journal of Diseases of Children*, vol. 97, no. 4, pp. 479–482, 1959.

[18] C. R. Fertleman and C. D. Ferrie, "What's in a name—familial rectal pain syndrome becomes paroxysmal extreme pain disorder," *Journal of Neurology, Neurosurgery and Psychiatry*, vol. 77, no. 11, pp. 1294–1295, 2006.

[19] J. P. H. Drenth, R. H. M. te Morsche, G. Guillet, A. Taieb, R. L. Kirby, and J. B. M. J. Jansen, "*SCN9A* mutations define primary erythermalgia as a neuropathic disorder of voltage gated sodium channels," *Journal of Investigative Dermatology*, vol. 124, no. 6, pp. 1333–1338, 2005.

[20] M. Eberhardt, J. Nakajima, A. B. Klinger et al., "Inherited pain sodium channel nav1.7 A1632T mutation causes erythromelalgia due to a shift of fast inactivation," *The Journal of Biological Chemistry*, vol. 289, no. 4, pp. 1971–1980, 2014.

[21] C. Han, J. G. J. Hoeijmakers, H.-S. Ahn et al., "Na_v1.7-related small fiber neuropathy: Impaired slow-inactivation and DRG neuron hyperexcitability," *Neurology*, vol. 78, no. 21, pp. 1635–1643, 2012.

[22] C. J. Klein, Y. Wu, D. H. Kilfoyle et al., "Infrequent SCN9A mutations in congenital insensitivity to pain and erythromelalgia," *Journal of Neurology, Neurosurgery and Psychiatry*, vol. 84, no. 4, pp. 386–391, 2013.

[23] C. Han, S. D. Dib-Hajj, Z. Lin et al., "Early- and late-onset inherited erythromelalgia: genotypephenotype correlation," *Brain*, vol. 132, no. 7, pp. 1711–1722, 2009.

[24] E. C. Emery, A. M. Habib, J. J. Cox et al., "Novel SCN9A mutations underlying extreme pain phenotypes: unexpected electrophysiological and clinical phenotype correlations," *The Journal of Neuroscience*, vol. 35, no. 20, pp. 7674–7681, 2015.

[25] M.-J. Lee, H.-S. Yu, S.-T. Hsieh, D. A. Stephenson, C.-J. Lu, and C.-C. Yang, "Characterization of a familial case with primary erythromelalgia from Taiwan," *Journal of Neurology*, vol. 254, no. 2, pp. 210–214, 2007.

[26] K. Takahashi, M. Saitoh, H. Hoshino et al., "A case of primary erythermalgia, wintry hypothermia and encephalopathy," *Neuropediatrics*, vol. 38, no. 3, pp. 157–159, 2007.

[27] T. P. Harty, S. D. Dib-Hajj, L. Tyrrell et al., "Na_v1.7 mutant A863P in erythromelalgia: effects of altered activation and steady-state inactivation on excitability of nociceptive dorsal root ganglion neurons," *The Journal of Neuroscience*, vol. 26, no. 48, pp. 12566–12575, 2006.

[28] N. Skeik, T. W. Rooke, M. D. Davis et al., "Severe case and literature review of primary erythromelalgia: novel *SCN9A* gene mutation," *Vascular Medicine*, vol. 17, no. 1, pp. 44–49, 2012.

[29] J.-S. Choi, F. Boralevi, O. Brissaud et al., "Paroxysmal extreme pain disorder: a molecular lesion of peripheral neurons," *Nature Reviews Neurology*, vol. 7, no. 1, pp. 51–55, 2011.

[30] M. R. Suter, Z. A. Bhuiyan, C. J. Laedermann et al., "P.L1612P, a novel voltage-gated sodium channel Nav1.7 mutation inducing a cold sensitive paroxysmal extreme pain disorder," *Anesthesiology*, vol. 122, no. 2, pp. 414–423, 2015.

[31] C. G. Faber, G. Lauria, I. S. J. Merkies et al., "Gain-of-function Na_v1.8 mutations in painful neuropathy," *Proceedings of the National Academy of Sciences of the United States of America*, vol. 109, no. 47, pp. 19444–19449, 2012.

[32] C. Han, D. Vasylyev, L. J. Macala et al., "The G1662S NaV1.8 mutation in small fibre neuropathy: impaired inactivation underlying DRG neuron hyperexcitability," *Journal of Neurology, Neurosurgery and Psychiatry*, vol. 85, no. 5, pp. 499–505, 2014.

[33] J. Huang, Y. Yang, P. Zhao et al., "Small-fiber neuropathy Nav1.8 mutation shifts activation to hyperpolarized potentials and increases excitability of dorsal root ganglion neurons," *Journal of Neuroscience*, vol. 33, no. 35, pp. 14087–14097, 2013.

[34] J. Huang, C. Han, M. Estacion et al., "Gain-of-function mutations in sodium channel NaV1.9 in painful neuropathy," *Brain*, vol. 137, no. 6, pp. 1627–1642, 2014.

[35] B. S. Galer and M. P. Jensen, "Development and preliminary validation of a pain measure specific to neuropathic pain: the Neuropathic Pain Scale," *Neurology*, vol. 48, no. 2, pp. 332–338, 1997.

[36] E. Battaglia, A. M. Serra, G. Buonafede et al., "Long-term study on the effects of visual biofeedback and muscle training as a therapeutic modality in pelvic floor dyssynergia and slow-transit constipation," *Diseases of the Colon & Rectum*, vol. 47, no. 1, pp. 90–95, 2004.

[37] C. J. Woolf and S. W. N. Thompson, "The induction and maintenance of central sensitization is dependent on N-methyl-d-aspartic acid receptor activation; implications for the treatment of post-injury pain hypersensitivity states," *Pain*, vol. 44, no. 3, pp. 293–299, 1991.

[38] J. F. Herrero, J. M. A. Laird, and J. A. Lopez-Garcia, "Wind-up of spinal cord neurones and pain sensation: much ado about something?" *Progress in Neurobiology*, vol. 61, no. 2, pp. 169–203, 2000.

[39] T. Minami, S. Matsumura, E. Okuda-Ashitaka et al., "Characterization of the glutamatergic system for induction and maintenance of allodynia," *Brain Research*, vol. 895, no. 1-2, pp. 178–185, 2001.

[40] A. B. Malmberg and T. L. Yaksh, "Hyperalgesia mediated by spinal glutamate or substance P receptor blocked by spinal cyclooxygenase inhibition," *Science*, vol. 257, no. 5074, pp. 1276–1279, 1992.

[41] G. Vargas-Alarcon, E. Alvarez-Leon, J.-M. Fragoso et al., "A SCN9A gene-encoded dorsal root ganglia sodium channel polymorphism associated with severe fibromyalgia," *BMC Musculoskeletal Disorders*, vol. 13, article 23, 2012.

[42] L. G. Biesecker and R. C. Green, "Diagnostic clinical genome and exome sequencing," *The New England Journal of Medicine*, vol. 371, no. 12, p. 1170, 2014.

Permissions

All chapters in this book were first published in CRNM, by Hindawi Publishing Corporation; hereby published with permission under the Creative Commons Attribution License or equivalent. Every chapter published in this book has been scrutinized by our experts. Their significance has been extensively debated. The topics covered herein carry significant findings which will fuel the growth of the discipline. They may even be implemented as practical applications or may be referred to as a beginning point for another development.

The contributors of this book come from diverse backgrounds, making this book a truly international effort. This book will bring forth new frontiers with its revolutionizing research information and detailed analysis of the nascent developments around the world.

We would like to thank all the contributing authors for lending their expertise to make the book truly unique. They have played a crucial role in the development of this book. Without their invaluable contributions this book wouldn't have been possible. They have made vital efforts to compile up to date information on the varied aspects of this subject to make this book a valuable addition to the collection of many professionals and students.

This book was conceptualized with the vision of imparting up-to-date information and advanced data in this field. To ensure the same, a matchless editorial board was set up. Every individual on the board went through rigorous rounds of assessment to prove their worth. After which they invested a large part of their time researching and compiling the most relevant data for our readers.

The editorial board has been involved in producing this book since its inception. They have spent rigorous hours researching and exploring the diverse topics which have resulted in the successful publishing of this book. They have passed on their knowledge of decades through this book. To expedite this challenging task, the publisher supported the team at every step. A small team of assistant editors was also appointed to further simplify the editing procedure and attain best results for the readers.

Apart from the editorial board, the designing team has also invested a significant amount of their time in understanding the subject and creating the most relevant covers. They scrutinized every image to scout for the most suitable representation of the subject and create an appropriate cover for the book.

The publishing team has been an ardent support to the editorial, designing and production team. Their endless efforts to recruit the best for this project, has resulted in the accomplishment of this book. They are a veteran in the field of academics and their pool of knowledge is as vast as their experience in printing. Their expertise and guidance has proved useful at every step. Their uncompromising quality standards have made this book an exceptional effort. Their encouragement from time to time has been an inspiration for everyone.

The publisher and the editorial board hope that this book will prove to be a valuable piece of knowledge for researchers, students, practitioners and scholars across the globe.

List of Contributors

Mangala Gopal
College of Osteopathic Medicine, Des Moines University, Des Moines, IA, USA

Melvin Parasram
Arizona College of Osteopathic Medicine, Midwestern University, Glendale, AZ, USA

Harsh Patel
Baroda Medical College, Vadodara, Gujarat, India

Chike Ilorah
Department of Neurology, University of Illinois College of Medicine at Peoria, Peoria, IL, USA

Hrachya Nersesyan
Department of Neurology, University of Illinois College of Medicine at Peoria, Peoria, IL, USA
Illinois Neurological Institute, OSF St. Francis Medical Center, Peoria, IL, USA

Paul L. M. de Kort
Department of Neurology, Elisabeth Tweesteden Hospital, Tilburg, Netherlands

Hugo P. Aben
Department of Neurology, Elisabeth Tweesteden Hospital, Tilburg, Netherlands
Department of Neurology, Brain Center Rudolf Magnus, University Medical Center Utrecht, Utrecht, Netherlands

Procras Study Group
Department of Neurology, Elisabeth Tweesteden Hospital, Tilburg, Netherlands
Department of Neurology, Brain Center Rudolf Magnus, University Medical Center Utrecht, Utrecht, Netherlands
Department of Rehabilitation Medicine, Brain Center Rudolf Magnus, University Medical Center Utrecht, Utrecht, Netherlands
Department of Clinical and Experimental Neuropsychology, University of Groningen, Groningen, Netherlands

Yael D. Reijmer and Geert Jan Biessels
Department of Neurology, Brain Center Rudolf Magnus, University Medical Center Utrecht, Utrecht, Netherlands

Johanna M. A. Visser-Meily
Department of Rehabilitation Medicine, Brain Center Rudolf Magnus, University Medical Center Utrecht, Utrecht, Netherlands

Jacoba M. Spikman
Department of Clinical and Experimental Neuropsychology, University of Groningen, Groningen, Netherlands

Shahvaiz Magsi, Adeel Khoja and Noman Ishaque
Aga Khan University, Karachi, Pakistan

Mansoor Ali Merchant Rameez and Ariba Khan
DOWUniversity of Health Sciences, Karachi, Pakistan

Mohammad Mousbah Al-Tabbaa
Visiting MD, University of Illinois College of Medicine at Peoria, Peoria, IL, USA

Hani Habal
Clinical Assistant Professor, University of Illinois College of Medicine at Peoria, Peoria, IL, USA

P. Natteru, P. Nattanmai and C. R. Newey
Department of Neurology, University of Missouri, 5 Hospital Drive, CE 540, Columbia, MO 65211, USA

George
Department of Neurology, Cerebrovascular Center, Cleveland Clinic, 9500 Euclid Avenue, Cleveland, OH 44125, USA

P. R. Bell
Department of Surgery, Division of Neurosurgery, University of Missouri, 1 Hospital Drive, Columbia, MO 65211, USA

Ahmed Al-Imam
Novel Psychoactive Substances Unit, Doctoral College, Hertfordshire University, Hertfordshire, UK
College of Medicine, University of Baghdad, Baghdad, Iraq

Shauna H. Yuan
Department of Neurosciences, University of California, San Diego, La Jolla, CA 92093, USA

Sonya G. Wang
Department of Neurology, University of Minnesota, Minneapolis, MN 55455, USA

A. Cucca, M. C. Biagioni, K. Sharma, R. M. Gilbert and A. Di Rocco
Department of Neurology, The Marlene and Paolo Fresco Institute for Parkinson's and Movement Disorders, New York University School of Medicine, NYU Langone Medical Center, New York, NY, USA

List of Contributors

J. Golomb
Department of Neurosurgery, Adult Hydrocephalus Program, NYU School of Medicine, New York, NY, USA

J. E. Fleisher
Department of Neurological Sciences, Rush University Medical Center, Chicago, IL, USA

Leigh A. Rettenmaier
University of Iowa Carver College of Medicine, 375 Newton Rd, Iowa City, IA 52242, USA

Marshall T. Holland and Taylor J. Abel
Department of Neurosurgery, University of Iowa, 200 Hawkins Drive, Iowa City, IA 52245, USA

E. Martínez, L. López-Mesonero, M. Ruiz and A. L. Guerrero
Neurology Department, Hospital Clínico Universitario, Valladolid, Spain

R. Moreno and I. Vidriales
2Clinical Analysis Department, Hospital Clínico Universitario, Valladolid, Spain

J. J. Tellería
IBGM, University of Valladolid, Valladolid, Spain

Murad Talahma, Vivek Sabharwal, Yana Bukovskaya, and Fawad Khan
Department of Neurocritical Care, Ochsner Health System, New Orleans, LA, USA

Juneki Kim and Jin-gyu Choi
Department of Neurosurgery, Seoul St. Mary's Hospital, College of Medicine, The Catholic University of Korea, Seoul, Republic of Korea

Byung-chul Son
Department of Neurosurgery, Seoul St. Mary's Hospital, College of Medicine, The Catholic University of Korea, Seoul, Republic of Korea
Catholic Neuroscience Institute, College of Medicine, The Catholic University of Korea, Seoul, Republic of Korea

Djaina Satoer and Arnaud Vincent
Department of Neurosurgery, Erasmus MC University Medical Center, Rotterdam, Netherlands

Evy Visch-Brink
Department of Neurosurgery, Erasmus MC University Medical Center, Rotterdam, Netherlands
Department of Neurology, Erasmus MC University Medical Center, Rotterdam, Netherlands

Elke De Witte
Department of Clinical and Experimental Neurolinguistics, Free University of Brussels, Brussels, Belgium

Peter Mariën
Department of Clinical and Experimental Neurolinguistics, Free University of Brussels, Brussels, Belgium
Department of Neurology and Memory Clinic, ZNA Middelheim, Antwerp, Belgium

Marion Smits
Department of Radiology, Erasmus MC University Medical Center, Rotterdam, Netherlands

Roelien Bastiaanse
Center for Language and Cognition Groningen (CLCG), University of Groningen, Groningen, Netherlands

Mark Bustoros, Joshua Frenster, Aram S. Modrek and N. Sumru Bayin
Department of Neurosurgery, NYU School of Medicine, New York, NY 10016, USA

Dimitris G. Placantonakis
Department of Neurosurgery, NYU School of Medicine, New York, NY 10016, USA
Perlmutter Cancer Center, NYU Langone Medical Center, New York, NY 10016, USA
Brain Tumor Center, NYU Langone Medical Center, New York, NY 10016, USA
Kimmel Center for Stem Cell Biology, NYU School of Medicine, New York, NY 10016, USA

Cheddhi Thomas
Department of Pathology, NYU School of Medicine, New York, NY 10016, USA

Matija Snuderl
Department of Pathology, NYU School of Medicine, New York, NY 10016, USA
Perlmutter Cancer Center, NYU Langone Medical Center, New York, NY 10016, USA
Brain Tumor Center, NYU Langone Medical Center, New York, NY 10016, USA

Gerald Rosen
Perlmutter Cancer Center, NYU Langone Medical Center, New York, NY 10016, USA
Department of Medicine, NYU School of Medicine, New York, NY 10016, USA

Peter B. Schiff
Perlmutter Cancer Center, NYU Langone Medical Center, New York, NY 10016, USA

Department of Radiation Oncology, NYU School of Medicine, New York, NY 10016, USA

Simonas Jesmanas and Kristina Norvainytė
Faculty of Medicine, Medical Academy, Lithuanian University of Health Sciences, Kaunas, Lithuania

Rymantė Gleiznienė
Department of Radiology, Medical Academy, Lithuanian University of Health Sciences, Kaunas, Lithuania

Algirdas Mačionis
Department of Neurology, Medical Academy, Lithuanian University of Health Sciences, Kaunas, Lithuania

Stéphane Mathis
Department of Neurology, Nerve-Muscle Unit, CHU Bordeaux (Groupe Hospitalier Pellegrin), place Am élie-Raba-Léon, 33000 Bordeaux, France

Laurent Magy, Karima Ghorab, Laurence Richard, Mathilde Duchesne and Jean-Michel Vallat
Department of Neurology, Centre de R´ef´erence "Neuropathies P´eriph´eriques Rares", CHU Limoges, 2 avenue Martin Luther King, 87042 Limoges, France

Philippe Corcia
Department of Neurology, CHU Bretonneau, 2 boulevard Tonnell´e, 37044 Tours, France

Jonathan Ciron
Department of Neurology, CHU Poitiers, 2 rue de la Mil´etrie, 86021 Poitiers, France

Judith Marcoux, Mark Angle and Jeanne Teitelbaum
Department of Neurology and Neurosurgery, Montreal Neurological Institute andHospital, McGill University, Montreal, QC, Canada

Hosam Al-Jehani
Department of Neurology and Neurosurgery, Montreal Neurological Institute andHospital, McGill University, Montreal, QC, Canada
Department of Neurosurgery and Critical Care Medicine, King Fahad Hospital of the University, Imam Abdulrahman bin Faisal University, Al-Khobar, Saudi Arabia

Kawthar Hadhiah and Faisal Alabbas
Department of Neurosurgery and Critical Care Medicine, King Fahad Hospital of the University, Imam Abdulrahman bin Faisal University, Al-Khobar, Saudi Arabia

Costantini Antonio
Universit`a Cattolica di Roma, Largo Agostino Gemelli, Roma, Italy
Centro Polispecialistico Giovanni Paolo I, Viterbo, Italy

Tiberi Massimo, Zarletti Gianpaolo and Trevi Erika
Centro Polispecialistico Giovanni Paolo I, Viterbo, Italy

Pala Maria Immacolata
Department of Neurological Rehabilitation, The "Villa Immacolata" Clinic, Viterbo, Italy

Aurelian Anghelescu
Neurorehabilitation Clinic, Teaching Emergency Hospital "Bagdasar-Arseni", Romania
"Carol Davila" University of Medicine and Pharmacy, Bucharest, Romania

Xijing Mao, Bochi Zhu and Gang Yao
Department of Neurology, The Second Hospital of Jilin University, China

Lifang Jin and Honghua Cui
Department of Hematology and Oncology, The Second Hospital of Jilin University, China

Min Yao
Department of Pathology, The Second Hospital of Jilin University, China

K. H. D. Thilini Hemachandra and Thamara Kannangara
Teaching Hospital Kandy, Kandy, Sri Lanka

M. B. Kavinda Chandimal Dayasiri
University Paediatrics Unit, Lady Ridgeway Hospital for Children, Colombo, Sri Lanka

Kedar R. Mahajan, Robin Dharia and Lori Sheehan
Department of Neurology, Thomas Jefferson University Hospital, Philadelphia, PA 19107, USA

Amity L. Roberts, Mark T. Curtis and Danielle Fortuna
Department of Pathology, Anatomy and Cell Biology, Thomas Jefferson University Hospital, Philadelphia, PA 19107, USA

Hiroshi Yamaguchi
Department of Emergency and Critical Care Medicine, Hyogo Prefectural Kobe Children's Hospital, 1-1-1 Takakuradai, Suma-Ku, Kobe, Hyogo 654-0081, Japan

Tsukasa Tanaka, Azusa Maruyama and Hiroaki Nagase
Department of Neurology, Hyogo Prefectural Kobe Children's Hospital, 1-1-1 Takakuradai, Suma-Ku, Kobe, Hyogo 654-0081, Japan

Angela Spurgeon, Sanjay Konakondla and N. Scott Litofsky
Division of Neurosurgery, University of Missouri School of Medicine, Columbia, MO 65212, USA

List of Contributors

Viet Le
University of Missouri School of Medicine, Columbia, MO 65212, USA

Douglas C. Miller
Department of Pathology and Anatomical Sciences, University of Missouri School of Medicine, Columbia, MO 65212, USA

Tamera Hopkins
Division of Hematology Oncology, University of Missouri School of Medicine, Columbia, MO 65212, USA

Jalal Othman, Marc Kühl, Annett Kunkel and Juergen Faiss
Department of Neurology, Asklepios Fachklinikum Teupitz, Teupitz, Germany

Tim Sinnecker
Department of Neurology, Asklepios Fachklinikum Teupitz, Teupitz, Germany
NeuroCure Clinical Research Center, Charité-Universitätsmedizin Berlin, Berlin, Germany
Department of Neurology, Universitätsspital Basel, Basel, Switzerland

Friedemann Paul
NeuroCure Clinical Research Center, Charité-Universitätsmedizin Berlin, Berlin, Germany
Experimental and Clinical Research Center, Charité-Universitätsmedizin Berlin and Max Delbrück Center for Molecular Medicine, Berlin, Germany
Clinical and Experimental Multiple Sclerosis Research Center, Charité-Universitätsmedizin Berlin, Berlin, Germany
Department of Neurology, Charité-Universitätsmedizin Berlin, Berlin, Germany

Jens Wuerfel
NeuroCure Clinical Research Center, Charité-Universitätsmedizin Berlin, Berlin, Germany
Medical Imaging Analysis Center AG, Basel, Switzerland

Imke Metz
Department of Neuropathology, Universitätsmedizin Göttingen, Göttingen, Germany

Thoralf Niendorf
Berlin Ultrahigh Field Facility, Max Delbrück Center for Molecular Medicine, Berlin, Germany
Experimental and Clinical Research Center, Charité-Universitätsmedizin Berlin and Max Delbrück Center for Molecular Medicine, Berlin, Germany

Shauna H. Yuan
Department of Neurosciences, University of California, San Diego, La Jolla, CA 92093, USA

Sonya G. Wang
Department of Neurology, University of Minnesota, Minneapolis, MN 55455, USA

Constantine L. Karras
The Ohio State University College of Medicine, Columbus, OH 43212, USA

Isaac Josh Abecassis
Department of Neurological Surgery, University of Washington, Seattle, WA 98122, USA

Zachary A. Abecassis
Feinberg School of Medicine, Northwestern University, Chicago, IL 60611, USA

Joseph G. Adel and Bernard R. Bendok
Feinberg School of Medicine, Northwestern University, Chicago, IL 60611, USA
Department of Neurological Surgery, Northwestern University, Chicago, IL, USA

Esther N. Bit-Ivan
Department of Pathology, Feinberg School of Medicine, Northwestern University, Chicago, IL 60611, USA

Rakesh K. Chandra
Department of Otolaryngology, Feinberg School of Medicine, Northwestern University, Chicago, IL 60611, USA

Vamshi K. Rao
Division of Neurology, Ann and Robert H. Lurie Children's Hospital of Chicago, Chicago, IL 60611, USA
Department of Pediatrics, Feinberg School of Medicine, Northwestern University, Chicago, IL 60611, USA

Christine J. DiDonato
Department of Pediatrics, Feinberg School of Medicine, Northwestern University, Chicago, IL 60611, USA
Human Molecular Genetics Program, Ann and Robert H. Lurie Children's Hospital, StanleyManne Research Institute, Chicago, IL 60611, USA

Paul D. Larsen
Division of Neurology, Department of Pediatrics, University of Nebraska Medical Center and Children's Hospital andMedical Center, Omaha, NE, USA

Homajoun Maslehaty
Department of Neurosurgery, Nordstadt Hospital, Hannover, Germany

Johannes Van de Nes and Sarah Teuber-Hanselmann
Institute of Neuropathology, Faculty of Medicine, University Duisburg-Essen, University Hospital Essen, Germany

Christoph Moenninghoff
Institute of Neuroradiology, Faculty of Medicine, University Duisburg-Essen, University Hospital Essen, Germany

Ulrich Sure and Neriman Oezkan
Department of Neurosurgery, University Duisburg-Essen, University Hospital Essen, Germany

Arito Yozu and Nobuhiko Haga
Department of Rehabilitation Medicine, The University of Tokyo Hospital, 7-3-1 Hongo, Bunkyo-ku, Tokyo 113-8655, Japan

Masahiko Sumitani
Department of Pain and Palliative Medicine, The University of Tokyo Hospital, 7-3-1 Hongo, Bunkyo-ku, Tokyo 113-8655, Japan

Masahiro Shin and Kazuhiko Ishi
Department of Neurosurgery, The University of Tokyo Hospital, 7-3-1 Hongo, Bunkyo-ku, Tokyo 113-8655, Japan

Michihiro Osumi
Neurorehabilitation Research Center, Kio University, 4-2-2 Umaminaka, Koryo-cho, Kitakatsuragi-gun, Nara 635-0832, Japan

Junji Katsuhira
Department of Prosthetics and Orthotics and Assistive Technology, Faculty of Medical Technology, Niigata University of Health andWelfare, 1398 Shimami-cho, Kita-ku, Niigata, Niigata 950-3198, Japan

Ryosuke Chiba
Research Center for Brain Function and Medical Engineering, Asahikawa Medical University, 1-1-1 Higashi-2-jyou, Midorigaoka, Asahikawa, Hokkaido 078-8510, Japan

Stephanie R. Mehr and Melissa Wiley
Department of Anesthesiology, Vanderbilt University, Nashville, TN 37212, USA

Roy C. Neeley and Avinash B. Kumar
Department of Anesthesiology, Division of Critical Care, Vanderbilt University, Nashville, TN 37212, USA

Laxmi Kokatnur and Mohan Rudrappa
Louisiana State University Health Sciences Center Shreveport, 1501 Kings Hwy, Shreveport, LA 71104, USA
Overton Brooks VA Medical Center, 510 E Stoner Ave, Shreveport, LA 71101, USA

Erol Akgul, Hasan Bilen Onan and Huseyin Tugsan Balli
Radiology Department of Medical Faculty, Cukurova University, Adana, Turkey

Nuri Eralp Cetinalp
Neurosurgery Department of Medical Faculty, Cukurova University, Adana, Turkey

Alan Lucerna, James Espinosa and Douglas Stranges
Department of Emergency Medicine, Rowan University SOM/Jefferson Health, Stratford, NJ, USA

Taimur Zaman
Department of Neurology, Jefferson Health, Stratford, NJ, USA

Risha Hertz
Penn Medicine, Gibbsboro, NJ, USA

Koji Tsuzaki, Naoko Tachibana and Toshiaki Hamano
Department of Neurology, Kansai Electric Power Hospital, Osaka, Japan

Takashi Nakamura
Department of Neurology, Kansai Electric Power Hospital, Osaka, Japan
Department of Neurology, National Cerebral and Cardiovascular Center, Osaka, Japan

Hiroyuki Okumura
Department of Neurology, Kansai Electric Power Hospital, Osaka, Japan
Okumura Clinic, Shiga, Japan

Ashley Cannon, Kimberly J. Guthrie and Douglas L. Riegert-Johnson
The Department of Medical Genetics, Mayo Clinic, Jacksonville, FL 32224, USA
Center for Individualized Medicine, Mayo Clinic, Jacksonville, FL 32224, USA

Svetlana Kurklinsky
Department of Pain Medicine, Mayo Clinic, Jacksonville, FL 32224, USA

Index

A
Abducens Nerve Palsy, 20, 122, 124-125
Acute Psychosis, 1, 6-7
Acute Psychotic Illness, 1, 4
Acute Stroke, 25, 114, 119, 191-193, 195
Acute Transverse Myelitis, 88, 91
Alzheimer's Dementia, 160-161
Ataxia, 2, 6, 18, 20, 56, 65, 94, 99, 111-112, 114, 132, 160, 172-176, 184-185
Autonomic Instability, 186-188

B
Bilateral Encephaloduroarteriosynangiosis, 14
Bilateral Moyamoya Disease, 14-15
Biphasic Seizure, 141
Bromocriptine, 22-25, 170

C
Cardiac Asystole, 186-187
Central Pontine Myelinolysis, 1, 5, 7
Cerebellopontine Area, 108
Cerebrospinal Fluid, 36-37, 40, 42, 57-59, 95, 102, 124, 131, 149, 152-153, 158, 207
Cervical Spinal Canal, 67, 88, 92
Cervical Spine, 46, 65-67, 69, 89-91, 147
Chordoma, 164-165, 170-171
Choreoathetosis, 4
Chronic Hydrocephalus, 131
Clival Ectopic, 164, 167, 170
Cluster Headache, 108-112
Combined Myositis, 94, 102
Compound Heterozygote, 172, 174
Cryptococcus Neoformans, 131, 133, 136-137

D
Disease Abnormality, 108

E
Electrocution, 191-193, 195
Emotional Lability, 20, 32, 35, 160, 163, 210
Encephalitis, 2, 20-21, 29, 114, 136, 146, 186-187, 190
Epidural Extraosseous, 80, 86
Epilepticus, 19, 58, 61-64, 138-139, 141-142
Etanercept Treatment, 207
Extrapontine, 1, 4, 6-7

F
Fingolimod, 152-155, 158

G
Glioma Surgery, 70, 78
Glucose Metabolism, 108, 111
Glucuronoxylomannan, 131

H
Hemiplegic Migraine, 56, 58-60
Hemorrhage, 8, 22-23, 25-26, 46, 52-54, 92, 105, 107, 114, 145, 170, 182, 192, 196, 204, 206
Hypermetabolism, 1-2, 7
Hypochloremia, 2
Hypokalemia, 2
Hyponatremia, 1-2, 4-7

I
Impaired Emotion Recognition, 8, 11-12
Inflammatory Polyneuropathy, 94
Intraparenchymal Bleeding, 203
Invasive Cerebral Perfusion, 105
Ischemia, 8, 11, 17, 107, 118, 125, 141, 195, 204-206

K
Ketamine Infusion, 61-63

L
Left Hemispheric Stroke, 8, 11
Ligamentum Flavum, 65-67, 69
Limb Pain, 203-206
Liver Failure, 1, 4
Lymphoma, 80-81, 102, 122-126, 144, 146, 165

M
Medulloblastoma, 177-178, 180
Middle Cerebral Artery, 15-17, 192, 196, 198
Moyamoya, 14-17
Moyamoya Disease, 14-17
Multifocal Leukoencephalopathy, 152, 157-159
Multiple Sclerosis, 29, 91-92, 146, 152, 158-159, 203
Myelinolysis, 1, 4-7

N
Natalizumab, 152, 157-159
Neurological Deficit, 92, 107

Nonconvulsive Status, 138, 142

O
Overlap Myasthenic Syndrome, 94, 103

P
Paranoia, 1, 4
Paroxysmal Extreme Pain Disorder, 212-213, 217-218
Pituitary Adenoma, 164-165, 167, 170-171
Psychological Processes, 8

R
Radiculomyelopathy, 65, 67
Refractory Bradycardia, 186
Rheumatoid Meningitis, 207, 210-211

S
Septic Encephalopathy, 138, 141
Social Cognition, 8, 12-13
Sphenoidal Sinus, 122-125
Status Epilepticus, 19, 58, 61-63, 138, 141-142
Subarachnoid Hemorrhage, 26, 46, 52-53, 105, 107, 196

T
Thalamic Pain, 181-184, 204
Thiamine, 108-112
Traumatic Brain Injury, 8, 11-12, 24-25, 29, 35, 142, 162-163
Traumatic Encephalopathy, 32-33, 35, 160, 162-163

V
Vasospasm, 105-107, 119, 121, 191-192, 195, 206
Viral Serology, 2

CPSIA information can be obtained
at www.ICGtesting.com
Printed in the USA
BVHW051000220519
549014BV00002B/202/P

9 781632 427212